Neuro-Infectious Diseases

Editors

RUSSELL BARTT
ALLEN AKSAMIT

NEUROLOGIC CLINICS

www.neurologic.theclinics.com

Consulting Editor
RANDOLPH W. EVANS

November 2018 • Volume 36 • Number 4

ELSEVIER

1600 John F. Kennedy Boulevard ● Suite 1800 ● Philadelphia, Pennsylvania, 19103-2899

http://www.theclinics.com

NEUROLOGIC CLINICS Volume 36, Number 4
November 2018 ISSN 0733-8619, ISBN-13: 978-0-323-64163-0

Editor: Stacy Eastman
Developmental Editor: Donald Mumford

Neurologic Clinics (ISSN 0733-8619) is published quarterly by Elsevier Inc., 360 Park Avenue South, New York, NY 10010–1710. Months of issue are February, May, August, and November. Periodicals postage paid at New York, NY, and additional mailing offices. Subscription prices are $312.00 per year for US individuals, $631.00 per year for US institutions, $100.00 per year for US students, $390.00 per year for Canadian individuals, $765.00 per year for Canadian institutions, $423.00 per year for international individuals, $765.00 per year for international institutions, and $210.00 for Canadian and foreign students/residents. To receive student/ resident rate, orders must be accompanied by name of affiliated institution, date of term, and the *signature* of program/residency coordinator on institution letterhead. Orders will be billed at individual rate until proof of status is received. Foreign air speed delivery is included in all *Clinics* subscription prices. All prices are subject to change without notice. **POSTMASTER:** Send address changes to *Neurologic Clinics*, Elsevier Health Sciences Division, Subscription Customer Service, 3251 Riverport Lane, Maryland Heights, MO 63043. **Customer Service: Telephone: 1-800-654-2452 (U.S. and Canada); 314-447-8871 (outside U.S. and Canada). Fax: 314-447-8029. E-mail: journalscustomerservice-usa@elsevier.com (for print support); journalsonlinesupport-usa@elsevier.com (for online support).**

Reprints. For copies of 100 or more of articles in this publication, please contact the Commercial Reprints Department, Elsevier Inc., 360 Park Avenue South, New York, New York, 10010-1710; Tel.: +1-212-633-3874; Fax: +1-212-633-3820, and E-mail: reprints@elsevier.com.

Neurologic Clinics is also published in Spanish by Nueva Editorial Interamericana S.A., Mexico City, Mexico.

Neurologic Clinics is covered in *Current Contents/Clinical Medicine, MEDLINE/PubMed (Index Medicus), EMBASE/Excerpta Medica, and PsycINFO, and ISI/BIOMED.*

Contributors

CONSULTING EDITOR

RANDOLPH W. EVANS, MD
Clinical Professor, Department of Neurology, Baylor College of Medicine, Houston, Texas, USA

EDITORS

RUSSELL BARTT, MD
Neurohospitalist, Blue Sky Neurology (a division of Carepoint Health), Greenwood Village, Colorado, USA

ALLEN AKSAMIT, MD
Professor of Neurology, Mayo Clinic College of Medicine, Consultant, Department of Neurology, Mayo Clinic, Rochester, Minnesota, USA

AUTHORS

JOSE DAVID AVILA, MD
Clinical Assistant Professor, Neurology Residency Associate Program Director, Geisinger Commonwealth School of Medicine, Danville, Pennsylvania, USA

KELLY J. BALDWIN, MD
Clinical Assistant Professor, Neurology Residency Program Director, Neuro-Infectious Disease Program Director, Geisinger Commonwealth School of Medicine, Danville, Pennsylvania, USA

FELIX BENNINGER, MD
Department of Neurology, Felsenstein Medical Research Institut, Rabin Medical Center, Beilinson Hospital, Petach Tikva, Israel; Sackler Faculty of Medicine, Tel Aviv University, Tel Aviv, Israel

JOSEPH R. BERGER, MD
Multiple Sclerosis Division, Department of Neurology, Perelman School of Medicine, University of Pennsylvania, Philadelphia, Pennsylvania, USA

BRUCE JAMES BREW, MBBS, DMedSci, DSc
Department of Neurology, HIV Medicine, Neurosciences Program, Peter Duncan Neurosciences Unit, St Vincent's Hospital, St Vincent's Centre for Applied Medical Research, University of New South Wales, University of Notre Dame, Sydney, Australia

MATTHIJS C. BROUWER, MD, PhD
Department of Neurology, Amsterdam UMC, University of Amsterdam, Amsterdam Neuroscience, Amsterdam, The Netherlands

TRACEY A. CHO, MD
Department of Neurology, University of Iowa Hospitals and Clinics, Iowa City, Iowa, USA

ANA HELENA A. FIGUEIREDO, MD
Department of Neurology, Amsterdam UMC, University of Amsterdam, Amsterdam Neuroscience, Amsterdam, The Netherlands

HECTOR H. GARCIA, MD, PhD
Cysticercosis Unit, Instituto Nacional de Ciencias Neurologicas, Center for Global Health, Universidad Peruana Cayetano Heredia, Lima, Peru

MICHAEL D. GESCHWIND, MD, PhD
Memory and Aging Center, Department of Neurology, University of California, San Francisco, San Francisco, California, USA

ELENA GREBENCIUCOVA, MD
Assistant Professor of Neurology, Multiple Sclerosis Division, The Ken & Ruth Davee Department of Neurology, Northwestern University Feinberg School of Medicine, Chicago, Illinois, USA

JOHN J. HALPERIN, MD
Chair, Department of Neurosciences, Overlook Medical Center, Summit, New Jersey, USA; Professor of Neurology and Medicine, Sidney Kimmel Medical College, Thomas Jefferson University, Philadelphia, Pennsylvania, USA

ERIKA MARIANA LONGORIA IBARROLA, MD
Global Brain Health Institute, University of California, San Francisco, San Francisco, California, USA; Dementia Department, National Institute of Neurology and Neurosurgery Manuel Velasco Suarez, La Fama, CDMX, Mexico

MAYRA MONTAVO, MD
Department of Neurology, Brown University, Rhode Island Hospital, Providence, Rhode Island, USA

OLWEN C. MURPHY, MBBCh, MRCPI
Division of Neuroimmunology and Neuroinfectious Diseases, Fellow, Department of Neurology, Johns Hopkins Encephalitis Center, Johns Hopkins School of Medicine, Baltimore, Maryland, USA

PRASHANTH S. RAMACHANDRAN, MBBS, BMedSci
Department of Neurology, UCSF Weill Institute for Neurosciences, University of California, San Francisco, San Francisco, California, USA

SAVINA REID, BS
Department of Neurology, Columbia University Medical Center, Milstein Hospital, New York, New York, USA

KATHRYN RIMMER, MD
Department of Neurology, Columbia University Medical Center, Milstein Hospital, New York, New York, USA

ISRAEL STEINER, MD
Department of Neurology, Felsenstein Medical Research Institut, Rabin Medical Center, Beilinson Hospital, Petach Tikva, Israel; Sackler Faculty of Medicine, Tel Aviv University, Tel Aviv, Israel

EMILY JANE SUTHERLAND, BMedSci (Hons), MBBS
Department of Neurology, University of New South Wales, University of Notre Dame,
Sydney, Australia

BOON LEAD TEE, MD, MS
Global Brain Health Institute, University of California, San Francisco, San Francisco,
California, USA; Department of Neurology, Buddhist Tzu Chi General Hospital, Hualien
City, Hualien County, Taiwan

KIRAN THAKUR, MD
Division of Critical Care and Hospitalist Neurology, Assistant Professor, Department of
Neurology, Columbia University Medical Center, Milstein Hospital, New York, New York,
USA

DIEDERIK VAN DE BEEK, MD, PhD
Department of Neurology, Amsterdam UMC, University of Amsterdam, Amsterdam
Neuroscience, Amsterdam, The Netherlands

ARUN VENKATESAN, MD, PhD
Division of Neuroimmunology and Neuroinfectious Diseases, Associate Professor,
Department of Neurology, Johns Hopkins Encephalitis Center, Johns Hopkins School
of Medicine, Baltimore, Maryland, USA

MICHAEL R. WILSON, MD, MAS
Department of Neurology, UCSF Weill Institute for Neurosciences, University of California,
San Francisco, San Francisco, California, USA

Contents

Neuro-Infectious diseases continue to cause morbidity and mortality worldwide, with many emerging or reemerging infections resulting in neurologic sequelae. Careful clinical evaluation coupled with appropriate laboratory investigations still forms the bedrock for making the correct etiologic diagnosis and implementing appropriate management. The treating physician needs to understand the individual test characteristics of each of the many conventional candidate-based diagnostics: culture, pathogen-specific polymerase chain reaction, antigen, antibody tests, used to diagnose the whole array of neuroinvasive infections. In addition, there is a growing need for more comprehensive, agnostic testing modalities that can identify a diversity of infections with a single assay.

Viruses are a frequent cause of encephalitis. Common or important viruses causing encephalitis include herpesviruses, arboviruses, enteroviruses, parechoviruses, mumps, measles, rabies, Ebola, lymphocytic choriomeningitis virus, and henipaviruses. Other viruses may cause an encephalopathy. Host factors and clinical features of infection are important to consider in identifying the cause for encephalitis. Cerebrospinal fluid evaluation, serologic/polymerase chain reaction studies, and neuroimaging are cornerstones of diagnostic evaluation in encephalitis. Treatable forms of encephalitis are important to consider in all cases. Central nervous system inflammation may also occur because of postinfectious autoimmunity, such as acute disseminated encephalomyelitis or antibody-mediated encephalitis after herpes simplex virus encephalitis.

The 3 neurotropic human herpes viruses, herpes simplex virus (HSV) type 1 and 2, and varicella-zoster virus (VZV) are capable of establishment of latent viral infection in trigeminal and dorsal root ganglia. HSV-1, and more rarely HSV-2, carries the potential to cause meningoencephalitis, with devastating clinical consequences. Immediate diagnosis, based on clinical presentation, MRI imaging, and molecular diagnosis by polymerase chain reaction, and initiation of therapy are mandatory to reduce mortality and neurologic permanent sequelae. VZV is associated with postprimary infection and reactivation disorders that may affect anywhere in the neuraxis. Early diagnosis and therapy are required.

> Progressive multifocal leukoencephalopathy (PML) is a rare opportunistic infection that occurs in patients whose immune system is compromised either because of an underlying illness or an immunosuppressive medication. John Cunningham virus, prevalent in 60% or more of the adult population as a latent or persistent infection, is responsible for the syndrome of PML. This article reviews PML in association with the most common immunotherapies and discusses risk mitigation and monitoring strategies.

> In the era of combination antiretroviral therapy, the diagnosis and management of HIV-associated neurocognitive disorders (HANDs) has arisen. Traditionally, severe HAND was seen in those with untreated HIV infection and had a guarded prognosis. Antiretroviral therapy has provided longevity and viral control to many living with the disease, revealing an increase in prevalence of less severe forms of HAND. Despite peripheral blood and cerebrospinal fluid viral suppression, cognitive impairment occurs and progresses for reasons that are unclear at present. This article provides a review of current theories behind the development of HAND, clinical and pathologic findings, recent developments, and future research opportunities.

> Zika virus (ZIKV) is an arthropod-borne virus that belongs to the Flaviviridae family. Although most cases are mild or go undetected, rare severe neurologic effects, including congenital ZIKV syndrome (CZS) and Guillain-Barré syndrome, have been identified. The serious neurologic complications associated with ZIKV prompted the declaration of the public health emergency of international concern by the World Health Organization. Overall, transmission occurred throughout South and Central America as well as the Caribbean, affecting 48 countries and territories from March 2015 to March 2017. Long-term management of CZS requires a comprehensive combination of supportive services throughout early development.

> Infectious diseases are an important cause of spinal cord dysfunction. Infectious myelopathies are of growing concern given increasing global travel and migration and expanding prevention and treatment with vaccinations, antibiotics, and antiretrovirals. Clinicians must recognize these pathologies because outcomes can dramatically improve with prompt diagnosis and management. We provide a complete review of the most frequent infectious agents that can affect the spinal cord. For each pathogen we describe epidemiology, pathophysiology, anatomic location, characteristic clinical syndromes, diagnostic approach, treatment, and prognosis. The review includes spinal imaging from selected cases.

Ana Helena A. Figueiredo, Matthijs C. Brouwer, and Diederik van de Beek

Community-acquired bacterial meningitis remains a disease with high impact. The epidemiology of this disease changed substantiality to large-scale introduction of conjugated vaccines. *Streptococcus pneumoniae* and *Neisseria meningitidis* are the main causative pathogens outside the neonatal age. Clinical presentation of patients with bacterial meningitis varies depending on age and underlying condition. A delay in diagnosis and antimicrobial therapy has been associated with increased risk of adverse clinical outcome. Empirical antibiotic treatment should be based on common bacterial species that cause the disease according to the patient's age group or clinical setting and on local antibiotic susceptibility patterns of the predominant pathogens.

John J. Halperin

Neurologic manifestations of nervous system infection with *Borrelia burgdorferi, Borrelia garinii,* and *Borrelia afzelii* are qualitatively similar, and include lymphocytic meningitis, cranial neuritis, radiculoneuritis, and other focal or multifocal mononeuropathies. Parenchymal central nervous system (CNS) infection occurs rarely. Neurobehavioral changes are common, but are rarely evidence of CNS infection. Diagnosis requires likely exposure and a finding with high diagnostic positive predictive value, specifically erythema migrans, or laboratory support, typically positive 2-tiered serologic testing. CNS infection is often evidenced by a cerebrospinal fluid pleocytosis and intrathecal production of specific antibody.

Kelly J. Baldwin and Jose David Avila

Chronic meningitis is defined as cerebrospinal fluid pleocytosis that persists for at least 4 weeks without spontaneous resolution. The differential diagnosis of chronic meningitis is broad, encompassing 4 main categories, including infectious, autoimmune, neoplastic, and idiopathic. Up to one-third of cases have no discernible cause, making chronic meningitis a diagnostic dilemma for many clinicians. This article suggests a diagnostic approach to chronic meningitis using clinical history, key examination findings, selective advanced testing, and neuroimaging. Case presentations demonstrate application of a diagnostic algorithm, followed by a brief discussion on common infectious pathogens, autoimmune conditions, and neoplastic disease with selected treatment regimens.

Hector H. Garcia

Neurocysticercosis (NCC) is a major contributor to the burden of seizure disorders and epilepsy in most of the world. NCC encompasses a variety of clinical presentations, depending on number, location, size, evolutionary stage of lesions, and the inflammatory response of the host, with late-onset seizures, headache, and intracranial hypertension the most frequent manifestations. Diagnosis and therapy depend on the type of

NEUROLOGIC CLINICS

THE CLINICS ARE AVAILABLE ONLINE!
Access your subscription at:
www.theclinics.com

Preface
Neurology gone 'Viral'

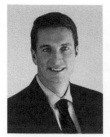 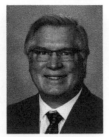

Russell Bartt, MD   Allen Aksamit, MD
Editors

It is with enthusiasm and gratitude that this issue of *Neurologic Clinics* is created to focus on the subspecialty of neuro-infectious diseases. The development of this field comes from the convergence of ideas that diverse microbes cause unique yet overlapping syndromes when they invade the nervous system, and without proper and timely treatment lead to devastating consequences for the affected patient. Though these disorders are relatively rare, specialized knowledge in both neurology and infectious disease is required for the neurologist to be well suited in the diagnosis and treatment of these patients. When confronted with a patient presenting with a neurologic infection, the possibilities may seem overwhelming. Some specialized knowledge helps to simplify the approach to these patients. Although there is variety in these disorders and their manifestations, principles of pathogenesis and host manifestations allow for a logical approach in clinical practice.

Remarkable are the advances in molecular and serologic techniques that have entered the armamentarium of the attending physician for patients affected by possible infections. In addition, advances have identified new causes for old neurologic syndromes, and new pathogens continue to emerge, changing the landscape of the differential diagnosis. With international travel and immigration, the world is as small as ever. As a result, diseases from other continents may appear in your or my hospital or clinic. And a new epidemic every few years continues to surprise us.

The aim of this issue is an attempt to survey, illustrate, and provide practical information about the investigation and treatment of patients with these diseases. With a clinical neurologic perspective, all of these articles provide an approach to these syndromes and pathogens. Armed with this knowledge, the diagnosis and best treatment are more attainable.

Neurol Clin 36 (2018) xiii–xiv
https://doi.org/10.1016/j.ncl.2018.08.001
0733-8619/18/© 2018 Published by Elsevier Inc.

The authors of these articles are all astute clinicians and respected educators in the field. In the past and present, they have taught us and been wonderful collaborators and friends. Our many thanks to all who have contributed.

Russell Bartt, MD
Blue Sky Neurology (a division of Carepoint Health)
Greenwood Village, CO 80111, USA

499 East Hampden Avenue, Suite 360
Englewood, CO 80113, USA

Allen Aksamit, MD
Mayo Clinic College of Medicine
Department of Neurology, Mayo Clinic
200 First Street Southwest
Rochester, MN 55905, USA

E-mail addresses:
russellbartt@gmail.com (R. Bartt)
aksamit@mayo.edu (A. Aksamit)

Diagnostic Testing of Neurologic Infections

Prashanth S. Ramachandran, MBBS, BMedSci, Michael R. Wilson, MD, MAS*

KEYWORDS

- Neuroinfectious diseases • Meningoencephalitis • Meningitis • Encephalitis
- Metagenomic next-generation sequencing • Neurosyphilis • Neurocysticercosis
- Neuroborreliosis

KEY POINTS

- A thorough clinical evaluation of a patient with meningoencephalitis should guide the physician toward a thoughtful differential diagnosis that will guide the selection of appropriate diagnostic tests to rule in or rule out suspected infections.
- Knowledge of the role and accuracy of each of the many diagnostic tests for identifying neurologic infections is crucial for accurate diagnosis.
- Multiplex assays, including unbiased metagenomic next-generation sequencing, promise to increase diagnostic yield in patients with meningitis and encephalitis.

Neuroinfectious diseases are a major cause of morbidity and mortality worldwide and have a sizable effect on local health care systems and economies.[1,2] A timely diagnosis and the institution of appropriate management can drastically improve mortality and morbidity when the precise organism is known.[3] In this review, the authors provide an overview of the current state of diagnostic techniques for neuroinvasive pathogens ranging from culture, polymerase chain reaction (PCR), to serology. The authors then review new diagnostic modalities, including unbiased metagenomic next-generation sequencing (mNGS). This overview is not meant to provide an exhaustive list of all possible diagnostics for all possible neuroinvasive pathogens. Instead, the authors hope that by reviewing the techniques in detail as they apply to particularly important and/or common neuroinvasive pathogens, including strengths and common pitfalls associated with each, the reader will be able to more judiciously select the most efficient and comprehensive diagnostic approach tailored to their particular patient.

Disclosure Statement: Dr Wilson is supported by the Rachleff Foundation, National Institute for Neurological Disorders and Stroke grant number K08NS096117, and the UCSF Center for Next-Gen Precision Diagnostics supported by the Sandler and William K. Bowes, Jr. Foundations. Dr Ramachandran is supported by the Australian Government Research Training Program Scholarship.
Department of Neurology, UCSF Weill Institute for Neurosciences, University of California, San Francisco, 675 Nelson Rising Lane, NS212A, Campus Box 3206, San Francisco, CA 94158, USA
* Corresponding author.
E-mail address: michael.wilson@ucsf.edu

CULTURE

Cerebrospinal fluid (CSF) culture is the gold standard for central nervous system (CNS) infections and can provide guidance for antimicrobial therapy. Bacterial cultures are critical in the management of meningitis with varying sensitivities depending on the causative organism. These range from 97% for *Haemophilus influenzae*, 87% for *Streptococcus pneumoniae*, and 80% for *Neisseria meningitidis*.[4] The timing of antibiotics in relation to the acquisition of CSF is crucial. A positive result decreases from 85% before antibiotics, to 73% when obtained less than 4 hours after therapy, 11% between 4 to 8 hours and 0% after 8 hours.[4,5] *Listeria monocytogenes* causes both meningitis and rhombencephalitis with associated abscess formation. Cultures are hampered by slow growth and are insensitive due to a low CSF bacterial load.[6,7] Sensitivities vary between studies and range from 55% to 90% and are as low as 41% in patients with rhombencephalitis.[6,8,9] Blood culture performs marginally better in cases of rhombencephalitis with rates reaching 61%.[9]

In general, larger CSF volumes improve the sensitivity of culture. However, even with large volumes of CSF, visualization of acid fast bacilli (AFB) by microscopy is only 15% sensitive, and *Mycobacterium tuberculosis* (TB) can take 2 to 4 weeks to culture with a sensitivity of only 50% to 60%. Therefore, AFB culture cannot be relied on for time critical TB meningitis diagnoses.[10] In addition, an estimated 480,000 people developed multidrug-resistant TB in 2015.[11] Despite its low yield, TB cultures remain the gold standard for identifying drug sensitivities.

Viral cultures are performed with cell lines, including rhesus monkey kidney, African green monkey kidney, A549, and MRC-5. The patient sample is added to the culture medium, and cytopathic changes are observed in positive cases. These changes can take up to 30 days to appear depending on the virus.[12] Shell vial culturing, antigen detection, and immunofluorescent antibodies to specific viruses have improved this previously slow turnaround.[13] Enteroviruses are the easiest viruses to culture with 75% sensitivity and a 3- to 8-day test turnaround.[14] Other viruses fail to display equivalent results. Herpes simplex virus (HSV) is only cultured from CSF in less than 5% of HSV encephalitis cases.[15] Fortunately, with the advent of advanced molecular techniques, the need for viral cultures as a diagnostic tool for CNS infections has diminished.[16]

Fungal cultures can be performed on specific fungal mediums. However, the 3 most frequent neuroinvasive fungi: *Cryptococcus* spp, *Candida* spp, and *Aspergillus* spp, can be cultured on standard bacterial mediums with variable sensitivity. When more rare fungi are being considered, as may be the case with chronic meningitis, specific culture mediums are required.[17]

SEROLOGY
Syphilis

Syphilis is caused by the bacteria *Treponema pallidum* and can manifest with a variety of neurologic syndromes depending on the duration of infection and the host's immune status.[18] The diagnostic gold standard is rabbit infectivity testing, but this is expensive and limited to research laboratories. Dark field microscopy is operator dependent, time consuming, and not routinely used in the diagnosis of neurosyphilis. Treponemal nucleic acid detection by PCR in CSF is insensitive.[19] Antibody testing is therefore the standard tool for diagnosis and is divided into 2 groups, treponemal and nontreponemal testing. Treponemal tests include fluorescent treponemal antibody absorption (FTA-ABS), *T pallidum* particle agglutination (TP-PA), and enzyme immunoassay (EIA).[20] These tests detect antibodies to specific antigenic components of the bacterium. The latter two tests are more sensitive and specific than the older

FTA-ABS test. These are opposed to nontreponemal tests, which detect antibodies to lipoidal material released from damaged host cells and cardiolipin-like material released by T pallidum.[21,22] The 2 most common nontreponemal tests are the Venereal Disease Research Laboratory (VDRL) slide test and the Rapid Plasma Reagin card test, in which reactive sera produce flocculation of the antigenic material.[21]

Treponemal tests remain positive for life after primary infection and are not used as a marker for treatment response. Nontreponemal tests are quantitative and are used to assess treatment response with the expectation that they will either revert to being negative or at least exhibit a 4-fold reduction in titer after successful treatment. However, the nontreponemal tests can be falsely negative either as a result of waning antibody titers in late latent syphilis, or conversely, as a result of very high antibody titers that interfere with the formation of the antigen-antibody lattice, called the prozone phenomenon. If the latter circumstance is suspected in a high-risk patient, the treating physician can ask the laboratory to dilute the biological sample and repeat the test. Because both treponemal and nontreponemal tests are susceptible to false positives and negatives, combined testing is recommended for an accurate diagnosis of syphilis (the syphilis testing algorithm for syphilis screening is outside the scope of this article).[23] A definitive diagnosis of neurosyphilis is based on a clinical syndrome suggestive of neurosyphilis, a positive serum TP-PA, and a positive CSF VDRL. However, CSF VDRL only has a sensitivity of roughly 70% and therefore cannot exclude neurosyphilis.[24] False positives can occur with traumatic taps resulting in contamination from peripheral blood. In the absence of a positive CSF VDRL, a probable diagnosis of neurosyphilis is made with a CSF white blood cell count >5 mm/μL or a protein greater than 45 mg/dL.[25] Treponemal tests are not routinely performed on the CSF despite some suggestions that the high sensitivity of the test should rule out syphilis.[26]

Varicella Zoster Virus

Varicella zoster virus (VZV) is a neurotropic virus that can cause a wide range of syndromes ranging from encephalomyelitis, multifocal polyradiculitis, and cranial neuritis to a vasculopathy affecting both small and large cerebral arteries leading to unifocal and multifocal strokes. Symptoms can present after a prolonged duration, and a rash can occur months before presentation and may not be present at all.[27] VZV serum immunoglobulin M (IgM) appears within 2 to 5 days of symptom onset. Levels begin to decrease by 3.5 weeks and cannot be detected by 1 year. IgG levels decrease with time but generally remain positive for life. Therefore, a positive serum IgM is usually indicative of active infection.[28] CSF evaluation displays a pleocytosis in two-thirds of patients, and the diagnosis is made with CSF VZV serology or PCR. VZV IgG levels have higher sensitivity in comparison to PCR, 93% versus 30%, respectively.[29] As most adults will have positive VZV IgG in serum, it is important to assess for a low-serum/CSF ratio to confirm intrathecal production.[27,29] CSF VZV IgM is also supportive of a diagnosis, despite its less robust sensitivity compared with IgG.[30,31] VZV PCR may also be dependent on the time of symptom onset and the time of CSF acquisition with decreasing sensitivity of PCR after 1 week. Time-dependent sensitivity is an important consideration given the protracted course and delayed presentation of most cases.[27,29]

Flaviviruses

Flaviviruses cause mosquito and tick-borne infections that are endemic to certain regions throughout the world. They can cause meningitis, meningoencephalitis, and anterior horn cell disease. West Nile virus (WNV) is endemic to Africa and Europe and arrived in North America in 1999. Viremia is detected as early as 1 to 2 days after the primary mosquito bite and persists for up to 1 week until the development of IgM neutralizing antibodies. Viremia is generally absent by the time neurologic symptoms appear in immunocompetent hosts, whereas immunocompromised patients demonstrate a prolonged viremia with a delay in antibody production.[32] The pathophysiology of WNV mirrors the yield of laboratory diagnostics. CSF PCR may be helpful very early in the disease but generally has a low sensitivity (57%).[33] IgM capture enzyme-linked immunosorbent assay (ELISA) in either blood or CSF during the acute phase is the gold standard for the diagnosis of neuroinvasive WNV and is generally always present by the time neurologic symptoms manifest. The large IgM pentamer does not cross the blood-brain barrier, and therefore, its presence in CSF is suggestive of intrathecal production.[34] IgM may be falsely negative in the early phase in immunocompromised patients who have not yet mounted an antibody response, and PCR or repeat CSF IgM assay 7 to 10 days into the illness may be more appropriate in this setting.[35] Despite the high sensitivity of ELISA, the assay has poor specificity because of cross-reactivity with other neuroinvasive flaviviruses (eg, Zika virus, yellow fever virus, St. Louis encephalitis virus, and dengue virus). Confirmatory testing can be performed using plaque reduction neutralization testing (PRNT) for WNV and other flaviviruses. It is also notable that WNV IgM titers can remain positive for up to 1 year in serum and 7 months in CSF.[36] Therefore, demonstration of a 4-fold or greater increase in virus-specific antibody titer or elevated virus-specific IgG antibodies in the acute or convalescent serum sample confirms acute infection.

In 2016, Zika virus spread rapidly through South America and led to an increased incidence of microcephaly, Guillain-Barré syndrome, encephalitis, and myelitis.[37] Once Zika virus was recognized as the etiologic agent 2 years after it was first introduced to Brazil,[38] pathogen-specific reverse transcription-PCR and Zika virus IgM serology were used on CSF to detect neuroinvasive disease. Zika virus serology suffered from the same drawbacks as most flavivirus serologies with false positives due to cross-reactivity. However, the Euroimmun anti–Zika fever IgG and IgM ELISA tests demonstrated high specificity for the Zika virus.[39] The Centers for Disease Control and Prevention no longer recommends the PRNT in regions with high prevalence of multiple flaviviruses due to its low accuracy in this setting.[40] Instead, patients are tested for dengue virus and Zika virus on CSF to rule out cross-reactivity.[41]

Lyme Disease

Lyme disease is a tick-borne illness secondary to the *Borrelia burgdorferi sensu lato* group and is endemic to North America, Europe, and Asia. *Borrelia burgdorferi sensu stricto* is the main species found in North America, whereas 5 known species are endemic to Europe. Lyme disease can present with a wide range of neurologic syndromes, including polyradiculitis, multiple cranial neuropathies, myelitis, meningitis, brainstem encephalitis, and optic neuritis.[42] Diagnostic difficulties are encountered due to poorly performing assays, insensitivity of US assays against European *Borrelia* species, delayed serologic response early in the disease, and the inability for serology to delineate past and active infection. Hence, it is important to conduct tests in patients with an appropriate history and examination for neuroborreliosis, therefore increasing the pretest probability and yield from laboratory investigations. Direct identification of the spirochete is difficult with resultant low sensitivities for cultures and PCR. A diagnosis is achieved through a 2-tier system with EIA followed by Western blot. EIA is highly sensitive, and if positive or equivocal, the Western blot is performed.[43] If the symptoms have been present for less than 1 month, then IgM and IgG are assayed. Two reactive bands constitute a positive IgM, and 5 or more out of 10 possible bands are a positive for IgG. If symptoms have occurred for longer than 1 month, then only IgG is performed, although like WNV, IgM antibodies to *B burgdorferi* can persist for months. IgM alone cannot be used to confirm a diagnosis, and evidence of seroconversion may be required.[43,44]

Both the EIA and the Western blot have significant flaws and may soon be superseded by newer assays. The current EIA was developed from whole cell sonicates of cultured *B burgdorferi* with no specific targeted antigen, which leads to a high degree of cross-reactivity. The Western blot has poor sensitivity; there are no bands that are more specific for the organism, and multiple antibodies with similar weights may colocate over the same band.[45] Both these tests perform very poorly with 50% sensitivity in early presentations, and serology may take up to 3 to 6 weeks to become positive.[46] Newer serologic tests target specific antigenic proteins, such as C6, on the "variable major protein–like sequence, expressed," a cell surface lipoprotein.[47,48] These new assays have demonstrated excellent sensitivity and specificity and may soon replace the Western blot in the 2-tier algorithm.[45,49] However, they suffer from similar issues of poor sensitivity in early disease, the inability to differentiate between active and past infection and false negatives in immunocompromised patients.[44,50,51]

A diagnosis of neuroborreliosis is made with a suggestive history and examination consistent with Lyme disease, positive serum serology, CSF pleocytosis, and evidence of intrathecal antibody production. Most patients will display a CSF pleocytosis and elevated protein, except in cases of polyneuropathies.[52] In early neurologic disease, elevated intrathecal antibody production is evident in only 75% of patients but increases to nearly 100% within several months. The IgG index is elevated in 100% of all late neuroborreliosis cases.[53,54] The index can remain elevated for several years after treatment and cannot be used as a marker for follow-up nor clinical activity.[54] Measurement of C6 on CSF has had variable results and sensitivities.[55] CXCL13 is a B-cell–attracting chemokine that has a high sensitivity even before detectable intrathecal antibodies with decreased levels after treatment.[56,57] False positives have also been found with CNS lymphoma, TB meningitis, and neurosyphilis.[56,58]

Neurocysticercosis

Neurocysticercosis (NCC) is caused by infection with *Taenia solium*, a pork tapeworm. NCC is endemic to Central America, South America, Sub-Saharan Africa, and Asia.[59] Diagnosis is made on clinical, exposure history, and radiological characteristics with confirmatory laboratory diagnosis. The lentil lectin glycoprotein enzyme-linked immunoelectrotransfer blot (EITB) is a Western blot assay that is considered the test of choice.[60] This assay uses 6 glycoprotein antigens on a strip to detect antibodies to *T solium*. Appearance of any of the 6 bands is consistent with a systemic infection by the parasite.[61] In patients with 2 or more noncalcified or enhancing lesions on brain imaging, serum EITB carries a sensitivity of 98% and 100% specificity for NCC.[62] However, the EITB performs poorly on samples from patients with single lesions (28%) and calcified lesions. This may be due to a lack of an antigenic response from dead calcified lesions compared with viable cysts. Serum carries a slightly higher sensitivity than CSF.[63]

Compared with the EITB, serum ELISA has poor sensitivity (89%) and specificity (93%) due to cross-reactivity with other helminthic infections.[64] This is less problematic in CSF due to fewer non-NCC antigenic components, allowing for a decreased test threshold and increased sensitivity.[63] CSF titers may also be higher in patients with subarachnoid, intraventricular, or malignant disease. ELISA also fares poorly with single or calcified brain lesions.[64–66]

The main drawback of serology is false positives in asymptomatic patients from endemic regions and an inability to differentiate between active and inactive infection. Some studies suggest that 40% of positive results in endemic regions are due to transient antibodies that become undetectable within 1 year.[67] For this reason, caution must be used when assessing patients from endemic regions, and weight should not be solely placed on serologic testing, but rather the entire clinical and neuroradiological information should be considered.

ANTIGEN TESTING

Antigen testing involves detection of antigenic proteins specific to a microbial source by immunologic methods, such as latex particle agglutination, coagglutination, and ELISA.

Neurocysticercosis

Monoclonal antibody-based antigen testing using ELISA is commonly used for NCC. Antigen levels are higher in patients with viable parasites, extraparenchymal disease, as well as the quantity and size of lesions. CSF samples have a higher sensitivity than serum. Sensitivity is again lower with calcified and single lesions.[68] Antigen testing is used to monitor treatment response because NCC antigen titers should normalize in successfully treated patients.[68–70]

Fungal Antigen Testing

Antigen testing is a rapid and accurate test for the diagnosis of Cryptococcus neoformans. This testing is done through latex particle agglutination or enzyme immunoassay. The test targets the cryptococcal polysaccharide capsule glucuronoxylomannan. The sensitivity of antigen testing is very high with 99% sensitivity and 97% specificity.[71] The introduction of the point of care lateral flow assay has allowed rapid and accurate diagnosis of Cryptococcus in resource limited settings. The lateral flow assay can be performed on serum, plasma, and CSF. It takes approximately 15 minutes for a result and has a higher sensitivity than standard latex particle agglutination.[72,73] Antigen titers decrease rapidly in response to treatment but may not normalize, with persisting low titers despite negative cultures, CSF normalization, and clinical improvement. Antigen testing should not be used to assess for cure.[74]

Galactomannan is a cell wall polysaccharide that is released by Aspergillus species during growth. Galactomannan antigen testing uses antibodies directed against b(1r5)-linked galactofuranosyl residues found on the side chains of galactomannan.[75] Its use for the detection of invasive aspergillosis in immunocompromised patients has been extensively studied in serum and recently in CSF with a sensitivity of 88% in the latter. Specificity is 96% due to cross-reactivity with Trichocomaceae family, Fusarium spp, and Histoplasma capsulatum.[76] Serum false positives can occur from antibiotic therapy (piperacillin-tazobactam), bacterial infections, blood transfusions, and dialysis. Sensitivity of the assay increases in patients with hematologic malignancy and severe neutropenia in comparison to solid organ transplant patients and those with mild immunosuppression.[75]

1,3-beta-D-Glucan (BDG) is the major cell wall component of most fungal species, and BDG antigen testing is used as a broad test for detection of fungal pathogens. Cryptococcus spp do not contain high levels of BDG in their cell walls and therefore are not detected. BDG antigen testing is helpful for detecting invasive aspergillosis and candidiasis. Most studies were conducted on serum that displayed 60% to 100% sensitivity with a recommended test cutoff of 60 to 80 pg/mL.[77] After a recent outbreak of fungal meningitis secondary to contaminated intrathecal methylprednisolone,[78] studies have suggested that CSF BDG at a cutoff of 138 pg/mL has a 100% sensitivity and 98% specificity for Aspergillus fumigatus, Exserohilum rostratum,

Cladosporium cladosporioides, Epicoccum nigrum, and with decreasing titers suggestive of an effective treatment response.[79,80]

POLYMERASE CHAIN REACTION
Herpes Simplex Viruses

Over the last 2 decades, the advent of PCR has revolutionized the diagnosis of infectious diseases. Its ability to detect common viral and bacterial pathogens has made it the gold standard in clinical diagnostics.[81–83] DNA is extracted from a biological sample and heated to separate the nucleic acid. Oligomeric primers for the organism-specific sequences are added with DNA polymerase, leading to transcription of new DNA, which is complementary to the target sequence. This process is repeated multiple times with each new strand undergoing the same process, leading to exponential amplification and increasing sensitivity. Labeled nucleotides are added during the final run to confirm the suspected genomic sequence.[84] The diagnosis of herpes simplex encephalitis (HSE) was revolutionized by the development of a CSF PCR assay.[81,85] Before this, diagnosing HSE required a brain biopsy because viral culture had only 5% sensitivity. HSV-1, 2 PCR has a sensitivity of 98% and 94% specificity.[86] False negatives may occur within the first 72 hours or after 7 to 10 days of antiviral treatment. If high clinical suspicion exists for HSE, then repeat lumbar puncture (LP) and PCR are required despite an early negative CSF HSV-1, 2 PCR.[87] PCR is available for numerous pathogens, including standard bacterial meningitis pathogens, VZV, enterovirus, human herpesvirus-6, Epstein-Barr virus, cytomegalovirus, JC virus, and WNV. Each PCR has different test performance characteristics, so both negative and positive results have to be interpreted in clinical context.[15]

Mycobacterium tuberculosis

The Xpert MTB/RIF is a rapid PCR used as the standard molecular test for the diagnosis of pulmonary TB. Xpert sensitivity for TB meningitis is approximately 50% depending on CSF volume and processing technique.[88] The Xpert MTB/RIF also allows detection of rifampicin resistance, a key drug in TB antimicrobial regimens. The new Xpert MTB/RIF Ultra is the next generation of the Xpert MTB/RIF and has recently been adopted by the World Health Organization as the test of choice for the diagnosis of TB meningitis.[89] Preliminary studies found a sensitivity of ~95% for TB meningitis when compared with Xpert MTB/RIF or TB cultures combined. However, when tested against the current uniform case definition for TB meningitis, Xpert MTB/RIF Ultra demonstrated a sensitivity of only 70%.[90]

Multiplex Polymerase Chain Reaction

Multiplex PCR is a technique in which multiple primers are used allowing detection of several organisms by a single assay. The FilmArray meningitis and encephalitis panel is a rapid, multiplex PCR panel that tests for 14 common viral, bacterial, and yeast pathogens. A recent prospective multicenter trial evaluating the FilmArray displayed a range in sensitivity of 85% to 100% depending on the organism. However, there was also a high rate of false positives and several false negatives.[91] The US Food and Drug Administration has approved this multiplex panel, and some hospitals are using it as a stand-alone test. Conventional agent-specific confirmation testing by PCR may be more appropriate in some circumstances.

Bacterial and Fungal Polymerase Chain Reaction

The 16s recombinant ribosomal RNA (rRNA) gene is a highly conserved genetic region that is found in all bacteria. The sequence is approximately 1550 base-pairs long and contains both hypervariable and conserved regions. Universal primers are used to complement either end of the conserved region. The hypervariable regions contain specific signature sequences useful for bacterial identification at a species level.[92] Fungal pathogens can be identified using a similar process with universal fungal primers targeting the ITS1 and ITS4 conserved regions on the 18s and 28s rRNA sequences, respectively. The amplified sequences include the variable ITS2 region for species identification.[93] The use of 16s rRNA PCR for bacterial meningitis has been encouraging. In culture-proven cases of meningitis, 16s rRNA PCR demonstrated a sensitivity of 94%, a specificity of 94% confirming a bacterial cause, and was positive in 30% of culture-negative cases.[94] In cases of suspected CNS infection with a CSF pleocytosis greater than 500 cells/μL (to increase likelihood of bacterial pathogens), universal primers to 16s and 18s had a 65% sensitivity compared with 35% by microscopy and culture. The main reason for discordance was pretreatment with antibiotics before LP leading to diminished culture results.[95]

BRAIN BIOPSY

Before the advent of advanced molecular and immunologic testing, brain biopsy was considered the gold standard for diagnosis for certain encephalitides. However, the yield from brain biopsies is moderate, and its ability to identify a clear cause in encephalitis is poor.[96] Indeed, a recent study demonstrated that the most common initial pathologic diagnosis after biopsy was "encephalitis of unclear origin." Despite this, diagnostic yield may be increased with re-review by a neuropathologist, careful clinical evaluation with appropriate follow-up, and more advance molecular and immunologic testing.[97] Neuropathology review adds to the hypotheses of what type of encephalitis might be present even if a specific cause is not identified.

HYPOTHESIS-FREE TESTING

The performance characteristics of a pathogen-specific test are irrelevant if that organism is not on the treating physician's differential diagnosis, and thus, the test is not ordered. The candidate-based diagnostic approach relies on the unrealistic expectation that a clinician will have complete knowledge of all pathogenic, local microorganisms and their clinical manifestations. Although certain pathogens are native and endemic to specific regions, a constant flux of novel and mutated microorganisms commonly occurs.[98] This ever changing microbial landscape is becoming increasingly evident in the era of globalization and climate change. Migration and travel have led to rapid spread of pathogens into new regions, increasing the potential for epidemics and pandemics. Zika virus is a recent example of a virus that spread rapidly, with 2 years elapsing before its neurologic manifestations became apparent.[38]

Over the last decade, the cost of whole genome sequencing has fallen drastically and can now be achieved for less than $1000 with the data being generated in a day rather than the 10 years and $3 billion it took to sequence the first draft of the human genome. Unbiased mNGS provides a hypothesis-free and agnostic approach to the diagnosis of infectious meningoencephalitis. Total DNA and RNA are extracted from a patient's biological sample (ie, CSF and/or brain biopsy material) and both host and nonhost nucleic acid are amplified and then sequenced in a massively parallel manner with NGS technologies. After human and environmental contaminant sequences are computationally filtered out, the remaining sequences are rapidly matched against publicly available databases to identify the infectious cause.[99] Instead of multiple, targeted PCR tests being performed, mNGS allows testing of thousands of pathogens including novel organisms within a short timeframe.[100] mNGS can identify early outbreaks and the arrival of novel organisms to a region before large epidemiologic studies can detect definitive trends.[101,102] The final promise of mNGS is to identify previously overlooked neurotropic pathogens that cause meningoencephalitis, thereby gradually discovering the organisms responsible for some of the large percentage of cases that are deemed as unknown origin.

Potential Drawbacks

As all the nucleic acid within a sample is amplified in the mNGS assay, invariably there will be amplification of host and environmental contaminant sequences. The latter can originate from the patient's skin flora, microbial nucleic acid present in the collection tube, and laboratory reagents. This significant "background noise," which frequently includes many bacterial and fungal species that have pathogenic potential, can make interpretation difficult. Thus, stringent measures should always be taken during sequencing library preparation to minimize cross-contamination. A mock sequence library is created from water samples and is used as a control, thereby characterizing the environmental and background microbiome.[103,104]

In addition to computational solutions to mitigate difficulties discriminating between signal and noise, molecular depletion and enrichment techniques have been developed. Commercially available human ribosomal and mitochondrial RNA depletion kits are not useful for CSF samples because of the very low RNA yields (typically picogram quantities). Therefore, depletion of abundant sequences by hybridization (DASH) is a tool now being utilized to remove unwanted sequences. DASH uses CRISPR (clustered regularly interspaced short palindromic repeats)-Cas9 technology to target human complementary DNA (cDNA) within an already amplified sequencing library to reduce background noise in a highly specific and programmable manner that is completely agnostic to the input sample type and quantity.[105]

Conversely, VirCapSeq-VERT is a method for enriching viral sequences in metagenomic sequencing libraries by up to 10,000-fold. Approximately 2 million oligonucleotide probes that are designed to bind to the coding site of all viral taxa known to infect vertebrae are hybridized to a cDNA library. Streptavidin magnetic beads are added to the probes and their associated cDNA components. The beads are magnetically captured, cDNA removed, followed by posthybridization PCR. However, this method only enriches for known viral pathogens.[106,107]

The delay in processing massive amounts of data used to be the bottleneck in the timely delivery of clinically pertinent information. However, with rapid development in bioinformatics pipelines, the time required to process these data has been reduced drastically. Several pipelines currently exist, including Sequence-based Ultrarapid Pathogen Identification (SURPI), which is a cloud-compatible, open-access, computational pipeline used for pathogen identification from complex mNGS data.[108] SURPI was tailored for clinical use, and its speed is suited for clinical application where results are required within hours. The algorithm initially matches the sequence library against viral and bacterial databases and can process 7 to 50 million reads within 10 to 30 minutes. If this is negative, a comprehensive review of all pathogens in GenBank is performed within in 1 to 5 hours. The simultaneous development of both mNGS and bioinformatics has allowed exponential progress in the field of infectious diagnostics with promise for ongoing advancements.

Clinical Application

The use of research-based mNGS in the sphere of meningoencephalitis gained momentum after several notable cases and case series.[35,104,109-113] Until recently, astrovirus was considered only as a gastrointestinal infection and was not a standard test in the investigation of meningoencephalitis. Several recent cases have demonstrated a divergent genotype of astrovirus (HAstV-VA1/HMO-C-UK1) that has highly neurotropic characteristics in immunocompromised patients.[100,114–116] Given this discovery, it is now recommended that astrovirus should be considered during the workup of patients with meningoencephalitis.[100] These cases demonstrate the ability of mNGS to discover new neuroinvasive organisms that have not been previously considered pathogenic.

The first evaluation of a clinically validated CSF mNGS assay whose results are reportable in the patient medical record has now been conducted. The Precision Diagnosis of Acute Infectious Diseases study enrolled 204 patients with idiopathic meningitis, encephalitis, or myelitis at 8 hospitals, and the study results are currently under review. This and other studies promise to guide clinicians and health policy experts as they seek to understand the proper context in which mNGS testing is most appropriate.

SUMMARY

Neuroinfectious diseases continue to play a major role in morbidity and mortality worldwide, with many emerging or reemerging infections resulting in neurologic sequelae.[117,118] There is a growing need for rapid and accurate diagnostics that can lead to meaningful results and curb the significant burden of these diseases. Careful clinical evaluation of the patient coupled with the appropriate laboratory investigations leads to the correct diagnosis and implementation of appropriate management. mNGS is a promising new tool as its ability to identify multiple pathogens in a single test leads to an unbiased and agnostic approach in the diagnosis of infectious diseases. Prospective studies are forthcoming and will help to answer urgent questions about the overall performance characteristics of mNGS relative to conventional diagnostic modalities. As with other direct detection assays, it is likely that CSF mNGS will be relatively insensitive for detecting pathogens that are traditionally diagnosed with serology (eg, WNV and syphilis), that are anatomically localized (ie, brain abscess), or that have very low titers in the CSF.

REFERENCES

1. George BP, Schneider EB, Venkatesan A. Encephalitis hospitalization rates and inpatient mortality in the United States, 2000-2010. PLoS One 2014;9(9): e104169.
2. Vora NM, Holman RC, Mehal JM, et al. Neurology 2014;82(5):443–51.
3. Whitley RJ, Alford CA, Hirsch MS, et al. Vidarabine versus acyclovir therapy in herpes simplex encephalitis. N Engl J Med 1986;314(3):144–9.
4. Bohr V, Rasmussen N, Hansen B, et al. 875 cases of bacterial meningitis: diagnostic procedures and the impact of preadmission antibiotic therapy Part III of a three-part series. J Infect 1983;7(3):193–202.
5. Michael B, Menezes B, Cunniffe J, et al. Effect of delayed lumbar punctures on the diagnosis of acute bacterial meningitis in adults. Emerg Med J 2010;27(6):433–8.
6. Arslan F, Meynet E, Sunbul M, et al. The clinical features, diagnosis, treatment, and prognosis of neuroinvasive listeriosis: a multinational study. Eur J Clin Microbiol Infect Dis 2015;34(6):1213–21.
7. Monnier A, Abachin E, Beretti JL, et al. Diagnosis of Listeria monocytogenes meningoencephalitis by real-time PCR for the hly gene. J Clin Microbiol 2011; 49(11):3917–23.

8. Mailles A, Lecuit M, Goulet V, et al, National Study on Listeriosis Encephalitis Steering Committee. Listeria monocytogenes encephalitis in France. Med Mal Infect 2011;41(11):594–601.
9. Armstrong RW, Diseases FP. Brainstem encephalitis (rhombencephalitis) due to listeria monocytogenes: case report and review. Clin Infect Dis 1993. https://doi.org/10.1093/clind/16.5.689.
10. Bahr N, Boulware D. Methods of rapid diagnosis for the etiology of meningitis in adults. Biomark Med 2014;8(9):1085–103.
11. World Health Organization. Global tuberculosis report 2016. Geneva (Switzerland): World Health Organization; 2016. Available at: http://apps.who.int/iris/bitstream/10665/250441/1/9789241565394-eng.pdf. Accessed January 14, 2018.
12. Hematian A, Sadeghifard N, Mohebi R, et al. Traditional and modern cell culture in virus diagnosis. Osong Public Health Res Perspect 2016;7(2):77–82.
13. Matthey S, Nicholson D, Ruhs S, et al. Rapid detection of respiratory viruses by shell vial culture and direct staining by using pooled and individual monoclonal antibodies. J Clin Microbiol 1992;30(3):540–4.
14. Ginocchio CC, Zhang F, Malhotra A, et al. Development, technical performance, and clinical evaluation of a NucliSens basic kit application for detection of enterovirus RNA in cerebrospinal fluid. J Clin Microbiol 2005;43(6):2616–23.
15. DeBiasi RL, Tyler KL. Molecular methods for diagnosis of viral encephalitis. Clin Microbiol Rev 2004;17(4):903–25.
16. Polage CR, Petti CA. Assessment of the utility of viral culture of cerebrospinal fluid. Clin Infect Dis 2006;43(12):1578–9.
17. Barenfanger J, Lawhorn J, Drake C. Nonvalue of culturing cerebrospinal fluid for fungi. J Clin Microbiol 2004;42(1):236–8.
18. Ghanem K. Review: neurosyphilis: a historical perspective and review. CNS Neurosci Ther 2010;16(5):e157–68.
19. Vanhaecke C, Grange P, Benhaddou N, et al. Clinical and biological characteristics of 40 patients with neurosyphilis and evaluation of treponema pallidum nested polymerase chain reaction in cerebrospinal fluid samples. Clin Infect Dis 2016;63(9).1180–6.
20. Ratnam S. The laboratory diagnosis of syphilis. Can J Infect Dis Med Microbiol 2005;16(1):45–51.
21. Long SS, Pickering LK, Prober CG. Principles and practice of pediatric infectious diseases. Philadelphia: Elsevier; 2012.
22. Morse S, Holmes K. Atlas of sexually transmitted diseases and AIDS. Philadelphia: Elsevier; 2010.
23. Association of Public Health Laboratories. Laboratory diagnostic testing for Treponema pallidum, Expert Consultation Meeting Summary Report. 2009. Available at: https://www.aphl.org/programs/infectious_disease/std/Documents/ID_2009Jan_Laboratory-Guidelines-Treponema-pallidum-Meeting-Report.pdf#search=Laboratory%20diagnostic%20testing%20for%20Treponema%20pallidum%2C. Accessed January, 2018.
24. Hooshmand H, Escobar MR, Kopf SW. Neurosyphilis: a study of 241 patients. JAMA 1972;219(6):726–9.
25. Workowski KA, Berman S. Sexually transmitted diseases treatment guidelines. MMWR Recomm Rep 2010;59:1–110.
26. Harding A, Ghanem K. The Performance of cerebrospinal fluid treponemal-specific antibody tests in neurosyphilis: a systematic review. Sex Transm Dis 2012;39(4):291.

27. Nagel MA, Cohrs RJ, Mahalingam R, et al. The varicella zoster virus vasculopathies Clinical, CSF, imaging, and virologic features. Neurology 2008;70(11): 853–60.

28. Min SW, Kim Y, Nahm F, et al. The positive duration of varicella zoster immunoglobulin M antibody test in herpes zoster. Medicine 2016;95(33):e4616.

29. Nagel M, Forghani B, Mahalingam R, et al. The value of detecting anti-VZV IgG antibody in CSF to diagnose VZV vasculopathy. Neurology 2007;68(13): 1069–73.

30. Mathiesen T, Linde A, Olding-Stenkvist E, et al. Antiviral IgM and IgG subclasses in varicella zoster associated neurological syndromes. J Neurol Neurosurg Psychiatry 1989;52(5):578–82.

31. Gilden D, Bennett J, Kleinschmidt-DeMasters B, et al. The value of cerebrospinal fluid antiviral antibody in the diagnosis of neurologic disease produced by varicella zoster virus. J Neurol Sci 1998;159(2):140–4.

32. Davis L, DeBiasi R, Goade D, et al. West Nile virus neuroinvasive disease. Ann Neurol 2006;60(3):286–300.

33. Lanciotti R, Kerst A. Nucleic acid sequence-based amplification assays for rapid detection of West Nile and St. Louis encephalitis viruses. J Clin Microbiol 2001;39(12):4506–13.

34. Shi PY, Wong SJ. Serologic diagnosis of West Nile virus infection. Expert Rev Mol Diagn 2003;3(6):733–41.

35. Wilson M, Zimmermann L, Crawford E, et al. Acute West Nile virus meningoencephalitis diagnosed via metagenomic deep sequencing of cerebrospinal fluid in a renal transplant patient. Am J Transplant 2017;17(3):803–8.

36. Roehrig J, Nash D, Maldin B, et al. Persistence of virus-reactive serum immunoglobulin m antibody in confirmed West Nile virus encephalitis cases. Emerg Infect Dis 2003;9(3):376–9.

37. White M, Wollebo H, Beckham J, et al. Zika virus: an emergent neuropathological agent. Ann Neurol 2016;80(4):479–89.

38. Faria NR, Azevedo RDSDS, Kraemer MUG, et al. Zika virus in the Americas: early epidemiological and genetic findings. Science 2016;352(6283):345–9.

39. Huzly D, Hanselmann I, Schmidt-Chanasit J, et al. High specificity of a novel Zika virus ELISA in European patients after exposure to different flaviviruses. Euro Surveill 2016;21(16). https://doi.org/10.2807/1560-7917.ES.2016.21.16. 30203.

40. Centers for Disease Control and Prevention. Fact sheet for healthcare providers: interpreting ZikaMAC-ELISA test results. Atlanta (GA): Centre for Disease Control and Prevention; 2017. Available at: https://www.cdc.gov/zika/pdfs/interpreting-zika-mac-elisa-results.pdf. Accessed January 14, 2018.

41. da Silva IRF, Frontera JA, Bispo de Filippis AM, et al, RIO-GBS-ZIKV Research Group. Neurologic complications associated with the Zika Virus in Brazilian adults. JAMA Neurol 2017;74(10):1190–8.

42. Koedel U, Pfister HW. Lyme neuroborreliosis. Curr Opin Infect Dis 2017;30(1): 101.

43. Center for Disease Control and Prevention. Recommendations for test performance and interpretation from the second national conference on serologic diagnosis of Lyme disease. MMWR Morb Mortal Wkly Rep 1995;44(31):590–1.

44. Kalish RA, McHugh G, Granquist J, et al. Persistence of immunoglobulin M or immunoglobulin G antibody responses to Borrelia burgdorferi 10-20 years after active Lyme disease. Clin Infect Dis 2001;33(6):780–5.

45. Branda JA, Body BA, Boyle J, et al. Advances in serodiagnostic testing for Lyme disease are at hand. Clin Infect Dis 2017. https://doi.org/10.1093/cid/cix943.
46. Aguero-Rosenfeld ME, Nowakowski J, Bittker S, et al. Evolution of the serologic response to Borrelia burgdorferi in treated patients with culture-confirmed erythema migrans. J Clin Microbiol 1996;34(1):1–9.
47. Crother TR, Champion CI, Wu XYY, et al. Antigenic composition of Borrelia burgdorferi during infection of SCID mice. Infect Immun 2003;71(6):3419–28.
48. Lawrenz MB, Hardham JM, Owens RT, et al. Human antibody responses to VlsE antigenic variation protein of Borrelia burgdorferi. J Clin Microbiol 1999;37(12): 3997–4004.
49. Wormser G, Schriefer M, Aguero-Rosenfeld M, et al. Single-tier testing with the C6 peptide ELISA kit compared with two-tier testing for Lyme disease. Diagn Microbiol Infect Dis 2013;75(1):9–15.
50. Embers M, Hasenkampf N, Barnes M, et al. Five-antigen fluorescent bead-based assay for diagnosis of Lyme disease. Clin Vaccine Immunol 2016; 23(4):294–303.
51. Maraspin V, Cimperman J, Lotric-Furlan S, et al. Erythema migrans in solid-organ transplant recipients. Clin Infect Dis 2006;42(12):1751–4.
52. Mygland Å, Ljøstad U, Fingerle V, et al. EFNS guidelines on the diagnosis and management of European Lyme neuroborreliosis. Eur J Neurol 2010;17(1): 8–16, e1–4.
53. Ljøstad U, Skarpaas T, Mygland Å. Clinical usefulness of intrathecal antibody testing in acute Lyme neuroborreliosis. Eur J Neurol 2007;14(8):873–6.
54. Blanc F, Jaulhac B, Fleury M, et al. Relevance of the antibody index to diagnose Lyme neuroborreliosis among seropositive patients. Neurology 2007;69(10): 953–8.
55. Burgel N, Brandenburg A, Gerritsen H, et al. High sensitivity and specificity of the C6-peptide ELISA on cerebrospinal fluid in Lyme neuroborreliosis patients. Clin Microbiol Infect 2011;17(10):1495–500.
56. Schmidt C, Plate A, Angele B, et al. A prospective study on the role of CXCL13 in Lyme neuroborreliosis. Neurology 2011;76(12):1051–8.
57. Burgel N, Bakels F, Kroes A, et al. Discriminating Lyme neuroborreliosis from other neuroinflammatory diseases by levels of CXCL13 in cerebrospinal fluid. J Clin Microbiol 2011;49(5):2027–30.
58. Mothapo K, Verbeek M, Velden L, et al. Has CXCL13 an added value in diagnosis of neurosyphilis? J Clin Microbiol 2015;53(5):1693–6.
59. Singhi P. Neurocysticercosis. Ther Adv Neurol Disord 2011;4(2):67–81.
60. Centre for Disease Control and Prevention. Parasites - Cysticercosis. Atlanta (GA): Center for Disease Control and Prevention; 2017. Available at: https://www.cdc.gov/parasites/cysticercosis/health_professionals/index.html. Accessed January 20, 2018.
61. Furrows S, McCroddan J, Bligh W, et al. Lack of specificity of a single positive 50-kDa band in the electroimmunotransfer blot (EITB) assay for cysticercosis. Clin Microbiol Infect 2006;12(5):459–62.
62. Tsang VC, Brand JA, Boyer AE. An enzyme-linked immunoelectrotransfer blot assay and glycoprotein antigens for diagnosing human cysticercosis (Taenia solium). J Infect Dis 1989;159(1):50–9.
63. Wilson M, Bryan RT, Fried JA, et al. Clinical evaluation of the cysticercosis enzyme-linked immunoelectrotransfer blot in patients with neurocysticercosis. J Infect Dis 1991;164(5):1007–9.

64. Odashima N, Takayanagui O, Figueiredo J, et al. Enzyme linked immunosorbent assay (ELISA) for the detection of IgG, IgM, IgE and IgA against Cysticercus cellulosae in cerebrospinal fluid of patients with neurocysticercosis. Arq Neuropsiquiatr 2002;60(2B):400–5.

65. Zini D, Farrell VJ, Wadee AA. The relationship of antibody levels to the clinical spectrum of human neurocysticercosis. J Neurol Neurosurg Psychiatry 1990; 53(8):656–61.

66. Rodriguez S, Wilkins P, Dorny P. Immunological and molecular diagnosis of cysticercosis. Pathog Glob Health 2013;106(5):286–98.

67. Garcia HH, Gonzalez AE, Gilman RH, et al. Short report: transient antibody response in Taenia solium infection in field conditions-a major contributor to high seroprevalence. Am J Trop Med Hyg 2001;65(1):31–2.

68. Rodriguez S, Dorny P, Tsang VC, et al. Detection of taenia solium antigens and Anti–T. solium antibodies in paired serum and cerebrospinal fluid samples from patients with intraparenchymal or extraparenchymal neurocysticercosis. J Infect Dis 2009;199(9):1345–52.

69. Wang CY, Zhang HH, Ge LY. A MAb-based ELISA for detecting circulating antigen in CSF of patients with neurocysticercosis. Hybridoma 1992;11:825–7.

70. Chen JP, Zhang XY, Tan W, et al. Determination of circulating antigen in cysticercosis patients using McAb-based ELISA. Chung Kuo Chi Sheng Chung Hsueh Yu Chi Sheng Chung Ping Tsa Chih 1991;9:122–5. In Chinese, with English summary.

71. Gade W, Hinnefeld SW, Babcock LS, et al. Comparison of the PREMIER cryptococcal antigen enzyme immunoassay and the latex agglutination assay for detection of cryptococcal antigens. J Clin Microbiol 1991;29(8):1616–9.

72. Hansen J, Slechta E, Gates-Hollingsworth M, et al. Large-Scale evaluation of the immuno-mycologics lateral flow and enzyme-linked immunoassays for detection of cryptococcal antigen in serum and cerebrospinal fluid. Clin Vaccin Immunol 2013;20(1):52–5.

73. Escandón P, Lizarazo J, Agudelo C, et al. Evaluation of a rapid lateral flow immunoassay for the detection of cryptococcal antigen for the early diagnosis of cryptococcosis in HIV patients in Colombia. Med Mycol 2013;51(7):765–8.

74. Lu H, Zhou Y, Yin Y, et al. Cryptococcal antigen test revisited: significance for cryptococcal meningitis therapy monitoring in a tertiary chinese hospital. J Clin Microbiol 2005;43(6):2989–90.

75. Lamoth F. Galactomannan and 1,3-β-d-Glucan Testing for the Diagnosis of Invasive Aspergillosis. J Fungi (Basel) 2016;2(3). https://doi.org/10.3390/jof2030022.

76. Chong G, Maertens J, Lagrou K, et al. Diagnostic performance of galactomannan antigen testing in cerebrospinal fluid. J Clin Microbiol 2016;54(2): 428–31.

77. Marchetti O, Lamoth F, Mikulska M, et al. ECIL recommendations for the use of biological markers for the diagnosis of invasive fungal diseases in leukemic patients and hematopoietic SCT recipients. Bone Marrow Transplant 2011;47(6): bmt2011178.

78. Malani A, Singal B, Wheat L, et al. (1,3)-β-d-glucan in cerebrospinal fluid for diagnosis of fungal meningitis associated with contaminated methylprednisolone injections. J Clin Microbiol 2015;53(3):799–803.

79. Litvintseva A, Lindsley M, Gade L, et al. Utility of (1–3)-β-d-glucan testing for diagnostics and monitoring response to treatment during the multistate outbreak of fungal meningitis and other infections. Clin Infect Dis 2014;58(5):622–30.

80. Lyons J, Thakur K, Lee R, et al. Utility of measuring (1,3)-β-d-glucan in cerebrospinal fluid for diagnosis of fungal central nervous system infection. J Clin Microbiol 2015;53(1):319–22.
81. Aurelius E, Johansson B, Sköldenberg B, et al. Rapid diagnosis of herpes simplex encephalitis by nested polymerase chain reaction assay of cerebrospinal fluid. Lancet 1991;337(8735):189–92.
82. Nicholson F, Meetoo G, Aiyar S, et al. Detection of enterovirus RNA in clinical samples by nested polymerase chain reaction for rapid diagnosis of enterovirus infection. J Virol Methods 1994;48(2–3):155–66.
83. Sawyer MH, Holland D, Aintablian N, et al. Diagnosis of enteroviral central nervous system infection by polymerase chain reaction during a large community outbreak. Pediatr Infect Dis J 1994;13(3):177.
84. Gibbs RA. DNA amplification by the polymerase chain reaction. Anal Chem 1990;62(13):1202–14.
85. Rowley AH, Wolinsky SM, Whitley RJ, et al. Rapid detection of herpes-simplex-virus DNA in cerebrospinal fluid of patients with herpes simplex encephalitis. Lancet 1990;335(8687):440–1.
86. Lakeman FD, Whitley RJ. Diagnosis of herpes simplex encephalitis: application of polymerase chain reaction to cerebrospinal fluid from brain-biopsied patients and correlation with disease. National Institute of Allergy and Infectious Diseases Collaborative Antiviral Study Group. J Infect Dis 1995;17(1):857–63.
87. Puchhammer-Stöckl E, Presterl E, Croÿ C, et al. Screening for possible failure of herpes simplex virus PCR in cerebrospinal fluid for the diagnosis of herpes simplex encephalitis. J Med Virol 2001;64(4):531–6.
88. Patel V, Theron G, Lenders L, et al. Diagnostic accuracy of quantitative PCR (Xpert MTB/RIF) for tuberculous meningitis in a high burden setting: a prospective study. PLoS Med 2013;10(10). https://doi.org/10.1371/journal.pmed.1001536.
89. World Health Organization. WHO meeting report of a technical expert consultation: non-inferiority analysis of Xpert MT. Geneva (Switzerland): World Health Organization; 2017. Available at: http://apps.who.int/iris/bitstream/10665/254792/1/WHO-HTM-TB-2017.04-eng.pdf. Accessed January 21, 2018.
90. Bahr N, Nuwagira E, Evans E, et al. Diagnostic accuracy of Xpert MTB/RIF Ultra for tuberculous meningitis in HIV-infected adults: a prospective cohort study. Lancet Infect Dis 2018;18(1):68–75.
91. Leber AL, Everhart K, Balada-Llasat JM, et al. Multicenter evaluation of biofire filmarray meningitis/encephalitis panel for detection of bacteria, viruses, and yeast in cerebrospinal fluid specimens. J Clin Microbiol 2016;54(9):2251–61.
92. Clarridge JE. Impact of 16S rRNA gene sequence analysis for identification of bacteria on clinical microbiology and infectious diseases. Clin Microbiol Rev 2004;17(4):840–62.
93. Lindsley M, Hurst S, Iqbal N, et al. Rapid identification of dimorphic and yeast-like fungal pathogens using specific DNA probes. J Clin Microbiol 2001;39(10):3505–11.
94. Srinivasan L, Pisapia JM, Shah SS, et al. Can broad-range 16S ribosomal ribonucleic acid gene polymerase chain reactions improve the diagnosis of bacterial meningitis? A systematic review and meta-analysis. Ann Emerg Med 2012;60(5):609–20.e2.
95. Meyer T, Franke G, Polywka SK, et al. Improved detection of bacterial central nervous system infections by use of a broad-range PCR assay. J Clin Microbiol 2014;52(5):1751–3.

96. Schuette AJ, Taub JS, Hadjipanayis CG, et al. Open biopsy in patients with acute progressive neurologic decline and absence of mass lesion. Neurology 2010;75(5):419–24.

97. Gelfand J, Genrich G, Green A, et al. Encephalitis of unclear origin diagnosed by brain biopsy: a diagnostic challenge. JAMA Neurol 2015;72(1):66–72.

98. Asnis DS, Conetta R, Waldman G, et al. The West Nile virus encephalitis outbreak in the United States (1999 2000). Ann N Y Acad Sci 2001 Dec;951: 161–71.

99. Schubert RD, Wilson MR. A tale of two approaches: how metagenomics and proteomics are shaping the future of encephalitis diagnostics. Curr Opin Neurol 2015;28(3):283–7.

100. Brown JR, Morfopoulou S, Hubb J, et al. Astrovirus VA1/HMO-C: an increasingly recognized neurotropic pathogen in immunocompromised patients. Clin Infect Dis 2015;60(6):881–8.

101. McMullan LK, Frace M, Sammons SA, et al. Using next generation sequencing to identify yellow fever virus in Uganda. Virology 2012;422(1):1–5.

102. Wilson M, Suan D, Duggins A, et al. A novel cause of chronic viral meningoen-cephalitis: Cache Valley virus. Ann Neurol 2017;82(1):105–14.

103. Strong MJ, Xu G, Morici L, et al. Microbial contamination in next generation sequencing: implications for sequence-based analysis of clinical samples. PLoS Pathog 2014;10(11):e1004437.

104. Wilson MR, O'Donovan BD, Gelfand JM, et al. Chronic meningitis investigated via metagenomic next-generation sequencing. JAMA Neurol 2018. https://doi.org/10.1001/jamaneurol.2018.0463.

105. Gu W, Crawford E. Depletion of Abundant Sequences by Hybridization (DASH): using Cas9 to remove unwanted high-abundance species in sequencing li-braries and molecular counting applications. Genome Biol 2016;17(41). https://doi.org/10.1186/s13059-016-0904-5.

106. Kennedy P, Quan PL, Lipkin W. Viral encephalitis of unknown cause: current perspective and recent advances. Viruses 2017;9(6):138. https://doi.org/10.3390/v9060138.

107. Briese T, Kapoor A, Mishra N, et al. Virome capture sequencing enables sensi-tive viral diagnosis and comprehensive virome analysis. MBio 2015;6(5): e01491–5.

108. Naccache SN, Federman S, Veeraraghavan N, et al. A cloud-compatible bioin-formatics pipeline for ultrarapid pathogen identification from next-generation sequencing of clinical samples. Genome Res 2014;24(7):1180–92.

109. Wilson MR, Shanbhag NM, Reid MJ, et al. Diagnosing Balamuthia mandrillaris Encephalitis With Metagenomic Deep Sequencing. Ann Neurol 2015;78(5): 722–30.

110. Wilson MR, Naccache SN, Samayoa E, et al. Actionable diagnosis of neurolep-tospirosis by next-generation sequencing. N Engl J Med 2014;370:2408–17.

111. Chiu C, Coffey L, Murkey J, et al. Diagnosis of fatal human case of St. Louis en-cephalitis virus infection by metagenomic sequencing, California, 2016. Emerg Infect Dis 2017;23(10). https://doi.org/10.3201/eid2310.161986.

112. Murkey J, Chew K, Carlson M, et al. Hepatitis E virus-associated meningoen-cephalitis in a lung transplant recipient diagnosed by clinical metagenomic sequencing. Open Forum Infect Dis 2017;4(3):ofx121.

113. Mongkolrattanothai K, Naccache SN, Bender JM, et al. Neurobrucellosis: unex-pected answer from metagenomic next-generation sequencing. J Pediatric Infect Dis Soc 2017;6(4):393–8.

114. Frémond ML, Perot P, Muth E, et al. Next-generation sequencing for diagnosis and tailored therapy: a case report of astrovirus-associated progressive encephalitis. J Pediatr Infect Dis Soc 2015;4(3):e53–7.
115. Naccache SN, Peggs KS, Mattes FM, et al. Diagnosis of neuroinvasive astrovirus infection in an immunocompromised adult with encephalitis by unbiased next-generation sequencing. Clin Infect Dis 2015;60(6):919–23.
116. Quan PL, Wagner TA, Briese T, et al. Astrovirus encephalitis in boy with X-linked agammaglobulinemia. Emerg Infect Dis 2010;16(6):918–25.
117. Nath A. Neuroinfectious diseases: a crisis in neurology and a call for action. JAMA Neurol 2015;72(2):143–4.
118. Wilson M, Tyler KL. Emerging diagnostic and therapeutic tools for central nervous system infections. JAMA Neurol 2016;73(12):1389–90.

Viral Encephalitis

Arun Venkatesan, MD, PhD*, Olwen C. Murphy, MBBCh, MRCPI

KEYWORDS

- Encephalitis • Infectious encephalitis • Viral encephalitis
- Herpes simplex encephalitis • Autoimmune encephalitis • NMDAR encephalitis
- Acute disseminated encephalomyelitis

KEY POINTS

- Viruses are the most frequent organisms causing infectious encephalitis.
- Clues to the causative organism include age, region, travel history, comorbidities, prodromal symptoms, systemic manifestations of infection, and neurologic manifestations.
- Virus-specific serology or PCR testing of the CSF and/or serum can confirm the diagnosis in most forms of viral encephalitis.
- A few causes of viral encephalitides are treated with antiviral therapy, most importantly herpes simplex virus with acyclovir.
- CNS inflammation may occur in the context of postinfectious autoimmunity, specifically in the case of acute disseminated encephalomyelitis or antibody-mediated encephalitis following HSV encephalitis.

INTRODUCTION

Encephalitis is defined as inflammation of brain parenchyma with associated neurologic dysfunction. The term cerebritis is used when the etiologic organism causes gross purulence. The most common etiologies of encephalitis are infectious, autoimmune, and postinfectious. In North America, the incidence of confirmed infectious encephalitis has been reported as 1.0 per 100,000 person-years, with viral encephalitis representing 60% of these cases.[1]

Viral encephalitis can occur as a rare complication of common infections (eg, herpes virus infections) or can occur as a characteristic presentation of rare viruses (eg, rabies virus infection). Encephalitis may be the only neurologic manifestation of infection, or may occur in association with meningitis, myelitis, radiculitis, or neuritis.

Disclosures: The authors report no disclosures.
Division of Neuroimmunology and Neuroinfectious Diseases, Department of Neurology, Johns Hopkins Encephalitis Center, Johns Hopkins University School of Medicine, 600 N Wolfe Street, Baltimore, MD 21287, USA
* Corresponding author.
E-mail address: avenkat2@jhmi.edu

Neurol Clin 36 (2018) 705–724
https://doi.org/10.1016/j.ncl.2018.07.001
0733-8619/18/© 2018 Elsevier Inc. All rights reserved.

Here we review the clinical features and diagnostic evaluation of viral encephalitis, along with a discussion of important causative organisms. We also address viral encephalopathy and postinfectious immune-mediated encephalitis.

GENERAL FEATURES AND CLINICAL PRESENTATION OF VIRAL ENCEPHALITIS

Encephalitis is most frequently infectious or autoimmune in etiology. The clinical features of encephalitis are common to both of these etiologies and are outlined in **Box 1**. Alternatively, infections may cause encephalopathy (manifesting with altered mental status, confusion, behavioral change, agitation, or disruption of sleep-wake cycle) without direct central nervous system (CNS) infection or inflammation of brain tissue. Diagnostic criteria for viral encephalitis outlined by the International Encephalitis Consortium in 2013 are summarized in **Box 2**.[2]

History taking in patients with suspected encephalitis should focus on several factors that are helpful in establishing the differential diagnosis. In terms of temporal profile, viral encephalitis typically presents acutely to subacutely, whereas chronic presentations should prompt consideration of other microorganisms, such as fungi or mycobacteria.[2] Geographic region and the patient's travel history can suggest certain endemic organisms, such as West Nile virus in the United States. Comorbidities, such as HIV, may increase the risk of primary or opportunistic infections. Prodromal symptoms or systemic manifestations of infections (eg, fever or skin rash) may provide a useful clue that favors an infectious rather than autoimmune cause of encephalitis.

Neurologic examination should include assessment of level of consciousness, mental status, speech, seizures, signs of meningism, or raised intracranial pressure, along with evaluation of the cranial nerves and limbs for other focal neurologic features. Physicians should remember that meningitis, myelitis, radiculitis, or neuritis may also be present.

Box 1
Neurologic features associated with viral encephalitis

Altered level of consciousness
- Agitation
- Inattentiveness
- Drowsiness
- Comatose

Impaired cognition
- Confusion
- Disorientation
- Amnesia
- Behavioral change

Dysphasia

Seizures

Cranial neuropathies

Focal deficits in limbs

Movement disorders

Meningism
- Photophobia
- Neck stiffness
- Headache

> **Box 2**
> **Diagnostic criteria for encephalitis**
>
> Major criterion (required): altered mental status consisting of altered level of consciousness, lethargy, or personality change for ≥24 hours with no alternate cause identified
>
> Minor criteria (2 required for possible; ≥3 required for probable/confirmed encephalitis)
> • Fever ≥38°C
> • New-onset seizures (not attributable to prior seizure disorder)
> • New onset of focal neurologic findings
> • Cerebrospinal fluid white blood cell count ≥5 cells/mm³
> • Neuroimaging demonstrates brain parenchymal abnormality suggestive of encephalitis
> • Electroencephalogram demonstrates abnormality consistent with encephalitis

IMPORTANT VIRUSES CAUSING ENCEPHALITIS

Various causes of viral encephalitis may have distinguishing epidemiologic or clinical features. Here we highlight the most frequent and important viruses known to cause encephalitis. Geographic distribution and characteristic clinical features associated with these viruses are outlined in **Table 1**, and recommended diagnostic tests and neuroimaging features are outlined in **Table 2**. Immunocompromised patients are susceptible to a broader array of viruses causing encephalitis, a topic that is beyond the scope of this review.

Herpesviruses

Herpes simplex virus

Herpes simplex virus (HSV) is the single most common nonepidemic cause of infectious encephalitis in most countries.[1,3] HSV encephalitis is almost exclusively caused by HSV-1, except in neonatal populations where HSV-2 predominates.[4] HSV encephalitis follows a bimodal age distribution with peaks in early childhood and older than the age of 50, with most cases occurring in this older age group.[5] Cases of HSV encephalitis may result from primary infection or viral reactivation, although the pathophysiology of CNS infection has not yet been fully elucidated.

HSV encephalitis usually begins unilaterally and has a predilection for selective brain areas of the anterior and medial temporal lobe, inferior frontal lobe, thalamus, and insular cortex.[6] Most patients present with nonspecific symptoms including fever, headache, confusion, and altered behavior. Less frequent neurologic features include dysphasia, seizures, cranial neuropathies, and other focal neurologic deficits.[6] Brainstem encephalitis is possible but uncommon.[7] Clinical manifestations usually evolve over a few days, with around one-third of patients becoming comatose.[6]

Intravenous acyclovir reduces morbidity and mortality in confirmed HSV encephalitis,[8,9] with early treatment conferring additional benefit. There is no definitive evidence that the routine addition of steroids is beneficial in HSV encephalitis, but anecdotally this approach may be helpful in cases with severe edema or mass effect.[5]

Outcome of HSV encephalitis has improved dramatically in the acyclovir era. Mortality is now reported as less than 15%, although many survivors experience epilepsy or long-term neuropsychiatric deficits.[5]

Varicella zoster virus

Varicella zoster virus (VZV) is the second leading cause of viral encephalitis after HSV.[3,10] In children, encephalitis typically occurs 1 week after primary chickenpox rash and manifests most commonly with cerebellar ataxia, but may also cause more diffuse encephalitis.[11] In adults, VZV encephalitis commonly occurs in elderly

Table 1
Clinical features and regions of endemicity of important causes of viral encephalitis

Virus	Regions of Highest Frequency	Characteristic Nonneurologic Features	Characteristic Neurologic Features
Herpes simplex virus-1	Worldwide	Fever	Frontotemporal predilection Seizures Altered behavior, confusion, amnesia Dysphasia, hemiparesis
Varicella zoster virus	Worldwide	Children: chickenpox in majority Adults: shingles in around two-thirds	Children: cerebellar ataxia more frequent than diffuse encephalitis
West Nile virus	United States, North Africa, Eastern Europe, France	Fever, myalgia, headache ± diffuse nonpruritic maculopapular rash	Movement disorders Cranial neuropathies Weakness/hyporeflexia Acute flaccid paralysis in 5%–10%
Dengue virus	India, China, South-East Asia, Africa, Central and South America	Fever, myalgia, maculopapular rash Hemorrhagic manifestations	Encephalitis or encephalopathy Acute flaccid paralysis Guillain-Barré syndrome
Rabies virus	Africa and Asia	-	Prodromal neuropathic pain Hydrophobia, aerophobia, agitation, inspiratory spasms, autonomic disturbance Flaccid paralysis
Lymphocytic choriomeningitis virus	Worldwide	First phase of illness Initial fever, headache, myalgia, nausea, malaise, lymphadenopathy ± rash	Second phase of illness Nonspecific meningitis or encephalitis
Enteroviruses	Worldwide EV-71 most frequently seen in Asia	Pharyngitis Gastrointestinal illness Hand-foot-and-mouth disease Herpangina	Usually mild encephalitis EV-71 causes severe brainstem encephalitis ± flaccid paralysis
Mumps	Worldwide (highest incidence in regions without universal immunization programs)	Fever, malaise, parotitis Orchitis, oopharitis Pancreatitis	Usually mild encephalitis Movement disorders and brainstem manifestations are possible

Measles	Worldwide (highest incidence in regions without universal immunization programs)	Prodrome: fever, coryza, cough, Koplik spots Exanthem: morbilliform rash (encephalitis usually occurs during this phase)	Severe encephalitis: seizures, coma, focal neurologic deficits, signs of intracranial hypertension
Nipah virus	Bangladesh, India, South-East Asia, Australia	Flulike or respiratory illness	Severe encephalitis: brainstem dysfunction, coma, seizures, autonomic disturbance, segmental myoclonus Cerebellar signs
Hendra virus	Australia	Flulike illness	Severe encephalitis, not well described
Ebola virus	West Africa	Fever, profuse vomiting and diarrhea, hypervolemic shock ± Hemorrhagic complications	Nonspecific encephalitis
Influenza	Worldwide distribution but encephalopathy most frequently reported in Japan and Australia	Fever Respiratory symptoms Vomiting	Encephalopathy, including acute necrotizing encephalopathy Seizures

Table 2
Laboratory testing and neuroimaging characteristics of certain viruses

Virus	Laboratory Testing	Characteristic Neuroimaging Findings
HSV-1	• CSF PCR (false negative can occur in first 72 h after onset of neurologic symptoms) • CSF IgG (if >1 wk of neurologic symptoms)	• MRI brain abnormal in most cases: asymmetric abnormalities in mesiotemporal lobes, orbitofrontal lobes, and insular cortex with associated edema, possible restricted diffusion, or hemorrhage.
VZV	• CSF PCR (becomes negative 1–3 wk after onset of neurologic symptoms) • CSF IgG and serum/CSF IgG ratio (if >1 wk of neurologic symptoms)	• Neuroimaging normal in most patients. • MRI brain: lesions in cerebellum, brainstem, temporal lobes. Vasculopathy suggested by ischemic or hemorrhagic lesions in white matter or grey-white matter junction.
EBV	• CSF PCR (may be nonspecific) • Serum viral capsid antigen IgM and IgG (IgM may be become negative before symptoms occur) • Serum anti–Epstein Barr nuclear antigen (negative in acute infection, positive late in disease and persists for life) • Serum heterophile antibodies (less specific than serum IgM) • Atypical lymphocytes in serum and occasionally in CSF	• MRI brain abnormalities may occur, without characteristic location and including white matter abnormalities. • Imaging abnormalities are frequently transient and resolve after acute infection, even if widespread.
HHV-6	• Serum and CSF PCR	• Abnormalities in medial temporal lobes, thalamus, hippocampus, and other regions. • Cerebral edema.
CMV	• Serum and CSF PCR • Serum and CSF IgM and IgG	• Not well described in immunocompetent individuals.
Arboviruses 　West Nile virus 　La Crosse encephalitis 　Eastern equine encephalitis 　Powassan virus 　Jamestown Canyon virus 　St. Louis encephalitis	• CSF IgM, serum IgM and IgG • CSF PCR (low sensitivity unless tested early in clinical course during initial viremia) • Note that serologic cross-reactivity with other arboviruses within the same family is possible (eg, flaviviruses, such as West Nile virus and dengue virus, may cross-react)	• Neuroimaging may be normal. • MRI brain: abnormalities in brainstem, thalamus, basal ganglia ± leptomeningeal enhancement. • MRI spine in acute flaccid paralysis: T2 hyperintensity of gray matter of anterior horn cells ± conus medullaris/nerve root enhancement.

(continued on next page)

Table 2
(continued)

Virus	Laboratory Testing	Characteristic Neuroimaging Findings
Rabies virus	• Viral isolation from CSF, saliva, skin biopsy • Serum rabies virus neutralizing antibodies (rapid fluorescent focus inhibition test)	• MRI brain: abnormalities in temporal cortices, hippocampi, thalamus, basal, ganglia, substantia nigra, brainstem, cerebral white matter. • MRI spine: early changes in nerve root and plexus at level of bitten limb, followed by widespread spinal cord and nerve root involvement.
Lymphocytic choriomeningitis virus	• Viral isolation from CSF • CSF viral PCR • CSF: lymphocytic pleocytosis > expected for viral meningitis/encephalitis (100s to 1000s of WBC), sometimes hypoglycorrhachia and elevated protein)	• None characteristic.
EVs	• CSF viral PCR • Viral isolation from CSF (low sensitivity) • Viral isolation from throat or rectal swab (note that viral shedding may continue for weeks after clinical infection) • EV-71 is particularly difficult to detect in CSF with PCR or culture	• Most enteroviruses: neuroimaging normal, or abnormalities in brainstem structures. • EV-71: characteristic lesions in posterior medulla, pons, and dentate nuclei of cerebellum. • HPeV: white matter abnormalities.
Mumps	• Serum IgM (may not be detectable in immunized individuals, but rising serum IgG may be an indicator in these patients) • CSF PCR (high sensitivity) or IgM and IgG • Viral isolation from CSF, saliva, urine (only within first week of symptoms)	• Brainstem, hippocampus, splenial lesions reported.
Measles	• Serum IgM (may not be detectable until 4 d after rash onset) • CSF PCR (high sensitivity) • PCR of nasopharyngeal, throat, or urine samples in early infection	• Cerebral edema. • Cerebral lesions.

Henipaviruses
  Nipah virus
  Hendra virus
	• Serum or CSF IgM (sensitivity peaks around Day 12 of illness in Nipah encephalitis)
	• PCR of CSF, serum, and urine
		• Widespread subcortical and deep white matter lesions (Nipah encephalitis).

(continued on next page)

Table 2 (continued)		
Virus	Laboratory Testing	Characteristic Neuroimaging Findings
Ebola virus	• PCR of CSF and serum (higher titer in CSF)	• Not well described.
Influenza virus	• PCR or antigen testing of respiratory secretions	• Neuroimaging usually normal. • Acute necrotizing encephalopathy with bilateral thalamic lesions. • Mild encephalopathy with reversible splenial lesion.

Abbreviations: CSF, cerebrospinal fluid; EBV, Epstein-Barr virus; EV, enterovirus; HHV, human herpesvirus; HPeV, human parechovirus 3; HSV, herpes simplex virus; PCR, polymerase chain reaction; VZV, varicella zoster virus; WBC, white blood cell.

patients or the immunocompromised as a manifestation of viral reactivation.[12] Typical symptoms are altered mental status, focal neurologic signs, cranial neuropathies, and sometimes seizures. Around two-thirds of adults demonstrate an associated zoster rash.[12] Although the pathophysiology of VZV encephalitis is not completely understood, it has been suggested that VZV encephalitis may primarily result from virus-associated vasculopathy.[13]

CNS complications of VZV infection should be treated with intravenous acyclovir.[13] Outcome studies suggest mortality rates of up to 20% with VZV encephalitis, and a favorable outcome in approximately half of patients.[14,15] VZV infection may be preventable with vaccination (**Table 3**).

Table 3 Selected viruses amenable to treatment with antiviral therapies or prevention with vaccination	
Virus	Treatment
HSV-1	Intravenous acyclovir for 14–21 d
VZV	Intravenous acyclovir for 14–21 d
West Nile virus	Possible role for intravenous immunoglobulin (particularly if pooled from endemic populations with high levels of anti–West Nile virus antibodies)
Virus	Vaccination
VZV	Live attenuated varicella vaccine for prevention of chickenpox in unvaccinated/unexposed individuals (mainly children): 2 doses, usually given around 12 mo and 4–6 y Recombinant zoster vaccine (Shingrix) for prevention of chickenpox in adults >50 y: 2 doses separated by 2–6 mo
Mumps and measles	MMR vaccine: 2 doses in early childhood and consider third dose in young adulthood
Rabies	Pre-exposure vaccination for those at risks, such as animal handlers or international travelers: 3 doses over 21–28 d Postexposure vaccination after an animal bite • If never vaccinated: 4 doses over 14 d and single dose of human rabies immunoglobulin • If prior vaccination: 2 doses over 3 d
Influenza	Seasonal influenza vaccination

Other herpesviruses
Epstein-Barr virus (EBV) encephalitis typically occurs during primary EBV infection in children or young adults, and is associated with nonspecific systemic symptoms, such as fever, or frank infectious mononucleosis.[16] A broad array of neurologic features have been reported including seizures, confusion, "Alice in Wonderland" syndrome, opercular syndrome, and hemorrhagic meningoencephalitis.[16–18] Clinical outcome is usually benign, and although some physicians treat with acyclovir there is no clear evidence that this is beneficial.[19]

Infection with human herpesvirus 6 (HHV-6) occurs in most individuals worldwide before the age of 2 years.[20] HHV-6 is a frequent cause of febrile seizures in this age group, but may also cause encephalitis with altered behavior, reduced consciousness, and sometimes brainstem manifestations.[21,22] Neurologic manifestations occur during the febrile period of infection, sometimes before development of the characteristic rash of roseola infantum.[21] Most children make a good recovery.[23] In adults, infection can occur in settings of substantial immunosuppression, with the best characterized example being HHV-6-associated post-transplant limbic encephalitis.[24] Although there have been no controlled trials of antiviral treatments in HHV-6 encephalitis, such agents as ganciclovir and foscarnet are frequently used in immunocompromised individuals, and have been reportedly used in some immunocompetent children with severe manifestations of encephalitis.[25]

Cytomegalovirus encephalitis is extremely rare in immunocompetent hosts, with few cases reported.[26,27] Some of these patients have been treated with antiviral therapy, such as ganciclovir, although the benefit of antiviral treatment in immunocompetent patients is unclear.

Arboviruses

Arboviruses are a large family of arthropod vector-borne viruses. Birds or small mammalian animals act as viral reservoirs. Human infection typically results from a bite of an infected mosquito or tick, with humans acting as a dead-end host.[28] Outbreaks may follow seasonal patterns according to vector activity. Human-to-human transmission of arboviruses is uncommon, but is possible with infected blood products or organ transplantation.[29,30] Arboviral infections may be asymptomatic, neuroinvasive, or nonneuroinvasive. Neurologic symptoms usually emerge after a systemic infectious prodrome. In general, arboviruses can cause meningitis and/or encephalitis, and less frequently can affect the peripheral nerves or spinal cord with a predilection for the anterior horn cells, manifesting as acute flaccid paralysis.

West Nile virus
The first cases of West Nile virus infection in the United States occurred in New York in 1999 and it is now the commonest cause of epidemic viral encephalitis in the United States, but also occurs in other regions including Europe and North Africa.[28] West Nile virus manifests with fever, fatigue, headache, and myalgia, with or without a diffuse nonpruritic maculopapular rash.[31] Elderly, male, diabetic, and immunocompromised patients are at highest risk of developing neuroinvasive disease.[28,32] Encephalitis is the most frequent neurologic presentation of West Nile virus, occurring in 50% to 60% of neuroinvasive infections.[28] The virus has a predilection for the brainstem predominantly with coma as an early manifestation, and also can affect the basal ganglia, thalamus, and cerebellum.[28] Movement disorders, such as tremor, dyskinesia, myoclonus, and parkinsonism, are frequent.[33] Mild weakness or hyporeflexia may be detectable even in patients without full-blown acute flaccid paralysis with anterior

horn cell infection.[34] Optic neuropathy and other cranial neuropathies may also occur.[35]

Mortality of up to 15% can occur with West Nile encephalitis, and chronic fatigue or persistent movement disorders may be seen in survivors.[34]

Other arboviruses seen in North America

Although West Nile virus is by far the most frequent arbovirus causing encephalitis in North America, several other historically older arboviruses may also cause sporadic cases or small outbreaks of encephalitis. La Crosse encephalitis most commonly occurs in children in the eastern half of the United States.[36] Clinical presentation is mild with low mortality, although seizures occur in almost half of patients.[37] St. Louis encephalitis occurs in an outbreak pattern throughout the United States.[38] Powassan virus occurs in North-Eastern and Midwest states, frequently in older age groups. It causes a severe encephalitis, with approximately 10% mortality rate and long-term neurologic deficits seen in around half of survivors.[39] Oculomotor abnormalities and hemiplegia are frequent focal neurologic findings.[39] Eastern equine encephalitis occurs predominantly in eastern regions of the United States. Clinical presentations of encephalitis are severe and mortality is around 40%.[40] Jamestown Canyon virus causes a mild encephalitis, often in older people.[40]

Arboviruses seen in geographic regions outside North America

Japanese encephalitis is the most common cause of infectious encephalitis worldwide, occurring in southern and eastern Asia and predominantly affecting children and young adults.[41] Seizures occur in most cases. Extrapyramidal features, such as masklike facies, tremor, and rigidity are also common as a subacute or chronic manifestation.[41] Tick-borne encephalitis occurs in Europe, East Asia, and Russia, and causes isolated meningitis more frequently than meningoencephalitis.[42]

Dengue virus is common in India, China, South-East Asia, Africa, and Central and South America.[43] Neurologic manifestations occur in less than 10% of patients with dengue fever, and may result in higher morbidity and mortality.[44] Chikungunya virus has a similar geographic distribution to dengue virus. CNS involvement is rare but encephalitis, encephalopathy, meningitis, and optic neuropathy have all been reported.[45] Encephalitis has also been reported with Zika virus, an important emerging virus.[46]

Enteroviruses and Parechoviruses

Neurologic manifestations of nonpolio enteroviruses (EVs) are rare complications of common infections, occurring most frequently in children. Viral strains that may cause encephalitis include EV-D68, -71, -75, -76, and -89; coxsackievirus A9 and A10; echovirus 4, 5, 9, 11, 19 and 30; and human parechovirus 3.[47] EV infections usually occur in outbreaks and spread by fecal-oral or respiratory routes.[34] Typical manifestations of infection are pharyngitis, gastrointestinal illness, hand-foot-and-mouth disease, or herpangina.

EVs usually cause a mild encephalitis, with seizures or focal neurologic deficits occurring in less than 30% of patients.[48] However, EV-71 and EV-D68 are associated with more severe neurologic manifestations than other EVs, typically in young children. EV-71 causes a severe brainstem encephalitis manifesting with cranial nerve palsies, myoclonus, ataxia, and respiratory depression.[49] Acute flaccid paralysis may occur in combination with encephalitis or in isolation. Mortality of around 14% has been reported.[49] Clusters of brainstem encephalitis and acute flaccid paralysis have also been reported with outbreaks of EV-D68, with most affected children experiencing residual neurologic deficits.[50]

Rabies Virus

Rabies virus is transmitted from an animal bite and travels to the CNS trans-synapti-cally.[51] Postexposure prophylaxis is available and outlined in **Table 3**.[51] Human rabies has become rare in developed nations but is still common in regions of Africa and Asia.

Clinically, rabies virus infection manifests as either furious rabies with early limbic encephalitis, or as paralytic rabies with early radiculomyelitis. As the infection pro-gresses encephalitis ensues in all patients. Patients may have prodromal symptoms of mild weakness and neuropathic pain in the bitten extremity.[52] Characteristic neuro-logic features include agitation, hydrophobia, aerophobia, fluctuating consciousness, inspiratory spasms, and autonomic disturbance.[52] As the disease evolves, patients become comatose with flaccid paralysis.

There is no proven treatment of human rabies and death usually occurs within days of presentation. Rare cases of survival have been reported with bat-variant infections.[53]

Lymphocytic Choriomeningitis Virus

Lymphocytic choriomeningitis virus use rodents, such as house mice and hamsters, as a viral reservoir. Humans acquire the infection through direct contact with contam-inated material (ie, urine, feces) or by inhalation of aerosolized virus.[54]

The clinical hallmark of lymphocytic choriomeningitis virus is a biphasic illness. Pa-tients develop fever, headache, malaise, nausea, myalgia (often severe), and lymph-adenopathy, with or without erythematous rash. These nonspecific symptoms are followed by temporary improvement, followed a few days later by the CNS phase of the illness consisting of meningitis or encephalitis.[34] Extra-CNS manifestations may also occur at this stage, such as pneumonitis, myocarditis, orchitis, and parotitis.[54]

Most lymphocytic choriomeningitis virus infections are mild, and it is likely that cases are underrecognized. However, mortality can rarely occur.[54]

Mumps and Measles

Mumps and measles predominantly affect children and young adults. Incidence of mumps and measles encephalitis have plummeted since the widespread availability of vaccination.[55]

Meningitis occurs in less than 10% of mumps infections, and encephalitis in around 0.1%.[56] Systemic features characteristic of mumps are usually present and include fe-ver, malaise, parotitis, orchitis, oophoritis, and rarely pancreatitis. Both meningitis and encephalitis are usually mild. However, rare severe presentations of mumps enceph-alitis may occur, involving seizures, movement disorders, brainstem manifestations, or cortical blindness.[56,57]

Acute measles encephalitis complicates less than 0.3% of primary measles infec-tions and typically occurs during the phase of morbilliform rash.[58] However, rash may not be present in all cases of encephalitis and other nonspecific symptoms, such as fever and cough, may be the only clues to measles infection.[59] Measles en-cephalitis is usually severe. Patients may experience seizures, coma, focal neurologic deficits, cerebral edema, and intracranial hypertension.[58] Mortality is up to 15%, and 25% of survivors experience residual neurologic problems including epilepsy and developmental delay.[58]

Subacute sclerosing panencephalitis is a chronic, progressive neurologic condition occurring 6 to 15 years after primary measles infection and is caused by persistent infection with defective measles virus.[58] It is almost always fatal.

Henipaviruses

Hendra and Nipah are zoonotic viruses that rarely cause human infection. Bats are the viral reservoir for both viruses. Hendra virus is transmitted from bats to horses and then acquired by humans from contact with secretions/excretions of infected horses.[60] Nipah virus is transmitted to humans in the same manner via pigs.[60] Outbreaks of Hendra virus have occurred in Australia, whereas outbreaks of Nipah virus have occurred in Bangladesh, India, and South-East Asia. Both viruses cause severe encephalitis, usually associated with influenza-like or respiratory illness. Abnormal brainstem reflexes, autonomic disturbance, segmental myoclonus, seizures, and cerebellar signs are characteristic features commonly observed with Nipah virus encephalitis.[61] Hendra virus encephalitis is rare and less well described. Mortality of 40% to 70% has occurred with outbreaks of these viruses.[60]

Ebola Virus

Ebola virus causes a severe and highly contagious infection. The largest epidemic to date occurred in West Africa between 2013 and 2016. Ebola virus is acquired via direct contact with bodily fluids or tissue of an infected animal or human premortem or postmortem.[62] Systemic illness is severe and manifests with fever, profuse diarrhea, and vomiting leading to hypovolemic shock. Some patients develop hemorrhagic complications. A range of neurologic symptoms have been reported in patients with Ebola including altered mental status, behavioral disturbance, hallucinations, headache, seizures, meningismus, tinnitus, hearing loss, and blindness.[63,64] Because of the severity of systemic illness, epidemics occurring in low resource settings, and poor surveillance systems, the frequency and characteristics of neurologic complications have not been well described. However, some confirmed cases of encephalitis or meningoencephalitis been reported, sometimes occurring late in the disease course.[64,65] Mortality of up to 90% may occur with Ebola outbreaks, but mortality is primarily caused by severe systemic disease.[62]

Influenza

Neurologic complications of influenza infection are rare and occur most frequently with influenza A.[66] Influenza-associated encephalopathy has most frequently been reported in children in East Asia and Australia, where annual incidence in the pediatric population has been calculated as approximately 3 per 1,000,000.[66,67] However, cases also occur in Europe, North America, and in the adult population, with those older than the age of 65 and patients with pre-existing neurologic disease seeming most susceptible.[66,68]

An acute viral illness usually precedes neurologic manifestations. Fever, altered consciousness, seizures, and vomiting and are the most frequently reported symptoms in patients with encephalopathy, followed by ataxia and focal neurologic deficits.[66,67] Some patients present with a more severe and specific syndrome of acute necrotizing encephalopathy characterized by bilateral, frequently hemorrhagic, thalamic lesions.[69] Genetic susceptibility to acute necrotizing encephalopathy is possible, with autosomal-dominant mutations in the RANBP2 gene identified in familial and recurrent cases.[70] Another recognized rare presentation of influenza is the syndrome of mild encephalopathy with reversible splenial lesion.[71]

Unlike with the other viruses discussed here, cerebrospinal fluid (CSF) rarely demonstrates pleocytosis in influenza-associated encephalopathy.[66] Furthermore, influenza virus is rarely identified in the CSF of affected patients (using either polymerase chain reaction or viral isolation).[72] Therefore most strains of influenza are not thought to be neurotropic, and encephalopathy may instead result from host immune response with excess proinflammatory cytokine production and vascular endothelial damage.[73]

Mortality with influenza-associated encephalopathy is 9% to 37%, with residual disability reported in an additional 30% to 43%.[66–68,74] Patients are treated with usual anti-influenza medications, such as oseltamivir, but it is unknown if treatment affects neurologic outcome.

DIAGNOSTIC APPROACH IN VIRAL ENCEPHALITIS

In general, encephalitis is either infectious or autoimmune in cause. In some cases, the clinical presentation favors infectious over autoimmune encephalitis, such as if there is associated fever, rash, gastrointestinal, or respiratory symptoms. However, such features as movement disorders or faciobrachial dystonic seizures may be characteristic of specific anti-LGI1 autoimmune encephalitis. However, in many cases the presentation is nonspecific and both categories of encephalitis need to be considered in the initial diagnostic evaluation.

A suggested diagnostic approach to the patient with encephalitis is outlined in **Fig. 1.** One caveat in the evaluation of patients with encephalitis is that CSF sampling may not be possible if there are signs of intracranial hypertension. CSF in viral encephalitis typically demonstrates mild to moderate pleocytosis (usually lymphocytic), sometimes with elevated protein, but these routine studies are not useful in discriminating between

CSF studies
- Opening pressure
- Cell counts & WBC differential
- Protein, glucose
- Gram stain & bacterial culture
- HSV-1/2, VZV, enterovirus PCR
- HSV-1/2, VZV IgG if >1 wk of symptoms
- Oligoclonal bands & IgG index
- Additional studies according to potential organisms
- Neural specific autoantibodies
- Freeze extra sample for later testing

Blood tests
- Bacterial blood cultures
- HIV serology
- Additional studies according to potential organisms
- Neural specific autoantibodies
- Store serum samples for later testing

Imaging
- Chest x-ray
- Brain imaging (MRI with and without contrast if possible)
- Consider spinal imaging if suspicion for associated myelopathy or radiculopathy

Adjunctive tests
- EEG
- Samples from associated sites of infection eg, throat swab, stool culture

Targeted testing of serum/CSF for suspected viruses
- EBV, HHV-6, CMV: children/young adults, immunocompromised
- Arboviruses: based on region, season and vector exposures
- Mumps, measles, influenza: suggestive clinical features or known sick-contacts
- Henipaviruses, rabies: based on region and animal exposures
- Ebola: outbreak situation
- Consider other bacterial or fungal causes of encephalitis

Fig. 1. Diagnostic evaluation in suspected viral encephalitis. CMV, cytomegalovirus; EEG, electroencephalogram; PCR, polymerase chain reaction; WBC, white blood cell.

causes of encephalitis.[34] Further CSF studies are guided by whether infectious, autoimmune, or both categories of encephalitis are being considered. Examination of organism-specific CSF and serologic markers is undertaken based on a range of factors including patient age, geographic location, travel history, immunocompromised state, and animal or vector exposures. The most useful diagnostic tests for identification of each virus are outlined in **Table 1**. Where autoimmune encephalitis is possible, serum and CSF evaluation should also include testing for the presence of a panel of neural autoantibodies including N-methyl-D-aspartate receptor (NMDAR), LGI1, AMPAR, GAD65, GABA-A, and GABA-B.[75] Finally, it is always prudent to freeze an initial sample of CSF to allow later broader evaluation if initial investigations are unrevealing.

MRI may be helpful in the etiologic diagnosis because it may show a pattern characteristic of certain infections (see **Table 1**) or a pattern commonly seen with autoimmune encephalitis, such as bilateral medial temporal lobe involvement.[75] Electroencephalogram frequently shows nonspecific features of encephalopathy and/or epileptiform activity. However, certain electroencephalogram patterns may have diagnostic utility, such as extreme delta brush seen in some cases of NMDAR encephalitis.[76] Fluorodeoxyglucose PET/computed tomography imaging may have a role in some patients with encephalitis to examine patterns of cerebral metabolism, look for systemic sources of infection, or assess for malignancies that are associated with autoimmune encephalitis.[77–80]

TREATMENT APPROACH IN VIRAL ENCEPHALITIS

Most presentations of encephalitis are nonspecific and the initial treatment approach should broadly cover treatable infections, with subsequent narrowing to the suspected diagnosis. All patients presenting with a syndrome suggestive of acute encephalitis should be treated empirically with acyclovir (for HSV and VZV encephalitis) and if there is any suspicion for a bacterial meningoencephalitis then vancomycin and third-generation cephalosporin as well.[81]

Viral encephalitides amenable to treatment with antiviral therapies are outlined in **Table 2**. For other viruses there are no specific treatments available. Supportive management may include management of cerebral edema; treatment of seizures; and prevention of complications, such as hospital-acquired infections. Many patients require physical and/or cognitive rehabilitation after an episode of encephalitis.

Where autoimmune encephalitis is suspected or confirmed after diagnostic evaluation, treatment approaches include immunotherapy, which is beyond the scope of this article.

POSTINFECTIOUS AUTOIMMUNITY
Acute Disseminated Encephalomyelitis

Acute disseminated encephalomyelitis (ADEM) is defined as a first episode of acute encephalopathy and multifocal CNS demyelination, with no new symptoms, signs, or MRI findings 3 months after onset.[82] It is predominantly a pediatric disorder, with highest frequency between ages 5 and 8.[82] Studies have shown that in most cases ADEM is temporally linked to infection, occurring days to weeks after an upper respiratory tract infection or acute febrile illness.[83] However, the infectious organism is rarely identified.[84]

The most frequent presenting symptoms of ADEM are altered mental status, altered behavior, fever, vomiting, malaise, headache, and focal neurologic deficits related to demyelinating lesion location. Reported focal neurologic features are numerous and include hemiparesis, ataxia, dysphasia, movement disorders, visual deficits, and cranial neuropathies.[83,85] Some patients develop seizures or coma. The spinal cord is involved in around one-quarter of patients.[85]

CSF studies usually show a mild lymphocytic pleocytosis.[86] MRI brain is the most useful investigation in ADEM. This typically shows multifocal T2-hyperintense irregular/poorly defined lesions measuring 5 mm to 50 mm,[83] with some or all lesions enhancing postcontrast in the acute phase. Lesions occur most frequently in the subcortical and central white matter of the frontal and temporal lobes, although other locations may also be involved.[83] Myelitis is usually longitudinally extensive.[84]

Although there are no randomized trials examining the treatment of ADEM, generally accepted and used treatments include high-dose intravenous steroids, intravenous immunoglobulin, and plasma exchange.[82] Most children recover substantially. Long-term neurocognitive deficits are most common in children affected younger than the age of 5 years.[84]

Relapsing or multiphasic ADEM occurs in up to 10% of cases, although this disease entity is an area of some debate.[84] Some multiphasic patients may actually have alternative distinct neuroimmunologic disorders, such as neuromyelitis optica, multiple sclerosis, or recently identified MOG-antibody-related syndromes.[87]

Herpes Simplex Virus Encephalitis Triggering N-Methyl-D-Aspartate Receptor Encephalitis

A minority of patients with HSV encephalitis follow a relapsing clinical course, with apparent deterioration or development of new neurologic symptoms in the weeks to months following their illness. In recent years evidence has emerged that relapsing symptoms post-HSV encephalitis in patients who have cleared the virus from CSF may be caused by autoimmune mechanisms. In 2012, Prüss and colleagues[88] reported that 30% of patients with HSV encephalitis developed NMDAR antibodies in the serum. Since then, NMDAR antibodies have been identified in many patients with relapsing symptoms post-HSV encephalitis. Cases occur most frequently in children who typically manifest with choreoathetosis, altered consciousness, or seizures.[89] Adults are more likely to manifest with psychiatric symptoms.[89]

In patients experiencing relapsing symptoms following treatment of HSV encephalitis, CSF study should be repeated for HSV polymerase chain reaction. Detectable HSV suggests ongoing infection and these patients should be retreated with acyclovir.[89] Undetectable HSV with a CSF pleocytosis supports an autoimmune mechanism and in these patients NMDAR antibody (and other routinely available neural autoantibodies) should be tested in the CSF and serum. Regardless of whether antibodies are actually detected at this stage, in patients who have cleared HSV an autoimmune mechanism should be suspected and immunotherapy should be strongly considered. Patients should be treated according to guidelines for NMDAR encephalitis, with first-line including high-dose steroids, plasma exchange, intravenous immunoglobulins, and second-line including rituximab, mycophenylate mofetil, and cyclophosphamide.[89]

Other antibodies including AMPAR, $GABA_AR$, and D2R have been detected in patients with relapsing symptoms post-HSV encephalitis. Similarly, it has been suggested that other viruses, such as VZV, EBV, EV, and HHV-6, may act as triggers for postinfectious NMDAR encephalitis.[89] Future research may elucidate further relationships between CNS infections and autoimmune syndromes.

SUMMARY

Viruses are a frequent cause of encephalitis. Causative viruses vary depending on host factors; geographic location; season; and exposure to vectors, animals, or sick-contacts. In addition, when evaluating a patient with possible encephalitis, other etiologies must also be considered, such as bacterial/fungal/parasitic infections or autoimmune encephalitis. Careful clinical evaluation may provide clues to the underlying cause of encephalitis and guide further diagnostic work-up. However, empiric treatment with acyclovir should still be considered in all cases, until HSV and/or VZV are excluded. Finally, recognition of CNS inflammation in the postinfectious period has important implications with respect to treatment.

REFERENCES

1. Dubey D, Pittock SJ, Kelly CR, et al. Autoimmune encephalitis epidemiology and a comparison to infectious encephalitis. Ann Neurol 2018. https://doi.org/10.1002/ana.25131.
2. Venkatesan A, Tunkel AR, Bloch KC, et al. Case definitions, diagnostic algorithms, and priorities in encephalitis: consensus statement of the international encephalitis consortium. Clin Infect Dis 2013;57(8):1114.
3. Mailles A, Stahl J. Infectious encephalitis in France in 2007: a national prospective study. Clin Infect Dis 2009;49(12):1838–47.
4. Whitley RJ. Herpes simplex virus infections of the central nervous system. Continuum (Minneap Minn) 2015;21(6 Neuroinfectious Disease):1704–13.
5. Bradshaw MJ, Venkatesan A. Herpes simplex virus-1 encephalitis in adults: pathophysiology, diagnosis, and management. Neurotherapeutics 2016;13(3):493–508.
6. Gnann JW, Whitley RJ. Herpes simplex encephalitis: an update. Curr Infect Dis Rep 2017;19(3):13.
7. Livorsi D, Anderson E, Qureshi S, et al. Brainstem encephalitis: an unusual presentation of herpes simplex virus infection. J Neurol 2010;257(9):1432–7.
8. Whitley RJ, Alford CA, Hirsch MS, et al. Vidarabine versus acyclovir therapy in herpes simplex encephalitis. N Engl J Med 1986;314(3):144–9.
9. Sköldenberg B, Forsgren M, Alestig K, et al. Acyclovir versus vidarabine in herpes simplex encephalitis. Randomised multicentre study in consecutive Swedish patients. Lancet 1984;2(8405):707–11.
10. Singh TD, Fugate JE, Rabinstein AA. The spectrum of acute encephalitis: causes, management, and predictors of outcome. Neurology 2015;84(4):359–66.
11. Science M, MacGregor D, Richardson SE, et al. Central nervous system complications of varicella-zoster virus. J Pediatr 2014;165(4):779–85.
12. Pahud BA, Glaser CA, Dekker CL, et al. Varicella zoster disease of the central nervous system: epidemiological, clinical, and laboratory features 10 years after the introduction of the varicella vaccine. J Infect Dis 2011;203(3):316–23.
13. Grahn A, Studahl M. Varicella-zoster virus infections of the central nervous system: prognosis, diagnostics and treatment. J Infect 2015;71(3):281–93.
14. Granerod J, Ambrose HE, Davies NW, et al. Causes of encephalitis and differences in their clinical presentations in England: a multicentre, population-based prospective study. Lancet Infect Dis 2010;10(12):835–44.
15. Mailles A, De Broucker T, Costanzo P, et al. Long-term outcome of patients presenting with acute infectious encephalitis of various causes in France. Clin Infect Dis 2012;54(10):1455–64.
16. Bathoorn E, Vlaminckx BJM, Schoondermark-Stolk S, et al. Primary Epstein–Barr virus infection with neurological complications. Scand J Infect Dis 2011;43(2):136–44.

17. Matsushima T, Nishioka K, Tanaka R, et al. Anterior opercular syndrome induced by Epstein-Barr virus encephalitis. Neurocase 2016;22(1):103–8.
18. Ascenção BB, Gonçalves AC, Luís N, et al. Epstein-Barr virus hemorrhagic meningoencephalitis: case report and review of the literature. J Neurovirol 2016;22(5):695–8.
19. Baskin HJ, Hedlund G. Neuroimaging of herpesvirus infections in children. Pediatr Radiol 2007;37(10):949.
20. Hill JA, Venna N. Human herpesvirus 6 and the nervous system. In: Tselis AC, Booss J, editors. Handbook of clinical neurology, vol. 123. Amsterdam (Netherlands): Elsevier; 2014. p. 327–55.
21. Suga S, Yoshikawa T, Asano Y, et al. Clinical and virological analyses of 21 infants with exanthem subitum (roseola infantum) and central nervous system complications. Ann Neurol 1993;33(6):597–603.
22. Crawford JR, Kadom N, Santi MR, et al. Human herpesvirus 6 rhombencephalitis in immunocompetent children. J Child Neurol 2007;22(11):1260–8.
23. Yoshikawa T, Asano Y. Central nervous system complications in human herpesvirus-6 infection. Brain Dev 2000;22(5):307–14.
24. Seeley WW, Marty FM, Holmes TM, et al. Post-transplant acute limbic encephalitis: clinical features and relationship to HHV6. Neurology 2007;69(2):156–65.
25. Olli-Lähdesmäki T, Haataja L, Parkkola R, et al. High-dose ganciclovir in HHV-6 encephalitis of an immunocompetent child. Pediatr Neurol 2010;43(1):53–6.
26. Prösch S, Schielke E, Reip A, et al. Human cytomegalovirus (HCMV) encephalitis in an immunocompetent young person and diagnostic reliability of HCMV DNA PCR using cerebrospinal fluid of nonimmunosuppressed patients. J Clin Microbiol 1998;36(12):3636–40.
27. Rafailidis PI, Mourtzoukou EG, Varbobitis IC, et al. Severe cytomegalovirus infection in apparently immunocompetent patients: a systematic review. Virol J 2008;5:47.
28. Beckham JD, Tyler KL. Arbovirus infections. Continuum (Minneap Minn) 2015; 21(6 Neuroinfectious Disease):1599–611.
29. Petersen LR, Busch MP. Transfusion-transmitted arboviruses. Vox Sang 2010; 98(4):495–503.
30. Nogueira ML, Estofolete CF, Terzian ACB, et al. Zika virus infection and solid organ transplantation: a new challenge. Am J Transplant 2017;17(3):791–5.
31. Sejvar JJ. Clinical manifestations and outcomes of West Nile virus infection. Viruses 2014;6(2):606–23.
32. Jean CM, Honarmand S, Louie JK, et al. Risk factors for West Nile virus neuroinvasive disease, California, 2005. Emerg Infect Dis 2007;13(12):1918.
33. Sejvar JJ, Haddad MB, Tierney BC, et al. Neurologic manifestations and outcome of West Nile virus infection. JAMA 2003;290(4):511–5.
34. DeBiasi RL, Tyler KL. Viral meningitis and encephalitis. Continuum (Minneap Minn) 2006;12(2, Infectious Diseases):58.
35. Watson NK, Bartt RE, Houff SA, et al. Focal neurological deficits and West Nile virus infection. Clin Infect Dis 2005;40(7):e62.
36. Centers for Disease Control and Prevention. Epidemiology & geographic distribution of La Crosse encephalitis. 2017. Available at: https://www.cdc.gov/lac/tech/epi.html. Accessed January 18, 2018.
37. McJunkin JE, de los Reyes EC, Irazuzta JE, et al. La Crosse encephalitis in children. N Engl J Med 2001;344(11):801–7.

38. Center for Disease Control and Prevention. Epidemiology & geographic distribution of Saint Louis encephalitis. 2017. Available at: https://www.cdc.gov/sle/technical/epi.html. Accessed January 18, 2018.
39. Hermance ME, Thangamani S. Powassan virus: an emerging arbovirus of public health concern in North America. Vector Borne Zoonotic Dis 2017;17(7):453–62.
40. Burakoff A, Lehman J, Fischer M, et al. West Nile virus and other nationally notifiable arboviral diseases—United States, 2016. MMWR Morb Mortal Wkly Rep 2018;67(1):13–7.
41. Solomon T, Dung NM, Kneen R, et al. Japanese encephalitis. J Neurol Neurosurg Psychiatry 2000;68(4):405–15.
42. Taba P, Schmutzhard E, Forsberg P, et al. EAN consensus review on prevention, diagnosis and management of tick-borne encephalitis. Eur J Neurol 2017;24(10): e61.
43. Bhatt S, Gething PW, Brady OJ, et al. The global distribution and burden of dengue. Nature 2013;496(7446):504–7.
44. Wasay M, Channa R, Jumani M, et al. Encephalitis and myelitis associated with dengue viral infection clinical and neuroimaging features. Clin Neurol Neurosurg 2008;110(6):635–40.
45. Cerny T, Schwarz M, Schwarz U, et al. The range of neurological complications in chikungunya fever. Neurocrit Care 2017;27(3):447–57.
46. Soares CN, Brasil P, Carrera RM, et al. Fatal encephalitis associated with Zika virus infection in an adult. J Clin Virol 2016;83:63–5.
47. Jain S, Patel B, Bhatt GC. Enteroviral encephalitis in children: clinical features, pathophysiology, and treatment advances. Pathog Glob Health 2014;108(5): 216–22.
48. Fowlkes AL, Honarmand S, Glaser C, et al. Enterovirus-associated encephalitis in the California encephalitis project, 1998–2005. J Infect Dis 2008;198(11): 1685–91.
49. Huang C, Liu C, Chang Y, et al. Neurologic complications in children with enterovirus 71 infection. N Engl J Med 1999;341(13):936–42.
50. Messacar K, Schreiner TL, Maloney JA, et al. A cluster of acute flaccid paralysis and cranial nerve dysfunction temporally associated with an outbreak of enterovirus D68 in children in Colorado, USA. Lancet 2015;385(9978):1662–71.
51. Jackson A. Human rabies: a 2016 update. Curr Infect Dis Rep 2016;18(11):1–6.
52. Hemachudha T, Ugolini G, Wacharapluesadee S, et al. Human rabies: neuropathogenesis, diagnosis, and management. Lancet Neurol 2013;12(5):498–513.
53. Hattwick MA, Weis TT, Stechschulte CJ, et al. Recovery from rabies. A case report. Ann Intern Med 1972;76(6):931–42.
54. Bonthius DJ. Lymphocytic choriomeningitis virus: an under-recognized cause of neurologic disease in the fetus, child, and adult. Semin Pediatr Neurol 2012; 19(3):89–95.
55. Iro MA, Sadarangani M, Goldacre R, et al. 30-year trends in admission rates for encephalitis in children in England and effect of improved diagnostics and measles-mumps-rubella vaccination: a population-based observational study. Lancet Infect Dis 2017;17(4):422–30.
56. Tyor W, Harrison T. Mumps and rubella [Chapter: 28]. In: Tselis AC, Booss J, editors. Handbook of clinical neurology, vol. 123. Elsevier; 2014. p. 591–600.
57. Suga K, Goji A, Shono M, et al. Mumps encephalitis with akinesia and mutism. Pediatr Int 2015;57(4):721–4.
58. Buchanan R, Bonthius DJ. Measles virus and associated central nervous system sequelae. Semin Pediatr Neurol 2012;19(3):107–14.

59. Zeng S, Zhang B, Zhang Y, et al. Identification of 12 cases of acute measles encephalitis without rash. Clin Infect Dis 2016;63(12):1630–3.

60. Abdullah S, Tan CT. Henipavirus encephalitis [Chapter: 32]. In: Tselis AC, Booss J, editors. Handbook of clinical neurology, vol. 123. Amsterdam (Netherlands): Elsevier; 2014. p. 663–70.

61. Goh KJ, Tan CT, Chew NK, et al. Clinical features of Nipah virus encephalitis among pig farmers in Malaysia. N Engl J Med 2000;342(17):1229–35.

62. Billioux BJ, Smith B, Nath A. Neurological complications of Ebola virus infection. Neurotherapeutics 2016;13(3):461–70.

63. Bwaka MA, Bonnet M, Calain P, et al. Ebola hemorrhagic fever in Kikwit, democratic republic of the Congo: clinical observations in 103 patients. J Infect Dis 1999;179(Supplement_1):S7.

64. de Greslan T, Billhot M, Rousseau C, et al. Ebola virus–related encephalitis. Clin Infect Dis 2016;63(8):1076–8.

65. Jacobs M, Rodger A, Bell DJ, et al. Late Ebola virus relapse causing meningoencephalitis: a case report. Lancet 2016;388(10043):498–503.

66. Okuno H, Yahata Y, Tanaka-Taya K, et al. Characteristics and outcomes of influenza-associated encephalopathy cases among children and adults in Japan, 2010-2015. Clin Infect Dis 2017. https://doi.org/10.1093/cid/cix1126.

67. Britton PN, Blyth CC, Macartney K, et al. The spectrum and burden of influenza-associated neurological disease in children: combined encephalitis and influenza sentinel site surveillance from Australia, 2013-2015. Clin Infect Dis 2017;65(4): 653–60.

68. Paksu MS, Aslan K, Kendirli T, et al. Neuroinfluenza: evaluation of seasonal influenza associated severe neurological complications in children (a multicenter study). Childs Nerv Syst 2018;34(2):335–47.

69. Araújo R, Gouveia P, Fineza I. Bilateral thalamic lesions in acute necrotizing encephalopathy due to H1N1 infection. Pediatr Neurol 2016;65:96–7.

70. Gika AD, Rich P, Gupta S, et al. Recurrent acute necrotizing encephalopathy following influenza A in a genetically predisposed family. Dev Med Child Neurol 2010;52(1):99–102.

71. Takatsu H, Ishimaru N, Ito M, et al. Mild encephalitis/encephalopathy with a reversible splenial lesion in an adult patient with influenza. Intern Med 2017; 56(22):3093–5.

72. Ekstrand JJ. Neurologic complications of influenza. Semin Pediatr Neurol 2012; 19(3):96–100.

73. Yamashita N. Neurotropic influenza virus infections. In: Reiss, Carol S, editors. Neurotropic viral infections. Cham (Switzerland): Springer; 2016. p. 295–314.

74. Morishima T, Togashi T, Yokota S, et al. Encephalitis and encephalopathy associated with an influenza epidemic in japan. Clin Infect Dis 2002;35(5):512–7.

75. Dubey D, Toledano M, McKeon A. Clinical presentation of autoimmune and viral encephalitides. Curr Opin Crit Care 2018. https://doi.org/10.1097/MCC. 0000000000000483.

76. Yildirim M, Konuskan B, Yalnizoglu D, et al. Electroencephalographic findings in anti-N-methyl-d-aspartate receptor encephalitis in children: a series of 12 patients. Epilepsy Behav 2018;78:118–23.

77. Probasco JC, Solnes L, Nalluri A, et al. Abnormal brain metabolism on FDG-PET/CT is a common early finding in autoimmune encephalitis. Neurol Neuroimmunol Neuroinflamm 2017;4(4):e352.

78. Probasco JC, Solnes L, Nalluri A, et al. Decreased occipital lobe metabolism by FDG-PET/CT: an anti-NMDA receptor encephalitis biomarker. Neurol Neuroimmunol Neuroinflamm 2018;5(1):e413.
79. Solnes LB, Jones KM, Rowe SP, et al. Diagnostic value of 18F-FDG PET/CT versus MRI in the setting of antibody-specific autoimmune encephalitis. J Nucl Med 2017;58(8):1307–13.
80. Kampe KKW, Rotermund R, Tienken M, et al. Diagnostic value of positron emission tomography combined with computed tomography for evaluating critically ill neurological patients. Front Neurol 2017;8:33.
81. Glaser C, Venkatesan A. Encephalitis. In: Scheld WM, Whitley RJ, Marra CM, editors. Infections of the central nervous system. 4th edition. Philadelphia: Wolters Kluwer Health Adis (ESP); 2014. p. 84–111.
82. Pohl D, Alper G, Van Haren K, et al. Acute disseminated encephalomyelitis: updates on an inflammatory CNS syndrome. Neurology 2016;87(9 Suppl 2):38.
83. Esposito S, Di Pietro GM, Madini B, et al. A spectrum of inflammation and demyelination in acute disseminated encephalomyelitis (ADEM) of children. Autoimmun Rev 2015;14(10):923–9.
84. Narula S, Banwell B. Pediatric demyelination. Continuum (Minneap Minn) 2016; 22(3):897–915.
85. Koelman DLH, Chahin S, Mar SS, et al. Acute disseminated encephalomyelitis in 228 patients: a retrospective, multicenter US study. Neurology 2016;86(22): 2085–93.
86. Gray MP, Gorelick MH. Acute disseminated encephalomyelitis. Pediatr Emerg Care 2016;32(6):395–400.
87. Jurynczyk M, Messina S, Woodhall MR, et al. Clinical presentation and prognosis in MOG-antibody disease: a UK study. Brain 2017;140(12):3128–38.
88. Prüss H, Finke C, Höltje M, et al. N-methyl-D-aspartate receptor antibodies in herpes simplex encephalitis. Ann Neurol 2012;72(6):902–11.
89. Prüss H. Postviral autoimmune encephalitis: manifestations in children and adults. Curr Opin Neurol 2017;30(3):327–33.

Manifestations of Herpes Virus Infections in the Nervous System

Israel Steiner, MD[a,b,*], Felix Benninger, MD[a,b]

KEYWORDS

- Herpes simplex virus • Varicella-zoster virus • Encephalitis • Meningoencephalitis
- Reactivation infection • Postinfection

KEY POINTS

- Intravenous acyclovir should be commenced as soon as a diagnosis of herpes simplex encephalitis (HSE) is suspected. A delay in starting acyclovir is associated with a worse prognosis.
- The role of steroid therapy in established HSE has yet to be established.
- Post–herpes zoster syndromes can involve anywhere in the neuraxis.

INTRODUCTION

Out of the 8 human herpes viruses, 3 are considered neurotropic. Herpes simplex virus (HSV) type 1 (HSV-1), HSV-2, and varicella-zoster virus (VZV) vary in their molecular structure but share the ability to establish latent infection for the lifetime of the human host in the peripheral nervous system (PNS) in the dorsal root ganglia (DRG). This state of latency can give rise to recurrent reactivations responsible for important morbidity and mortality.

HSV-I is the cause of encephalitis, corneal blindness, and several disorders of the PNS; HSV-2 is mainly responsible for meningoencephalitis in neonates and meningitis in adults. Reactivation of VZV, the pathogen of varicella (chickenpox), is associated with herpes zoster (shingles) and central nervous system (CNS) complications such as myelitis and focal vasculopathies.

Disclosure: The authors have no relevant disclosure.
a Department of Neurology, Felsenstein Medical Research Institut, Rabin Medical Center, Beilinson Hospital, Beilinson Campus, Petach Tikva 49100, Israel; b Sackler Faculty of Medicine, Tel Aviv University, Tel Aviv 6997801, Israel
* Corresponding author. Department of Neurology, Beilinson Hospital, Rabin Medical Center, Petach Tikva 49100, Israel.
E-mail address: israels2@clalit.org.il

Neurol Clin 36 (2018) 725–738
https://doi.org/10.1016/j.ncl.2018.06.005
neurologic.theclinics.com

The name herpes stems from the ancient Greek and means to creep or crawl.[1] The herpes viruses were the focus of intense research and study for more than a century, because they are important human pathogens in the realms of dermatology, pediatrics, infectious diseases, obstetrics and gynecology, and neurology.

STRUCTURE, LATENCY, AND REACTIVATION

The Herpesviridae family of DNA viruses has a double-stranded DNA molecule located within an icosapentahedral capsid that contains 162 capsomers. The capsid is surrounded by the tegument, an amorphous proteinic material, which is in turn encapsulated by an envelope.

HSV-I and HSV-2 are closely related, with nearly 70% genomic homology. Differences in antigen expression and biological properties serve as methods for differentiation. VZV differs from the two herpes simplex viruses because it replicates only in human cells and tissues and is therefore difficult to study.

Latent viral infection is defined as the presence of the viral genome in the host tissue without production of infective viral particles.[2] During latency the pathogen maintains the potential to reactivate, resume replication, and cause recurrent disease. The 3 neurotropic herpes viruses establish latent infection mainly in the trigeminal ganglion and in DRG. They share several features that affect the course of infection in the human nervous system: (1) the primary infection involves the mucocutaneous surfaces, which serve as the portal of entry of the viral particles into the PNS; (2) the primary and the infectious recurrent diseases caused by the same virus take place within the same cutaneous distribution; (3) under normal, immunocompetent conditions, the reactivated infection usually does not spread beyond the cutaneous anatomic distribution of a single DRG; (4) although primary infection usually takes place during the first 2 to 3 decades of life, reactivation can occur at any time in the patient's life, sometimes at a very advanced age. These features can be grouped under a unifying hypothesis in herpes virology[3,4]: after primary infection, the virus gains access to axon endings after mucocutaneous infection and is transported to the DRG, where it is maintained in a latent state for the entire life of the human host. Under certain circumstances the virus can reactivate and travel to regions innervated by the respective DRG, causing the recurrent disease symptoms.

By contrast with its replication in DRG, HSV-1 replication in cells in culture results in lysis of the infected cell. Replication in the individual neuron at the peripheral site of primary infection or in the DRG is not required for the establishment of latency.[5] Lack of replication carries obvious advantages for the virus because the destruction of the host cell would prevent its ability to establish latent infection.[6] Viral particles are transported from the peripheral site of primary infection by retrograde axonal transport to the DRG, where they establish latent infection in neuronal cells in a nonintegrated (episomal) circular/concatemeric form.[7] During latency in human DRG, restricted HSV-1 gene expression produces 2 colinear latency-associated transcripts (LATs) 2.0 and 1.5 kb in size. The 2.0-kb LAT is a stable intron and the 1.5-kb LAT is its splicing product. The LATs might be beneficial to HSV-1 reactivation ability.

HSV-2 is also transcriptionally active during latency,[8] and a mutant lacking HSV-2 LATs has a defective reactivation phenotype.[9]

HSV-1 reactivation, even when multiple and recurrent, is not accompanied by permanent sensory deficit, suggesting that reactivation is not accompanied by neuronal cell destruction.

Understanding of VZV latency is more limited because of its species-specific nature. As with HSV-I, the genome is maintained in a nonintegrated circular concatemeric form[10] and has limited gene expression.[11] Neurons are the main cellular site of VZV latency. There is also a highly restricted pattern of viral gene expression during VZV latency.

Several hypothetical explanations were put forward to explain the clinical and biological differences in latency and reactivation between HSV and VZV.[12] Viral replication during VZV reactivation seems to spread to the entire ganglion and many neurons are infected, culminating in a peripheral disease within the dermatologic distribution of the entire DRG. Unlike HSV-I, where reactivation takes place within 1 neuron, and is therefore likely to evade the host immunologic response, VZV reactivation involves the spread of virus throughout the tissue and can be altered by cellular and humoral immune responses. Because VZV nucleic acids detected in DRG during latency are considerably less than those present during HSV-1 latent infection, VZV might be less capable of reactivation, whereas reactivation of HSV-1 might be favored. When VZV reactivation occurs, there is associated cellular death with reduction in the number of cells harboring latent viral copies; the remaining amounts of virus within DRG could be so reduced that its ability to reactivate is effectively impaired. In immunocompetent individuals, local cell-mediated immune responses might inhibit the cell-to-cell spread, thereby preventing VZV reactivation. This theory could explain why the incidence of herpes zoster increases with age, because VZV-specific T-cell responses have been shown to diminish with advancing age.

INFECTION AND REACTIVATION
Herpes Simplex Viruses

HSV infects mucosal surfaces or damaged skin. The first, or primary, infection is usually asymptomatic and depends on the immunologic status of the host. HSV-1 and HSV-2 are usually transmitted via different routes. Most cases of genital herpes are caused by HSV-2, whereas HSV-1 is typically transmitted during childhood via the orolabial route. There are several exceptions to this rule. HSV-1 has become a principal causative agent of genital herpes in some developed countries, including the United States, whereas HSV-2 can also cause recurrent herpes labialis. In less developed countries, HSV-I primary infection with seroconversion usually takes place within the first 2 decades of life. In developed countries, about half of seroconversion occurs at 20 to 40 years of age. HSV-1 seropositivity changes according to geography, race, age, sex, and social class, and has reached 80% to 90% worldwide,[13] whereas the reported increase in HSV-2 seroprevalence of the 1980s seems now to have been reversed and decreased to less than 20% in the United States.

HSV reactivations can either be symptomatic (termed recrudescence) or asymptomatic; asymptomatic reactivation can contribute to inadvertent HSV transmission.

Besides recurrent mucocutaneous disease, both viruses are responsible for infrequent but serious diseases, such as meningoencephalitis, blindness, and neonatal infections.

Varicella-Zoster Virus

VZV causes varicella (chickenpox) during primary infection and herpes zoster during reactivation.[14] Varicella, mainly a childhood disease with the highest incidence between 1 and 9 years of age, usually results in mild to moderate illness in immunocompetent patients but is also associated with serious complications, such as CNS involvement, pneumonia, secondary bacterial infections, and death.[14] In most temperate climates more than 90% of people are infected before adolescence, with an incidence of 13 to 16 cases per 1000, peak incidence during winter and spring, and a tendency for epidemics every 2 to 5 years. Older age, immune-compromised state, and possibly pregnancy are risk factors associated with higher severity of varicella. The danger of dying from varicella is highest in infants and in elderly individuals. Although varicella is more severe in immune-compromised people, most cases of severe morbidity and mortality are seen in healthy people.

The VZV vaccination resulted in decrease in the incidence, morbidity, and mortality caused by varicella. It is currently recommended for children 12 to 15 months old, and all healthy persons aged 13 years and older without evidence of anti-VZV immunity. The Society of Independent European Vaccination Experts (SIEVE) recommends immunization of susceptible adolescents, high-risk patients, their close contacts with a negative history of varicella, and seronegative health-care workers. However, considerable care needs to be taken with vaccination in immunocompromised patients.

NEUROLOGIC DISORDERS CAUSED BY THE NEUROTROPIC HERPESVIRUSES
Herpes Simplex Encephalitis

Herpes simplex encephalitis HSE, the most common cause of sporadic fatal viral encephalitis, has an incidence of between 1 and 3 cases per million without seasonal or sex-related variability.[15] It is associated with 70% mortality in untreated patients and with up to 30% mortality and a high incidence of severe and permanent neurologic sequelae in treated cases. There is a bimodal age distribution of the disease: most patients are either less than 20 years of age or more than 51 years of age, with the peak between 60 and 64 years. In immunocompetent adults, more than 90% of HSE cases are caused by HSV-I. Whether HSE is caused by viral reactivation or primary infection is uncertain. Likewise, the mechanism of HSV entry into the brain is still undetermined and could be caused by (1) reactivation of the viral genome in the trigeminal ganglion, a natural reservoir of HSV-I latent infection, with resultant axonal spread via the trigeminal nerve into the frontal and temporal lobes[16]; (2) in situ reactivation of the latent virus from CNS tissue, where it can occasionally be identified; or (3) primary infection of the nervous system. Pathways for entry of HSV to the brain include both the olfactory and the trigeminal nerves. Herpes virus particles were seen in the olfactory tract in some patients with HSE, and in animal models this tract has been shown to enable viral access to the CNS.[17] The primary infection option is supported by the finding that at least half of cases of HSE are caused by a different viral strain from the one responsible for cold sores in the same individual[18] because, in some patients, the disease affects the 2 cerebral hemispheres simultaneously and because neuronal cells expressing the latency-associated gene are protected from HSV-1 superinfection.[19]

Despite anecdotal reports, HSE is generally not a disorder of the immunocompromised host, except in the context of bone marrow transplant and in patients with acquired immunodeficiency syndrome (AIDS). However, deficiency of an intracellular protein, UNC93B, resulting in impaired cellular interferon alfa/beta and lambda antiviral responses as the probable underlying pathogenesis of herpes encephalitis has been reported.[20]

Several studies delineated the clinical presentation and the characteristic features of HSE in the era before the routine use of polymerase chain reaction (PCR) for diagnosis, when the ultimate confirmation of the clinical diagnosis by brain histology was missing. PCR technology as a major diagnostic tool enlarged and modified understanding of the clinical spectrum of HSE.[21] The symptoms and signs of HSE are related to nonspecific meningoencephalitis: headache, fever, and sometimes neck stiffness associated with signs of brain dysfunction and convulsions, including alterations of consciousness, personality and behavior, focal neurologic signs, cognitive disturbances, and seizures. More specific to HSE are prodromal symptoms of upper respiratory tract infection and neurologic findings related to dysfunction of the frontotemporal lobes, sometimes mimicking acute psychiatric conditions because of the characteristic limbic system involvement.

Several points should be emphasized: (1) milder, less severe forms of encephalitis that do not conform with the classic frontotemporal syndrome occur; (2) fever is one of the most frequent features at presentation, and its absence should cast doubt on the diagnosis in the immunopreserved; (3) headache is present in up to 90% of HSE cases; (4) the disease is of acute onset, usually less than a week; (5) in the clinical series of the pre-PCR era, gray matter dysfunction was a dominant feature (personality changes, confusion, and disorientation were present in about three-quarters of patients and seizures in half), and focal neurologic signs (eg, hemiparesis) were less frequent and were present in about a third of all patients; (6) preferential involvement of brainstem structures is rare.

HSE is a medical emergency. Because prognosis depends mainly on early initiation of treatment, the need for immediate and accurate diagnosis cannot be overemphasized. Thus, in one study on 42 patients with HSE, the time from admission to the start of acyclovir treatment was longer in patients with a poor outcome, with 1.8 days in the good-outcome group and 4.0 days for the poor-outcome group.[22]

The differential diagnosis should usually be limited to infectious, parainfectious, and acute inflammatory conditions, and final diagnosis is eventually based on analysis of cerebrospinal fluid (CSF) and neuroimaging.

In the presence of focal neurologic signs, neuroimaging before lumbar puncture might be indicated, provided that it can be obtained immediately. Because neuroimaging can sometimes delay diagnosis when immediate therapy is mandatory,[23] lumbar puncture should be postponed only when strict contraindications are present. In the context of a contraindication, antiherpetic therapy should be introduced and eventually be amended according to neuroimaging and CSF findings when those are available. CSF is abnormal in more than 95% of patients with HSE and contains moderate pleocytosis (usually 10–200 cells/mm^3), typically mononuclear white and red blood cells, reflecting the hemorrhagic nature of the infectious process within brain parenchyma. A moderate increase in CSF protein level is present in more than 80% of cases, and hypoglycorrhachia is the exception, detected in less than 5% of patients with biopsy-proven HSE. Demonstration of intrathecal production of anti-HSV antibodies, for many years the main noninvasive diagnostic tool, has been replaced by PCR for HSV-I DNA that is very sensitive (98%) and specific (94%) compared with the gold standard of histology, obtained by brain biopsy.[22] False-negative results might be present during the first days of disease, and, when in doubt, a repeat lumbar puncture after 1 to 2 days is indicated. The optimum time-frame in which to obtain a positive CSF PCR in HSE is probably 2 to 10 days after the onset of the illness. Computed tomography (CT) scanning is usually normal within the first 4 to 6 days of disease. Electroencephalogram, although sensitive, is a nonspecific diagnostic aid but could enable localization of disorder to frontotemporal brain regions before any abnormality can be visualized on imaging (mainly CT) studies. The findings are usually those of periodic sharp and slow wave complexes referred to as periodic lateralized epileptiform discharges. Both have therefore been supplanted by MRI, which is more sensitive, showing high-signal-intensity lesions on T2-weighted, diffusion-weighted, and fluid-attenuated inversion recovery (FLAIR) images early in the disease.

MRI is virtually never normal, usually showing edema and/or abnormal T2 signal and sometimes T1 postcontrast enhancement in one or both medial and anterior temporal and inferior frontal lobes, insular cortex, and the thalamus. Brain biopsy, needed in the preacyclovir/pre-PCR era, is now seldom done but might be indicated in cases unresponsive to antiherpetic therapy, in the investigation of a relapsing encephalitic illness, and where there is serious diagnostic uncertainty.

To reduce permanent sequelae, treatment should be introduced as soon as possible. Therefore, when the clinical setting is suspicious, therapy should be initiated immediately and modified according to radiologic, serologic, and molecular results. The mainstay of treatment is still acyclovir,[24] which prevents viral replication by inhibiting the viral (as well as the cellular) DNA polymerase in infected cells, which is activated only in cells that contain replicating virus. HSE is treated with acyclovir 10 mg/kg intravenously every 8 hours. In cases of poor response after a 10-day course of acyclovir therapy, the current recommended protocol has increased from 10 days of therapy to 2 to 3 weeks. Although for how long HSV DNA can be detected in the CSF after initiation of therapy is unclear, a consensus report[25] and a retrospective assessment[26] suggest that, when in doubt, identification of viral DNA by PCR on reexamination of the CSF could indicate the need for an additional 1 to 2 weeks of acyclovir therapy or reconsideration of the initial diagnosis. In immunocompromised patients, or in children less than 12 years old, acyclovir should be continued for at least 21 days.[27]

The emergence of drug-resistant HSV and VZV that carry alterations in the viral thymidine kinase gene, which is required to metabolize acyclovir into its active compound, affects an estimated 5% to 25% of immunocompromised patients receiving long-term prophylactic treatment with acyclovir. For such patients, foscarnet, which requires no metabolic activation, and cidofovir, a nucleoside analogue that is phosphorylated to its active compound by cellular enzymes, have become the second-line drugs. With the long intracellular half-life of its metabolites, cidofovir can be administered once weekly; however, the drug should be administered with probenecid to decrease nephrotoxicity, and its use is restricted to the treatment of acyclovir-resistant HSV isolates. Because acyclovir has only a 15% to 39% oral absorption, valacyclovir, an acyclovir prodrug for oral administration with a better bioavailability, was introduced. Penciclovir achieves higher intracellular concentrations than acyclovir, and famciclovir is a prodrug of penciclovir with better oral bioavailability. However, none of these drugs is currently indicated for the treatment of HSE because there are no prospective trials to prove efficacy; intravenous acyclovir remains the therapy of choice for HSE. Penciclovir is poorly absorbed when given orally and is therefore formulated for intravenous and topical use.

The use of corticosteroids as an adjunct treatment of HSE is controversial. However, when encephalitis is complicated by severe, vasogenic cerebral edema with neuroimaging evidence of midline shift, high-dose steroids (dexamethasone) might have a role in therapy.

Survival is dramatically improved by therapy, but the quality of survival is still unsatisfactory. Although acyclovir has reduced mortality from HSE, most survivors have persistent neurologic symptoms, signs, or both. Cognitive impairment remains the main problem despite early diagnosis, treatment, and a promising early beneficial outcome.

Neonatal Herpes Simplex Virus-2 Encephalitis

About 80% of neonatal encephalitis cases are caused by HSV-2, and most are acquired from a mother who has active genital herpes infection (either primary infection or recurrent disease) at the time of delivery.[28] Neonates present with systemic findings (alterations in body temperature, lethargy, respiratory distress, anorexia, vomiting, cyanosis) and neurologic signs (irritability, bulging fontanels, seizures, opisthotonus, and coma). The infection can take one of 3 patterns: disseminated infection; an isolated CNS disease; or a focal infection confined to the skin, eye, or mouth. The skin, eye, and mouth findings are present in about 80% of all cases, but, although they are highly suggestive of the diagnosis, the condition can also resemble bacterial sepsis or meningitis, and therefore laboratory diagnosis is mandatory. Such diagnosis can be achieved rapidly by PCR identification of the virus from maternal genital lesions and secretions or from vesicles, peripheral blood, and CSF of the newborn. Staining of samples for viral antigen or PCR analysis establishes diagnosis within several hours. Both acyclovir and vidarabine have been shown to reduce the morbidity and mortality of HSV infection in neonates, but acyclovir is preferred because of its safety profile and convenient dosing regimen. Acyclovir is given at 30 mg/kg/d intravenously in divided doses every 8 hours for 14 days in infants with disease localized to skin, eyes, and mouth, and for 21 days when the infection is disseminated or involves the CNS. Because the drug can cause neutropenia and nephrotoxicity, the available data do not support the routine use of oral suppressive acyclovir therapy following treatment of acute neonatal HSV disease.

Even with appropriate treatment, prognosis of neonatal encephalitis is very poor. Between a third and half of all treated babies with disseminated disease die, and about two-thirds of survivors have neurologic sequelae. This prognosis raises 2 unresolved issues. First, should a neonate who was discovered postnatally to have been delivered via an HSV-lesioned or culture-positive birth canal be treated prophylactically? In view of the serious consequences of untreated neonatal HSV infection, the authors and others recommend prophylactic intravenous acyclovir (60 mg/kg/d in 3 divided doses) for 10 days. Second, is cesarean section recommended in all cases of mothers with a history of HSV genital infection? Because asymptomatic HSV-2 shedding is a frequent occurrence in seropositive individuals, and cesarean section seems to decrease the risk of HSV transmission, our policy has been to avoid vaginal delivery in women with a history of genital HSV infection. However, this approach might be too cautious, but, for women who present with a first episode of genital herpes lesions within 6 weeks of the expected date of delivery or onset of preterm labor, elective cesarean section could be considered at term.[29]

Mollaret Meningitis

Mollaret meningitis is characterized by recurrent self-limited lymphocytic meningitis in otherwise healthy individuals. Recurrence takes place at intervals of several weeks to months and has been documented after up to 28 years. CSF contains from 200 to several thousand lymphocytes per cubic millimeter, and large endothelial cells identified on cytologic examination, called Mollaret cells, are sometimes present. CSF protein levels are increased, and glucose level can sometimes be low. Complete recovery occurs within several days. Diagnosis is established after other causes of lymphocytic meningitis have been ruled out. The most frequent causative agent is HSV-2,[30] although other pathogens have also been reported. Although some reports suggested either shorter episodes or resolution of the syndrome with antiherpetic treatment, it could be argued that the therapy does not affect the viral reservoir in DRG and is not associated with prevention of future mucocutaneous disease.

NEUROLOGIC COMPLICATIONS OF VARICELLA-ZOSTER VIRUS INFECTION

The neurologic complications of VZV infections can be categorized into those caused by primary infection and those that are associated with and follow reactivation. Similar syndromes might be related to both, but usually they are of different frequency and features (eg, vasculopathy or myelitis).

Herpes Zoster

This is mainly a disease of older individuals (people >60 years old have an 8-fold to 10-fold increased incidence of herpes zoster compared with those <60 years old) and of immunocompromised patients. Bone marrow transplant recipients and HIV-seropositive patients are also at particular risk. Waning cell-mediated immunity is likely a major factor in the increased incidence of herpes zoster in elderly individuals, especially because antibody titers remain unchanged or can even increase with age.

Although any level of the neuraxis can be affected, herpes zoster tends to involve the cutaneous sites where the highest burden of lesions containing viral particles was present during varicella: the thorax and the face within the distribution of the trigeminal nerve. In immunocompetent individuals, herpes zoster usually presents as a single episode and more than 3 recurrences are extremely rare. Typical herpes zoster takes the form of vesicular eruptions distributed unilaterally within a dermatome. The vesicles are clear, become turbid, and crust within 5 to 10 days. Resolution can leave scars. The rash is frequently preceded by paresthesia, itching, and pain: a condition termed preherpetic neuralgia. Sensory symptoms can be severe enough to suggest an alternative cause, such as coronary ischemia or an abdominal condition. Pain and itching are usual concomitants of the eruption and can follow the rash and become a chronic disorder termed postherpetic neuralgia. Dissemination of the eruption to neighboring dermatomes can occur. Occasionally, a typical herpes zoster pain is not associated with skin lesions but is accompanied by an increase in VZV antibody titers, a condition known as zoster sine herpete.

Herpes zoster can be associated with subtle signs of aseptic meningitis (mild CSF mononuclear pleocytosis with slight increase in protein levels) in up to 50% of patients. Only seldom is this associated with isolation of the causative virus from the CSF.

Predisposing factors and triggers for herpes zoster include diabetes mellitus, malignancies, and conditions associated with immune suppression, such as lymphoma, steroid therapy, immunosuppressive agents, and AIDS. However, a search for an underlying malignancy is not warranted in otherwise healthy patients who develop herpes zoster.[31] Although varicella can follow exposure to herpes zoster, the opposite (ie, occurrence of herpes zoster after exposure to a patient with varicella) is extremely rare and the underlying mechanism unclear. In a population at risk, the occurrence of herpes zoster increases the possibility of HIV infection and is regarded as a poor prognostic sign.

The dermatologic appearance of herpes zoster is, in most cases, sufficiently distinctive for accurate diagnosis. When laboratory confirmation is required, viral culture has a low yield, whereas direct immunofluorescence assay and PCR are much more sensitive.

The therapeutic approach differs according to the immune state of the patient. For the immunocompetent, acyclovir (800 mg 5 times orally daily, for 7–10 days), valacyclovir (1000 mg every 8 hours orally, for 7 days), or famciclovir (500 mg every 8 hours orally, for 7 days) are approved in the United States for the treatment of herpes zoster. Valacyclovir and famciclovir are preferable because they have better pharmacokinetic profiles and simpler dosing regimens. All three drugs are safe and well tolerated without contraindications, although dose adjustment is required in patients with renal insufficiency. With the risk of relapsing infection in these patients, therapy is given until all lesions have resolved.

Acute Cerebellar Ataxia

This entity develops in 1 in 4000 children less than 15 years of age who have varicella and usually follows the rash within a week, although it can take up to 3 weeks to manifest. It has not been reported following herpes zoster. Whether it is a truly an infectious state, a possibility backed by the finding of VZV DNA in the CSF of pediatric patients,[31] or an immune-mediated, postinfectious condition is uncertain. Clinically, acute cerebellar ataxia manifests as gait ataxia, tremor, vomiting, and headache, and findings consist of mild cerebellar dysfunction sometimes with meningeal irritation and CSF pleocytosis with increased protein levels. Imaging is usually normal and recovery is the rule. Intravenous acyclovir at doses of 10 mg/kg every 8 hours for adults, and 500 mg/m^2 body surface area for children for a week, might be considered in patients with CSF evidence for active infection backed by PCR, although controlled clinical trials are missing.

Guillain-Barré Syndrome

Guillain-Barré syndrome (GBS) accounts for about 7% of all complications of varicella. Nevertheless, in all patients with varicella, it is a rare complication (eg, 8 of 2534 patients in one study).[32] There are no characteristic features to distinguish this polyradiculopathy from any other acute inflammatory demyelinating polyneuropathy that follows other infections. GBS variants, such as cranial nerve palsies (extraocular nerve paralysis with diplopia, facial diplegia, bulbar involvement), have been reported. GBS has also been associated with herpes zoster. The true incidence of this disorder is unknown. Cranial nerve involvement is present in 50% of patients.

Reye Syndrome

Reye syndrome is a condition of unknown cause and pathogenesis that follows mainly influenza or varicella, primarily in the pediatric age group. It has not been reported following herpes zoster. The use of aspirin increases the risk of the disorder, which is characterized by intractable vomiting that heralds seizures, lethargy, and coma. Liver dysfunction is associated with massive brain edema that leads to permanent neurologic deficit or death in up to 30% of patients. Recommended therapeutic measures, hyperventilation and mannitol, are designed to decrease the increased intracranial pressure. Notably, the incidence of this condition has dramatically declined over the past 2 decades.

Myelitis

Myelitis is a rare complication of varicella and much more common following herpes zoster. The authors identified unsuspected spinal cord involvement in more than 50% of patients with spinal herpes zoster[33] consisting of paraparesis, impaired sensation with a level compatible with the segment of VZV reactivation, and sphincter dysfunction. In most patients, spinal cord involvement is subtle and asymptomatic, and complete recovery is the rule. The pathogenesis of the condition is unknown, but the authors proposed that it is caused by spread of viral infection from the respective DRG into the spinal cord and therefore acyclovir therapy is indicated. Myelitis might be subacute or even chronic in immunocompromised individuals and might lead to death. Autopsy reveals active infection of the spinal cord, justifying therapy with acyclovir in such patients.

Optic Neuritis

Optic neuritis can follow varicella in rare instances and is usually, but not exclusively, unilateral. In immunocompetent individuals it is considered an immune-mediated abnormality, responsive to intravenous steroid therapy, and with good prognosis. Of interest are several reports of optic neuritis associated with myelitis following varicella, suggesting a possible link to neuromyelitis optica. In immunocompromised patients, optic neuritis can follow varicella or herpes zoster or can appear in the absence of any cutaneous lesions. Sometimes it is associated with the presence of VZV DNA in the CSF, suggesting a possible infectious process, supporting the possibility that in such patients a course of acyclovir therapy might be warranted.

Meningoencephalitis

The introduction of PCR diagnosis has increased the spectrum of VZV-induced neurologic complications to include unsuspected cases of meningitis or encephalitis that follow either varicella or herpes zoster in immunocompetent or immunosuppressed patients. Some of the cases can be categorized as acute disseminated encephalomyelitis (ADEM), although they can overlap with acute cerebellar ataxia. Other cases might be of a benign and nonspecific nature. Some can also represent a vasculopathy' that is, a disorder caused by VZV infection of blood vessels. There are no evidence-based data to recommend either antiviral therapy or high-dose steroids, and therapy has to rely on the context of immunocompetence, the possible putative pathogenesis such as vasculitis, and disease severity.

Vasculitis

Two clinicopathologic entities have been delineated from the size of the involved blood vessels: large vessel unifocal granulomatous arteritis and small vessel multifocal vasculopathy. Large vessel unifocal granulomatous arteritis is usually a disorder of immunocompetent host and follows varicella, herpes zoster, or VZV infection without skin lesions. It is mainly a disorder of elderly individuals, in whom a brain infarction develops weeks to months following ipsilateral trigeminal zoster, and is associated with a mortality of up to 25%. The CSF shows mild lymphocytic pleocytosis, increased protein level, and sometimes oligoclonal bands, and PCR is positive for VZV nucleic acid. Diagnosis is best supported by detection of anti-VZV immunoglobulin G antibody in the CSF at a level that suggests intrathecal synthesis. Angiography reveals focal narrowing or occlusion of the blood vessel, which on autopsy displays arterial inflammation with multinucleated giant cells, VZV antigens, Cowdry type A inclusion bodies, and VZV nucleic acids. Although no results of therapeutic trials are available, empiric treatment with intravenous acyclovir is typically used (60 mg/kg/d in 3 divided doses for 10 to 14 days). Some experts also add a short course of steroids.

Small vessel multifocal vasculopathy usually occurs in immunocompromised patients. It typically presents without skin lesions and consists of subacute multifocal neurologic deficits accompanied by headache, fever, mental status changes, and seizures. History of herpes zoster might precede the symptoms by several weeks to months. CSF analysis shows mild pleocytosis with slightly increased or normal levels of protein and VZV DNA as well as anti-VZV antibodies. MRI reveals multifocal infarcts and, on autopsy, ovoid mixed necrotic and demyelinative lesions with small vessel vasculopathy and demyelination are present. Cowdry A intranuclear viral inclusions can be present in glial cells at the edge of the smaller ovoid, demyelinative lesions.

In the context of immunosuppression, which predisposes individuals to a range of opportunistic infections, a lack of a history of antecedent VZV infection or rash requires a high index of suspicion to establish the diagnosis. On diagnosis, therapy with intravenous acyclovir, although not based on controlled clinical trials, seems appropriate and is recommended.

Stroke in Children

VZV-associated stroke in children is a rare complication that can occur from days to months after the primary VZV infection. In young children with ischemic stroke there is a 3-fold increase in preceding varicella infection. At present, no common pathogenic mechanism or histopathologic picture of this disorder has been identified. The mechanisms underlying cerebrovascular events after VZV infection can be vasculitis, thrombosis caused by direct endothelial damage, and acquired protein S deficiency. The rarity of this entity and the lack of controlled clinical trials in children for the therapy for thromboembolic disease have thus far prevented the development of adequate antithrombotic therapy protocols for pediatric stroke, VZV-associated stroke inclusive.

Motor Weakness

Focal motor weakness in herpes zoster is exceptional. Motor impairment might follow herpes zoster within 1 day to 4 months and usually involves the same dermatome that is affected by the rash. Cranial nerve variants are peripheral facial weakness with herpes zoster oticus and eruption within the ear canal and the adjacent skin (Ramsay-Hunt syndrome), or ophthalmoplegia, mainly of the third cranial nerve and usually associated with meningitis. Myotomal involvement includes arm weakness in association with herpes zoster within cervical dermatomes (sometimes also responsible for diaphragmatic paresis), and lumbosacral herpes zoster leading to leg weakness associated with lumbar dermatomal rash. Neurogenic bladder and loss of anal sphincter control can follow sacral herpes zoster, again often with a meningitis. The prognosis of the motor weakness is generally good and more than half of patients regain full motor power. In another third the improvement is significant.

Postherpetic Neuralgia

Postherpetic neuralgia is the most common neurologic complication of herpes zoster.[34] It is defined as pain in the distribution of the rash that persists beyond 4 to 6 weeks following herpes zoster. The risk for postherpetic neuralgia increases with age, and almost half of patients more than 60 years old who experience herpes zoster develop it, immunocompromised patients being more susceptible. The pain involves the affected dermatome and is usually severe, burning, lancinating, and constant, and can be so disturbing as to lead to severe depression and even suicide. The pathogenesis of postherpetic neuralgia is not well understood. Whether it is the outcome of persistence of the viral infection following herpes zoster, as might be suggested by the presence of VZV-specific proteins in peripheral mononuclear cells of patients with postherpetic neuralgia,[35] or is caused by structural changes within the DRG following infection and injury is not clear. Central mechanisms can also contribute to this and other neuropathic pain syndromes, including long-term induction of central sensitization, reactive alterations of spinal cord cell excitability, and altered interneuron control mechanisms permitting hyperexcitability.

Treatment of postherpetic neuralgia is usually very difficult and the pain in many cases can be intractable. Regimens that have been tried include the combination of local application of cold, analgesics, and 3 main drug classes: antidepressants (eg, tricyclic antidepressants, preferably amitriptyline), anticonvulsants (gabapentin, pregabalin), and opioids (eg, tramadol, oxycodone, morphine). Topical application of capsaicin or lidocaine can also render a temporary ameliorating effect. Although carbamazepine is commonly used for the treatment of postherpetic neuralgia, there is currently no strong evidence for its use. When considering more drastic measures (eg, surgery of the dorsal root entry zone or ganglionotomy), clinicians should always keep in mind that postherpetic neuralgia is a self-limited condition and that, when it resolves, it does not relapse.

A study showed that vaccination with an attenuated VZV vaccine reduced the incidence of herpes zoster by more than half and that of postherpetic neuralgia by about two-thirds. No information on long-term safety and duration of relative protection against herpes zoster is currently available. From this study, it seems logical and safe to recommend the vaccine for general use for patients beyond 60 years of age, but with close and extended monitoring and scrutiny for the effect of the vaccine on anti-VZV cell-mediated immunity and on protection from herpes zoster.

The Association of Herpes Simplex Virus with Other Neurologic Diseases

Several neurologic conditions have been associated with acute, chronic, or reactivated HSV or VZV infections. In some, there is presently insufficient evidence to implicate the virus in the cause and pathogenesis of the disease. In some conditions the data seem to be more intriguing and could support the possibility that, in a subgroup of patients, HSV-I has a causative role in pathogenesis.

Of special note is the speculation that, in some sporadic cases of Alzheimer disease, HSV-I might be the trigger that initiates or contributes to the pathogenic cascade.[36,37]

From the assumption that HSV-I resides in the geniculate ganglion, in a similar fashion to colonization of other DRG, it was postulated that HSV might be the causative agent of idiopathic peripheral facial nerve paralysis (Bell palsy). However, in humans, HSV-I reactivation is not usually associated with motor impairment and HSV-I causes recurrent reactivation, whereas Bell palsy, in most cases, is a single episode and a rare condition compared with the incidence of cold sores. The indication to treat Bell palsy with anti–HSV-1 therapy is therefore questionable.[38]

Giant cell arteritis (GCA), the most prevalent vasculitis, is of elusive pathogenesis. It was hypothesized that the condition is caused by VZV reactivation based on the similarities between the disorder of GCA and that of VZV vasculitis.[39] Three studies from the same group found VZV nucleic acids and antigens in a large proportion of patients with GCA. However, this was not reproduced, and we found that VZV vaccination, which is linked with reduced herpes zoster, was associated with increased rate of GCA, refuting the possibility of a causative relationship between VZV and GCA.[40]

REFERENCES

1. Cumston CG. The history of herpes from the earliest times to the nineteenth century. Ann Med Hist 1926;8:284–91.
2. Steiner I, Kennedy PG. Herpes simplex virus latent infection in the nervous system. J Neurovirol 1995;1(1):19–29.
3. Goodpastur EW. Herpetic Infection, with especial reference to involvement of the nervous system. Medicine 1929;8(2):223.
4. Hope-Simpson RE. The nature of herpes zoster: a long-term study and a new hypothesis. Proc R Soc Med 1965;58(1):9–20.
5. Steiner I, Spivack JG, Deshmane SL, et al. A herpes simplex virus type 1 mutant containing a nontransinducing Vmw65 protein establishes latent infection in vivo in the absence of viral replication and reactivates efficiently from explanted trigeminal ganglia. J Virol 1990;64(4):1630–8.
6. Steiner I, Kennedy PG. Herpes simplex virus latency in the nervous system–a new model. Neuropathol Appl Neurobiol 1991;17(6):433–40.

7. Rock DL, Fraser NW. Detection of HSV-1 genome in central nervous system of latently infected mice. Nature 1983;302(5908):523–5.
8. Croen KD, Ostrove JM, Dragovic L, et al. Characterization of herpes simplex virus type 2 latency-associated transcription in human sacral ganglia and in cell culture. J Infect Dis 1991;163(1):23–8.
9. Krause PR, Stanberry LR, Bourne N, et al. Expression of the herpes simplex virus type 2 latency-associated transcript enhances spontaneous reactivation of genital herpes in latently infected guinea pigs. J Exp Med 1995;181(1):297–306.
10. Clarke P, Beer T, Cohrs R, et al. Configuration of latent varicella-zoster virus DNA. J Virol 1995;69(12):8151–4.
11. Kennedy PG, Grinfeld E, Bell JE. Varicella-zoster virus gene expression in latently infected and explanted human ganglia. J Virol 2000;74(24):11893–8.
12. Kennedy PGE, Steiner I. A molecular and cellular model to explain the differences in reactivation from latency by herpes simplex and varicella-zoster viruses. Neuropathol Appl Neurobiol 1994;20(4):368–74.
13. Smith JS, Robinson NJ. Age-specific prevalence of infection with herpes simplex virus types 2 and 1: a global review. J Infect Dis 2002;186(Suppl 1):S3–28.
14. Heininger U, Seward JF. Varicella. Lancet 2006;368(9544):1365–76.
15. Kennedy PGE, Chaudhuri A. Herpes simplex encephalitis. J Neurol Neurosurg Psychiatry 2002;73(3):237–8.
16. Davis LE, Johnson RT. An explanation for the localization of herpes simplex encephalitis? Ann Neurol 1979;5(1):2–5.
17. Stroop WG, Schaefer DC. Production of encephalitis restricted to the temporal lobes by experimental reactivation of herpes simplex virus. J Infect Dis 1986;153(4):721–31.
18. Whitley R, Lakeman AD, Nahmias A, et al. DNA restriction-enzyme analysis of herpes simplex virus isolates obtained from patients with encephalitis. N Engl J Med 1982;307(17):1060–2.
19. Mador N, Goldenberg D, Cohen O, et al. Herpes simplex virus type 1 latency-associated transcripts suppress viral replication and reduce immediate-early gene mRNA levels in a neuronal cell line. J Virol 1998;72(6):5067–75.
20. Casrouge A, Zhang S-Y, Eidenschenk C, et al. Herpes simplex virus encephalitis in human UNC-93B deficiency. Science 2006;314(5797):308–12.
21. Steiner I, Schmutzhard E, Sellner J, et al. EFNS-ENS guidelines for the use of PCR technology for the diagnosis of infections of the nervous system. Eur J Neurol 2012;19(10):1278–91.
22. McGrath N, Anderson NE, Croxson MC, et al. Herpes simplex encephalitis treated with acyclovir: diagnosis and long term outcome. J Neurol Neurosurg Psychiatry 1997;63(3):321–6.
23. Hasbun R, Abrahams J, Jekel J, et al. Computed tomography of the head before lumbar puncture in adults with suspected meningitis. N Engl J Med 2001;345(24):1727–33.
24. Whitley R, Arvin A, Prober C, et al. A controlled trial comparing vidarabine with acyclovir in neonatal herpes simplex virus infection. Infectious Diseases Collaborative Antiviral Study Group. N Engl J Med 1991;324(7):444–9.
25. Cinque P, Cleator GM, Weber T, et al. The role of laboratory investigation in the diagnosis and management of patients with suspected herpes simplex encephalitis: a consensus report. The EU concerted action on virus meningitis and encephalitis. J Neurol Neurosurg Psychiatry 1996;61(4):339–45.
26. Ito Y, Kimura H, Yabuta Y, et al. Exacerbation of herpes simplex encephalitis after successful treatment with acyclovir. Clin Infect Dis 2000;30(1):185–7.

27. Solomon T, Michael BD, Smith PE, et al. Management of suspected viral encephalitis in adults – Association of British Neurologists and British Infection Association national guidelines. J Infect 2012;64(4):347–73.
28. Whitley R, Arvin A, Prober C, et al. Predictors of morbidity and mortality in neonates with herpes simplex virus infections. The national Institute of Allergy and Infectious Diseases Collaborative Antiviral Study Group. N Engl J Med 1991;324(7): 450–4.
29. Patel R, Kennedy OJ, Clarke E, et al. 2017 European guidelines for the management of genital herpes. Int J STD AIDS 2017;28(14):1366–79.
30. Berger JR. Benign aseptic (Mollaret's) meningitis after genital herpes. Lancet 1991;337(8753):1360–1.
31. Ragozzino MW, Melton LJ, Kurland LT, et al. Risk of cancer after herpes zoster: a population-based study. N Engl J Med 1982;307(7):393–7.
32. Kennedy PGE. Neurological complications of varicella-zoster virus. In: Kennedy PGE, Johnson RD, editors. Infections of the nervous system. Oxford (England): Butterworth-Heinemann; 2000. p. 177–208.
33. Steiner I, Steiner-Birmanns B, Levin N, et al. Spinal cord involvement in uncomplicated herpes zoster. Clin Diagn Lab Immunol 2001;8(4):850–1.
34. Kost RG, Straus SE. Postherpetic neuralgia — pathogenesis, treatment, and prevention. N Engl J Med 1996;335(1):32–42.
35. Vafai A, Wellish M, Gilden DH. Expression of varicella-zoster virus in blood mononuclear cells of patients with postherpetic neuralgia. Proc Natl Acad Sci U S A 1988;85(8):2767–70.
36. Itzhaki RF. Herpes simplex virus type 1 and Alzheimer's disease: possible mechanisms and signposts. FASEB J 2017;31(8):3216–26.
37. Itzhaki RF, Lin W-R, Shang D, et al. Herpes simplex virus type 1 in brain and risk of Alzheimer's disease. Lancet 1997;349(9047):241–4.
38. Steiner I, Mattan Y. Bell's palsy and herpes viruses: to (acyclo)vir or not to (acyclo)vir? J Neurol Sci 1999;170(1):19–23.
39. Gilden D, White T, Khmeleva N, et al. Prevalence and distribution of VZV in temporal arteries of patients with giant cell arteritis. Neurology 2015;84(19):1948–55.
40. Lotan I, Steiner I. Giant cell arteritis following varicella zoster vaccination. J Neurol Sci 2017;375:158–9.

Progressive Multifocal Leukoencephalopathy

Elena Grebenciucova, MD[a],*, Joseph R. Berger, MD[b]

KEYWORDS

- John Cunningham virus • Progressive multifocal leukoencephalopathy
- Opportunistic infection

KEY POINTS

- Progressive multifocal leukoencephalopathy (PML) is a rare central nervous system infection with a high risk of morbidity and mortality.
- Neurologists may encounter PML in patients with underlying immune deficiencies, HIV, solid and hematologic malignances, transplant medicine, certain rheumatologic disorders, and in association with immunotherapies used in the treatment of cancers, rheumatologic conditions, and multiple sclerosis.
- Diagnosis of PML requires a high level of clinical suspicion and radiologic vigilance.

INTRODUCTION

Although previously considered an opportunistic infection primarily associated with acquired immunodeficiency syndrome (AIDS), in the past decade, the epidemiology of progressive multifocal leukoencephalopathy (PML) has significantly changed, reigniting the awareness of the infection among general neurologists.

Initially described in 1958 in 3 patients with hematologic malignancies (Hodgkin lymphoma and chronic lymphocytic leukemia),[1] PML became widely known in the 1980s at the time of the AIDS epidemic. Over the following decade, as the antiretroviral therapies became widely available, PML became rarer, but re-emerged in the past decade in association with monoclonal antibody therapies used in the treatment of cancers and rheumatologic disorders and several disease-modifying therapies used in the treatment of multiple sclerosis.

BASIC EPIDEMIOLOGY

PML is a viral infection of the central nervous system that typically occurs secondary to reactivation of John Cunningham (JC) virus in those whose cellular immunity is

[a] Multiple Sclerosis Division, Davee Department of Neurology, Northwestern University Feinberg School of Medicine, 675 St. Clair, Chicago, IL 60611, USA; [b] Multiple Sclerosis Division, The Department of Neurology, Perelman School of Medicine, The University of Pennsylvania, 3400 Convention Avenue, Philadelphia, PA 19104, USA
* Corresponding author.
E-mail address: elena.grebenciucova@northwestern.edu

Neurol Clin 36 (2018) 739–750
https://doi.org/10.1016/j.ncl.2018.06.002
0733-8619/18/© 2018 Elsevier Inc. All rights reserved.

neurologic.theclinics.com

compromised, either because of an underlying disorder or secondary to iatrogenic immunosuppression or immunomodulation. Hematologic and solid malignancies, several rheumatologic disorders that alter immunity (eg, systemic lupus erythematosus [SLE], sarcoidosis), primary immune deficiencies (idiopathic CD4 lymphopenia or severe combined immunodeficiency [SCID]), and HIV infection are some of the more common conditions that predispose to PML. Incidence of PML per 100,000 patient-years is estimated at 2.4 cases for SLE, 10.8 cases for autoimmune vasculitis, 8.3 cases for non-Hodgkin lymphoma, 11.1 cases for CLL, and 35.4 cases for bone marrow transplant patients.[2] In a survey of 9675 cases of PML, 8.7% were caused by hematologic malignancies; 80% were caused by HIV. Additionally, 2.83% were caused by solid cancers; 0.44% were reported in SLE patients, and 0.25% were reported in rheumatoid arthritis patients.[3]

Therapies such as natalizumab, fingolimod, dimethyl fumarate, rituximab, alemtuzumab, efalizumab, and other immunosuppressive medications have been associated with cases of PML with a variable magnitude of risk, ranging from an estimated 1 case 30,000 population for rituximab to 1 case per 100 population in JCV antibody-positive patients with prior exposure to immunosuppressive medications, receiving natalizumab for over 2 years.[4]

PROGRESSIVE MULTIFOCAL LEUKOENCEPHALOPATHY PATHOGENESIS

JCV is a polyoma virus that is ubiquitously present, with seroepidemiological studies indicating that 30% to 90% of the worldwide adult population harbors anti-JCV antibodies. A recent study of 7724 patients from 10 countries confirmed this estimate, highlighting the association of increased seropositivity with advanced age.[5] The virus exists in 8 molecular subtypes. Its capsid binding protein (VP1) type (Type 4 common in Europe and 2B common in Eurasia) may confer a different degree of virulence, resulting in geographic incidence variability.[6]

Primary infection usually occurs via a fecal-oral or respiratory route.[7] The virus remains predominantly latent/persistent in the kidneys, but may be seen in other tissues, usually in low copy numbers.[8] In fact, up to 40% of healthy adults shed JCV in their urine.[9] However, the virus does not become pathogenic until it transforms into a neurotropic strain, and the host's immune defenses are severely compromised. There appear to be multiple barriers to the development of PML, and several key steps need to occur in order for JCV to establish a productive central nervous system (CNS) infection:

1. Primary infection
2. Reactivation of the virus in the setting of immune compromise
3. Genetic rearrangement into a neurotropic strain (if the primary infection occurred with an archetype strain)
4. Entry of the virus into the CNS and infection of oligodendrocytes
5. Failure of the immune surveillance within the CNS compartment, allowing for an uncontrolled viral replication

CLINICAL PRESENTATION

Reflecting its diffuse, usually multifocal involvement of the central nervous system, PML can present with variable symptoms such as cognitive deficits, visual symptoms, gait impairment, hemiparesis, and speech disturbances. The virus does not affect the optic nerve, and although it rarely can be found in the spinal cord on biopsy, it has not been known to produce clinical myelitis symptoms. Interestingly, PML presentation may vary depending on the medication/condition associated. For example, HIV-associated PML frequently presents with limb weakness in up to 50% patients,[10] while natalizumab-associated PML frequently presents with cognitive disturbances in 48% patients, language impairment in 31% of patients, and visual symptoms in 26% of patients.[11]

DIAGNOSIS OF PROGRESSIVE MULTIFOCAL LEUKOENCEPHALOPATHY

Diagnosing PML relies on a high degree of clinical suspicion in patients whose immune system is compromised. Many other disorders, including multiple sclerosis (MS), can mimic symptoms of PML. MRI is the most sensitive and will typically demonstrate abnormalities before they become clinically apparent, but is by no means diagnostic by itself. Cerebrospinal fluid (CSF) analysis is essential for the diagnosis of PML. CSF cell count usually does not exceed 20 white blood cells, reflecting an immunocompromised state of the CNS compartment.[10] In fact, 70% of patients with PML have normal cell count in the CSF. The sensitivity of the newer polymerase chain reaction (PCR) methods is at least 95%, with most laboratories being able to detect values as low as 50 copies and some as low as 10.[12] However, in the absence of the appropriate clinical picture and radiologic findings, a low number of JCV DNA copies in CSF does not necessarily imply that the patient has PML. In fact, out of 515 samples of CSF in patients without PML, JCV DNA was detected in 2 samples, alerting clinicians to a small possibility of false-positive results.[13] When PCR in CSF is negative, but the clinical picture and radiologic findings are concerning, a biopsy of the brain tissue remains the gold standard for diagnosis. Histopathological triad of demyelination, bizarre astrocytes, and large oligodendroglial nuclei are characteristic of PML, which should be coupled with confirmatory tests for the presence of JCV in the tissue.[12]

RADIOLOGY OF PROGRESSIVE MULTIFOCAL LEUKOENCEPHALOPATHY

MRI is a modality of choice and may show either single or multiple asymmetric diffuse areas of demyelination without significant edema or mass effect and typically without significant enhancement, although mild enhancement may be present in some cases and generally purports a more favorable prognosis, often indicating the presence of PML-IRIS (immune reconstitution inflammatory syndrome). Although in HIV-associated PML, enhancement is observed in 10% to 15% of cases,[10] it is more common in natalizumab-associated PML and occurs in up to 40% of PML patients.[11] The lesions are hypointense on T1 sequence and hyperintense on T2 and FLAIR sequences (**Fig. 1**) and occur most commonly in the frontal and fronto-parietal lobes; however, they can also be found in the basal ganglia, brainstem, and cerebellum.[14] Diffusion-weighted imaging (DWI) may infrequently show restricted diffusion. Given PML predilection for subcortical white matter, lesions frequently have a scalloped appearance toward the cortex and a more poorly defined appearance toward the white matter. On susceptibility-weighted sequences, hypointense rims that involve U fibers can occur.[15]

In time, as the infection progresses, multifocal lesions may coalesce into large diffuse areas of signal abnormality. One must note, that chronic ischemic strokes, multiple sclerosis lesions, and low-grade gliomas can frequently mimic PML lesions, and care must be taken to consider these in the differential diagnosis of PML.

CLINICAL SURVEILLANCE AND RISK MITIGATION

As the risk of PML depends on a predisposing condition or therapy, various risk mitigation strategies can be considered. Testing for seropositivity to JCV is often

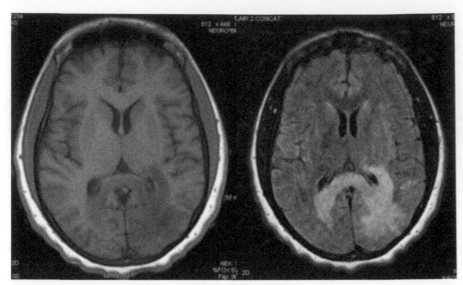

Fig. 1. T1 sequence showing hypointense signal of PML lesions (*left*) and FLAIR sequence showing hyperintense white matter signal of PML lesion (*right*).

performed in patients who are at high risk of PML because of an underlying condition or therapy, but has only been validated as a risk for natalizumab-associated PML. This allows for further risk stratification and the appropriate degree of vigilance. In those who have been exposed to JCV and have circulating antibodies, clinical and radiologic (MRI) monitoring may be warranted to detect the disorder early depending on the magnitude of the risk of PML associated with a given medication/condition.

NATALIZUMAB

The highest number of PML cases in association with any singular medication (>700 confirmed cases) has occurred in association with natalizumab therapy. Postmarketing surveillance estimates the incidence at 4.2 cases of PML per 1000 patients treated with natalizumab.

Natalizumab is a humanized monoclonal antibody that binds to α4β1-integrin (very late antigen 4 [VLA-4]), an adhesion molecule on the surface of leukocytes. The drug inhibits white cell transmigration through the blood-brain barrier.[16,17] As white cells' access to the central nervous system becomes diminished, virologic surveillance and control in the CNS compartment are undermined. Significant reductions in CD4/CD8 lymphocyte ratios occur in the serum[18] and in the CSF[19] as a result of natalizumab treatment. These CD4/CD8 ratio changes are reminiscent of the alterations in the ratio that occur in acquired immunodeficiency syndrome (AIDS), a disorder most strongly associated with PML. Additionally, natalizumab is associated with an increase in certain B cell populations, including CD34 + cells that may harbor the virus.[20]

Natalizumab increases the risk of PML altered CD4/CD8+ T lymphocytes ratios in the CNS, leading to an impaired CNS immunosurveillance, and increased egress of CD34 + B cells, reservoirs of JCV, from the bone marrow.[20]

JCV antibody positivity, prior use of immunosuppressive medications, and duration of natalizumab therapy are helpful in defining the risk of PML.

Enzyme-linked immunosorbent assay (ELISA) testing for JCV antibody has a false-negative rate of 2.2%.[21] Rechecking JCV antibody status every 3 to 4 months while on therapy is strongly advised.

The risk of PML for those who are JCV antibody positive without any history of prior immunosuppression is estimated at 1 case per 1000 patients during the first 2 years, and then precipitously rises to 3 cases per 1000 patients between year 2 and 4. For those patients who are JCV antibody positive with prior history of immunosuppression, the risk of PML is estimated at 12 cases per 1000 patients between year 2 and 4 on therapy. Higher risk estimates have been calculated.[22,23]

The JCV antibody index became available in 2014 and has been useful in monitoring the risk of PML. Elevations in JCV index reflect an increase in the viral burden. In natalizumab-associated cases of PML, higher levels of the serum anti-JCV antibody index were associated with a higher risk of PML. In the first 24 months on natalizumab, the risk of PML in patients who were JCV antibody positive and had no history of prior immunosuppression was estimated at 0.1 case per 1000 patients with index value between 0.9 and 1.5 and increased tenfold for patients with the index values greater than 1.5.[24] Patients with index values less than or equal to 0.9 and greater than 1.5 are considered to be at a lower and higher risk respectively.[25]

A recent study analyzed data from over 37,249 patients from 4 clinical studies (Stratify-2, Strata, TOP, Tygris) showing that for anti-JCV antibody negative patients on Tysabri, the risk of PML during the first 6 years was less than 0.07 cases per 1000 patients. For those who were anti-JCV antibody positive, the risk at 6 years was estimated at 1.7% for those without prior use of immunossupressive medications and 2.7% in those previously exposed to prior immunosuppressants. When further stratified based on JCV antibody index, the cummulative risk of PML per 1000 patients not previously exposed to immunosuppressive therapies was estimated at 0.01 case at year 1, 0.06 case at year 2, and 1.6 cases at year 6 for those with index value less than or equal to 0.9; for those with index value greater than 1.5, the cumulative risk per 1000 patients was estimated at 0.2 case at year 1, 1.1 cases at year 2, and 28.0 cases at year 6. For patients previously exposed to immunosuppressive therapies, the risk of PML per 1000 patients was estimated at 0.4 case at 12 months, 0.8 case at 2 years and 27 cases at 6 years.[26]

Despite the usefulness of JCV antibody positivity and index, on rare occasion, PML may occur in patients whose JCV antibody index had been recently negative.[27]

In addition, transient elevations of JCV antibody index, which may not necessarily reflect true JCV activity, can be seen following a recent vaccination or other infection, and, in these settings, JCV index should be rechecked within 1 to 2 months to confirm the elevation.[28]

FINGOLIMOD

Fingolimod was approved for the treatment of RRMS in 2009. Fingolimod prevents egress of specific lymphocyte subsets from the primary lymphoid organs, resulting in significant peripheral lymphopenia. Fingolimod affects CD4 T cell counts to a greater extent and, in patients on fingolimod long-term, results in significantly altered peripheral CD4/CD8 ratios (1:2), reminiscent of the same reversal in patients with AIDS.[29] To date, at least 15 cases of PML have occurred in association with fingolimod in the absence of recent prior natalizumab administration. The utility of the JCV antibody index in predicting the risk of PML has been studied predominantly in natalizumab-associated cases. Although its usefulness in monitoring the risk of PML in association with other therapies and conditions can be extrapolated, currently there are no data to show that the same index numbers hold true predictive value for patients on fingolimod, dimethyl fumarate, and other immunomodulatory therapies. Currently, no specific recommendation for JCV antibody/index monitoring exists in association with fingolimod. Based on the total exposure of over greater than 170,000, the incidence of PML continues to be low at approximately 1 case per 11,000 population.

DIMETHYL FUMARATE

Dimethyl fumarate (DMF) is an oral therapy used in the treatment of RRMS, approved in 2013. This medication activates nuclear (erythroid derived 2)-related factor (NRF2), an anti-inflammatory transcriptional pathway.[30] DMF induces apoptosis of T lymphocytes [26], with a preference for CD8+ subset.[31] Five cases of PML have been reported in patients on DMF therapy. Interestingly, the average age of these cases was 60.8 years (54, 59, 61, 64, and 66 years [Biogen, personal communication, 2017]), pointing to the likelihood of the importance of the natural effects of immunosenescence in relationship to the risk of PML.

DMF use is associated with various degrees of lymphopenia, preferably affecting CD8+ subset of T lymphocytes. CD8+ T cells are the main effector cells in the control of viral infections.[32] DMF increases the risk of PML via CD8 lymphopenia, which is a risk factor for PML, as well as other viral infections or decrease in VCAM-1 by 33%,[33] resulting in the egress of CD34 + B lymphocytes, reservoirs of JCV, from the bone marrow. The authors recommend DMF should be discontinued in patients with lymphopenia below $0.5X10^9$/L sustained for 6 months or more. Checking JCV antibody status in patients about to initiate DMF may be helpful in discussing the risk of PML with the patient. The authors recommend periodic monitoring for seroconversion, in those initially negative, which can be of value in discussion of theoretic risk.

The utility of monitoring JCV antibody index has not been evaluated in patients on DMF, primarily because of the paucity of cases; however, in a theoretic patient with sustained lymphopenia, irrespective of the grade, with a precipitous increase in JCV antibody index, the risk versus benefit of continuing DMF may need to be reevaluated. This may be particularly of value in patients of age greater than 50 years, who may be at higher risk. No specific guidelines for monitoring JCV antibody status and index in patients on DMF currently exist.

RITUXIMAB

Rituximab is an anti-CD20 B cell-depleting therapy that has been available since 1997 for the treatment of B cell-mediated malignancies and rheumatoid arthritis. Rituximab is also used in the treatment of neuromyelitis optica spectrum disorders, autoimmune encephalitis, and off label for the treatment of multiple sclerosis. The precise risk of PML in association with rituximab is difficult to estimate, as most conditions in which rituximab is used (eg, chronic lymphocytic leukemia [CLL], lymphoma, or rheumatoid arthritis) are associated with various degrees of immune system impairment and carry an independent risk of PML. Current literature suggests that the overall risk is about 1 case per 30,000 population,[4] but that may significantly vary based on the prior use of immunosuppression and concurrent use of other immunosuppressive medications. To date, no cases of PML have been reported in patients receiving rituximab off label for MS or neuromyelitis optica. In a 5-year follow-up study that included 30 patients with neuromyelitis optica spectrum disorder (NMOSD) on rituximab, no cases of PML were reported.[34] In a Korean study of 78 patients with NMOSD, 69% of whom were JCV antibody positive prior to rituximab initiation, no cases of PML were reported during the 4 years on treatment.[35] No cases of PML in patients with autoimmune encephalitis treated with rituximab have been reported to date.

OCRELIZUMAB

Ocrelizumab is a novel anti-CD20 B cell-depleting therapy approved in April 2017 for the treatment of relapsing remitting and primary progressive MS. During clinical trials (Opera I, Opera II, Oratorio), no cases of PML were reported over the average duration of 2 years. A case of PML was reported in a patient who was transitioned from a long-term natalizumab onto ocrelizumab, within the first month after the infusion.[36] This case was felt to be strongly related to the carry-over risk of PML from natalizumab, given a duration of therapy greater than 3 years. When transitioning patients from natalizumab to ocrelizumab or any other disease-modifying therapy with a risk of PML, it is important to be aware of an existing carry-over risk of PML, within at least the first 6 months after cessation of natalizumab.[37] Given that cases of PML have been reported with rituximab, PML should be considered in any patient who exhibits concerning clinical or radiologic changes while on ocrelizumab. Currently no specific clinical guidelines for PML surveillance and risk stratification in patients on ocrelizumab exist.

ALEMTUZUMAB

Alemtuzumab is an anti-CD52 agent that results in a prolonged depletion of lymphocytes, with a mean recovery of 7.1, 35, and 20 months for B cells, and CD4 and CD8 lymphocytes, respectively.[38] Over 9200 patients have been exposed to alemtuzumab since its approval. Although cases of PML have been reported in patients receiving alemtuzumab for myeloproliferative disorders,[39–41] to date, no cases of PML have occurred in MS patients who received alemtuzumab. Because of the potential risk of PML in association with alemtuzumab, a high level of clinical and radiologic suspicion should be maintained in patients receiving alemtuzumab. As no cases of PML in MS patients receiving alemtuzumab have occurred, there are no established practice guidelines regarding PML monitoring.

MYCOPHENOLATE MOFETIL

Mycophenolate mofetil (MMF) is a noncompetitive and reversible inhibitor of inosine-5′-monophosphate (IMP) dehydrogenase that leads to the inhibition of lymphocyte proliferation. In renal transplant patients, out of 33,000 patients, the incidence of PML associated with MMF use is 14.4 cases per 100,000 population.[42] In neurology clinics, MMF is used in the treatment of myasthenia gravis, NMOSD, and sarcoidosis. Physicians should be aware of the possibility of PML in association with MMF.

OTHER IMMUNE-ALTERING THERAPIES

Other medications such as cyclosporine, belatacept, efalizumab, cladribine, leflunomide, infliximab, and other immunosuppressive medications have been associated with cases of PML.

IMMUNOSENESCENCE AND THE RISK OF PROGRESSIVE MULTIFOCAL LEUKOENCEPHALOPATHY

Immunosenescence is a cumulative term for the many subtle changes occurring in the immune system with advanced age. People of older age are at an increased risk of infection.[43] With age, both CD4+ and CD8+ compartments undergo profound changes. The changes are most profound in CD8+ compartment, consisting predominantly of terminally differentiated effector memory cells with features of replicative immunosenescence, resulting in a poorer response to antigens and lower ability to proliferate.[44] A recent study of risk factors associated with earlier onset of PML in association with natalizumab therapy found that an age greater than 50 years at therapy start doubled the risk of earlier PML onset.[45] Among fingolimod-associated PML cases, average age was 54 years (range 32–63 years) based on cases as of May 2017, and for dimethyl fumarate-associated PML cases, the average age was 60.8 years (range 54–66 years).[43] As with most infections, age may be an important risk factor to consider when discussing the risk of PML versus the benefit of a specific medication.

TREATMENT

Currently, there are no highly effective treatments that can reliably control and reverse PML. The basis of PML management is the removal of the offending agent/therapy and supportive measures while allowing for the reconstitution of the immune system. In AIDS-associated PML, initiation of antiretroviral therapy is critical. In natalizumab-associated PML, immediate cessation of infusions, discontinuation of any other immune suppressive medications, and initiation of plasma exchanges is indicated, although the value of the latter has been questioned.[46]

Nucleoside analogs inhibiting viral DNA synthesis (cytosine arabinoside (cytarabine, ARA-C) have been shown in vitro to inhibit JCV replication; however, AIDS-associated PML trial of ARA-C failed to show any benefit.[47]

The use of 5HT2A (one of the routes for JCV entry into cells) blockers such as ziprasidone, olanzapine and risperidone showed some efficacy in vivo, but failed to show efficacy in clinical trials either individually or in combination with antiretrovirals.[48] Mirtazapine likewise has been used with variable level of success through mainly anecdotal evidence.[49–51] Mefloquine, an anti-malarial medication, with excellent blood-brain-barrier penetration was studied in a 38-week long open-label randomized trial, which found no evidence of efficacy.[52] Anecdotal evidence suggested that maraviroc, a CCR5 antagonist, might be helpful in the treatment of IRIS; however, a larger study did not show any significant benefit.[53]

JCV-specific T cells adaptive therapy is being investigated in an ongoing immunotherapeutic trial (NCT02694783). This trial employs ex vivo generated polyomavirus-specific T cells injected into patients with PML.

PROGNOSIS

Prognosis of PML vastly depends on the underlying predisposing condition, the timing of diagnosis and the ability to restore any associated immune defect, for example, by the discontinuation of natalizumab for natalizumab-associated PML. Thus, a multiple sclerosis patient on natalizumab, whose PML is promptly diagnosed, may have better outcomes than a patient with non-Hodgkin's lymphoma or CLL, whose immune system is irreversibly compromised and who is receiving cancer treatments that further undermine his/her immune system. At the heart of PML prognosis lies the ability of the patient's cellular immune system to mount a JCV-specific T cell response.[54] In natalizumab-associated PML, mortality is estimated at 20% to 25%. In this scenario, PML has the best prognosis when detected early, natalizumab is stopped and plasma exchange is initiated. Nevertheless, 1/3 of survivors have severe neurologic deficits, 1/3 moderate deficits and 1/3 mild deficits.[11] IRIS arises as a result of immune system restoration. As JCV-specific CD8+ lymphocytes rise in numbers, they mount an attack on the infected cells, resulting in clinical and radiological worsening. IRIS is not specific to PML, and can happen with a variety of other infections in the setting of immune reconstitution. In HIV-associated PML, IRIS can occur within 4 to 8 weeks after antiretroviral therapy is initiated. In natalizumab-associated PML cases, IRIS can occur at the time of the diagnosis of PML, reflecting a more intact level of the immune system. Treatment of natalizumab-associated PML with plasma exchange nearly always results in IRIS.[55] IRIS is treated with steroid administration with a prolonged taper,[56] but there are no randomized controlled trials demonstrating the value of this approach to PML-IRIS.

SUMMARY

Various novel immunotherapies used in the treatment of rheumatologic disorders, cancers, multiple sclerosis, myasthenia gravis, neuromyelitis optica spectrum disorder, and neurosarcoidosis can predispose patients to PML. It is important to remember that those of older age may have an even higher risk of PML, as is the trend with virtually all other infections, reflecting the immunosenescent state. High clinical vigilance is recommended for patients at risk. Knowing JCV antibody status and monitoring JCV index values can be helpful in a subset of patients at risk for PML. Patient education lies at the heart of clinical surveillance.

REFERENCES

1. Astrom KE, Mancall EL, Richardson EP Jr. Progressive multifocal leuko-encephalopathy; a hitherto unrecognized complication of chronic lymphatic leukaemia and Hodgkin's disease. Brain 1958;81(1):93–111.
2. Amend KL, Turnbull B, Foskett N, et al. Incidence of progressive multifocal leu-koencephalopathy in patients without HIV. Neurology 2010;75(15):1326–32.
3. Molloy ES, Calabrese LH. Progressive multifocal leukoencephalopathy: a national estimate of frequency in systemic lupus erythematosus and other rheumatic diseases. Arthritis Rheum 2009;60(12):3761–5.
4. Berger JR. Classifying PML risk with disease modifying therapies. Mult Scler Relat Disord 2017;12:59–63.
5. Bozic C, Subramanyam M, Richman S, et al. Anti-JC virus (JCV) antibody prevalence in the JCV Epidemiology in MS (JEMS) trial. Eur J Neurol 2014;21(2):299–304.
6. Ferenczy MW, Marshall LJ, Nelson CD, et al. Molecular biology, epidemiology, and pathogenesis of progressive multifocal leukoencephalopathy, the JC virus-induced demyelinating disease of the human brain. Clin Microbiol Rev 2012;25(3):471–506.
7. Bofill-Mas S, Formiga-Cruz M, Clemente-Casares P, et al. Potential transmission of human polyomaviruses through the gastrointestinal tract after exposure to virions or viral DNA. J Virol 2001;75(21):10290–9.
8. Berger JR, Miller CS, Danaher RJ, et al. Distribution and quantity of sites of John Cunningham virus persistence in immunologically healthy patients: correlation with JC virus antibody and urine JC virus DNA. JAMA Neurol 2017;74:437–44.
9. Rossi A, Delbue S, Mazziotti R, et al. Presence, quantitation and characterization of JC virus in the urine of Italian immunocompetent subjects. J Med Virol 2007;79(4):408–12.
10. Berger JR, Pall L, Lanska D, et al. Progressive multifocal leukoencephalopathy in patients with HIV infection. J Neurovirol 1998;4(1):59–68.

11. Clifford DB, De Luca A, Simpson DM, et al. Natalizumab-associated progressive multifocal leukoencephalopathy in patients with multiple sclerosis: lessons from 28 cases. Lancet Neurol 2010;9:438–46.
12. Berger JR, Aksamit AJ, Clifford DB, et al. PML diagnostic criteria: consensus statement from the AAN Neuroinfectious Disease Section. Neurology 2013; 80(15):1430–8.
13. Iacobaeus E, Ryschkewitsch C, Gravell M, et al. Analysis of cerebrospinal fluid and cerebrospinal fluid cells from patients with multiple sclerosis for detection of JC virus DNA. Mult Scler 2009;15:28–35.
14. Whiteman ML, Post MJ, Berger JR, et al. Progressive multifocal leukoencephalopathy in 47 HIV-seropositive patients: neuroimaging with clinical and pathologic correlation. Radiology 1993;187:233–40.
15. Miyagawa M, Maeda M, Umino M, et al. Low signal intensity in U-fiber identified by susceptibility-weighted imaging in two cases of progressive multifocal leukoencephalopathy. J Neurol Sci 2014;344(1–2):198–202.
16. Elices MJ, Osborn L, Takada Y, et al. VCAM-1 on activated endothelium interacts with the leukocyte integrin VLA-4 at a site distinct from the VLA-4/fibronectin binding site. Cell 1990;60:577–84.
17. Lobb RR, Hemler ME. The pathophysiologic role of α4 integrins in vivo. J Clin Invest 1994;94:1722–8.
18. Carotenuto A, Scalia G, Ausiello F, et al. CD4/CD8 ratio during natalizumab treatment in multiple sclerosis patients. J Neuroimmunol 2017;309:47–50.
19. Stüve O, Marra CM, Bar-Or A, et al. Altered CD4+/CD8+ T-cell ratios in cerebrospinal fluid of natalizumab-treated patients with multiple sclerosis. Arch Neurol 2006;63(10):1383–7.
20. Frohman EM, Monaco MC, Remington G, et al. JC virus in CD34+ and CD19+ cells in patients with multiple sclerosis treated with natalizumab. JAMA Neurol 2014;71(5):596–602.
21. Lee P, Plavina T, Castro A, et al. A second-generation ELISA (STRATIFY JCV™ DxSelect™) for detection of JC virus antibodies in human serum and plasma to support progressive multifocal leukoencephalopathy risk stratification. J Clin Virol 2013;57(2):141–6.
22. Berger JR, Fox RJ. Reassessing the risk of natalizumab-associated PML. J Neurovirol 2016;22:533.
23. Borchardt J, Berger JR. Re-evaluating the incidence of natalizumab-associated progressive multifocal leukoencephalopathy. Mult Scler Relat Disord 2016;8: 145–50.
24. Plavina T, Subramanyam M, Bloomgren G, et al. Anti–JC virus antibody levels in serum or plasma further define risk of natalizumab-associated progressive multifocal leukoencephalopathy. Ann Neurol 2014;76(6):802–12.
25. Schwab N, Schneider-Hohendorf T, Melzer N, et al. Challenges with incidence, resulting risk, and risk stratification. Neurology 2017;88(12):1197–205.
26. Ho PR, Koendgen H, Campbell N, et al. Risk of natalizumab-associated progressive multifocal leukoencephalopathy in patients with multiple sclerosis: a retrospective analysis of data from four clinical studies. Lancet Neurol 2017;16(11): 925–33.
27. Gagne Brosseau MS, Stobbe G, Wundes A. Natalizumab-related PML 2 weeks after negative anti-JCV antibody assay. Neurology 2016;86(5):484–6.
28. Miranda Acuña JA, Weinstock-Guttman B. Influenza vaccination increases anti-JC virus antibody levels during treatment with Natalizumab: case report. Mult Scler Relat Disord 2016;9:54–5.

29. Schwanitz N, Boldt A, Stoppe M, et al. Treatment, safety, and tolerance: longterm fingolimod treatment of multiple sclerosis induces phenotypical immunsenescence (P2.082). Neurology 2016;86(16 Supplement):P2.082.
30. Scannevin RH, Chollate S, Jung MY, et al. Fumarates promote cytoprotection of central nervous system cells against oxidative stress via the nuclear factor (erythroid-derived 2)-like 2 pathway. J Pharmacol Exp Ther 2012;341(1):274–84.
31. Ghadiri M, Rezk A, Li R, et al. Dimethyl fumarate-induced lymphopenia in MS due to differential T-cell subset apoptosis. Neurol Neuroimmunol Neuroinflamm 2017; 4(3):e340.
32. Khatri BO, Garland J, Berger J, et al. The effect of dimethyl fumarate (Tecfidera) on lymphocyte counts: a potential contributor to progressive multifocal leukoencephalopathy risk. Mult Scler Relat Disord 2015;4:377–9.
33. Rubant SA, Ludwig RJ, Diehl S, et al. Dimethyl fumarate reduces leukocyte rolling in vivo through modulation of adhesion molecule expression. J Invest Dermatol 2008;128(2):326–31.
34. Kim SH, Huh SY, Lee SJ, et al. A 5-year follow-up of rituximab treatment in patients with neuromyelitis optica spectrum disorder. JAMA Neurol 2013;70(9): 1110–7.
35. Kim SH, Hyun JW, Jeong IH, et al. Anti-JC virus antibodies in rituximab-treated patients with neuromyelitis optica spectrum disorder. J Neurol 2015;262(3): 696–700.
36. Hughes S. PML Reported in patient receiving ocrelizumab. Medscape 2017. Available at: http://www.medscape.com/viewarticle/880654. Accessed July 10, 2017.
37. Fine AJ, Sorbello A, Kortepeter C, et al. Progressive multifocal leukoencephalopathy after natalizumab discontinuation. Ann Neurol 2014;75(1):108–15.
38. Hill-Cawthorne GA, Button T, Tuohy O, et al. Long term lymphocyte reconstitution after alemtuzumab treatment of multiple sclerosis. J Neurol Neurosurg Psychiatry 2012;83(3):298–304.
39. Martin SI, Marty FM, Fiumara K, et al. Infectious complications associated with alemtuzumab use for lymphoproliferative disorders. Clin Infect Dis 2006;43(1): 16–24.
40. Isidoro L, Pires P, Rito L, et al. Progressive multifocal leukoencephalopathy in a patient with chronic lymphocytic leukaemia treated with alemtuzumab. BMJ Case Rep 2014;2014 [pii:bcr2013201781].
41. Keene DL, Legare C, Taylor E, et al. Monoclonal antibodies and progressive multifocal leukoencephalopathy. Can J Neurol Sci 2011;38(4):565–71.
42. Neff R, Hurst F, Falta E, et al. Progressive multifocal leukoencephalopathy and use of mycophenolate mofetil after kidney transplantation. Transplantation 2008;86:1474–8.
43. Grebenciucova E, Berger JR. Immunosenescence: the role of aging in the predisposition to neuro-infectious complications arising from the treatment of multiple sclerosis. Curr Neurol Neurosci Rep 2017;17(8):61.
44. Nikolich-Zugich J, Li G, Uhrlaub JL, et al. Age-related changes in CD8 T cell homeostasis and immunity to infection. Semin Immunol 2012;24:356–64.
45. Prosperini L, Scarpazza C, Imberti L, et al. Age as a risk factor for early onset of natalizumab-related progressive multifocal leukoencephalopathy. J Neurovirol 2017;23(5):742–9.
46. Scarpazza C, Prosperini L, De Rossi N, et al, Italian PML Group. To do or not to do? Plasma exchange and timing of steroid administration in progressive multifocal leukoencephalopathy. Ann Neurol 2017;82(5):697–705.

47. Hall CD, Dafni U, Simpson D, et al. Failure of cytarabine in progressive multifocal leukoencephalopathy associated with human immunodeficiency virus infection. AIDS Clinical Trials Group 243 Team. N Engl J Med 1998;338(19):1345–51.
48. Altschuler EL, Kast RE. The atypical antipsychotic agents ziprasidone [correction of zisprasidone], risperdone and olanzapine as treatment for and prophylaxis against progressive multifocal leukoencephalopathy. Med Hypotheses 2005; 65(3):585–6.
49. Trentalange A, Calcagno A, Ghisetti V, et al. Clearance of cerebrospinal fluid JCV DNA with mirtazapine in a patient with progressive multifocal leukoencephalopathy and sarcoidosis. Antivir Ther 2016;21(7):633–5.
50. Jamilloux Y, Kerever S, Ferry T, et al. Treatment of Progressive Multifocal Leukoencephalopathy with Mirtazapine. Clin Drug Investig 2016;36(10):783–9.
51. Cettomai D, McArthur JC. Mirtazapine use in human immunodeficiency virus-infected patients with progressive multifocal leukoencephalopathy. Arch Neurol 2009;66(2):255–8.
52. Clifford DB, Nath A, Cinque P, et al. A study of mefloquine treatment for progressive multifocal leukoencephalopathy: results and exploration of predictors of PML outcomes. J Neurovirol 2013;19(4):351–8.
53. Sierra-Madero JG, Ellenberg SS, Rassool MS, et al. CADIRIS study team. Effect of the CCR5 antagonist maraviroc on the occurrence of immune reconstitution inflammatory syndrome in HIV (CADIRIS): a double-blind, randomised, placebo-controlled trial. Lancet HIV 2014;1(2):e60–7.
54. Koralnik IJ, Du Pasquier RA, Letvin NL. JC virus-specific cytotoxic T lymphocytes in individuals with progressive multifocal leukoencephalopathy. J Virol 2001; 75(7):3483–7.
55. Tan IL, McArthur JC, Clifford DB, et al. Immune reconstitution inflammatory syndrome in natalizumab-associated PML. Neurology 2011;77(11):1061–7.
56. Johnson T, Nath A. Neurological complications of immune reconstitution in HIV-infected populations. Ann N Y Acad Sci 2010;1184:106–20.

Human Immunodeficiency Virus and the Nervous System

Emily Jane Sutherland, MBBS[a],
Bruce James Brew, MBBS, DMedSci, DSc[b],*

KEYWORDS

- Human Immunodeficiency Virus • HAND • HIV Dementia

KEY POINTS

- In the era of combination antiretroviral therapy (cART), the diagnostic and management issue of HIV-associated neurocognitive disorders (HANDs) has arisen.
- Traditionally, severe HAND, known as HIV-associated dementia (HAD), was seen in those with untreated HIV infection and had a guarded prognosis.
- The introduction of antiretroviral therapy has provided longevity and viral control to many of those living with the disease, in turn revealing an overall increase in prevalence of the less severe forms of HAND: asymptomatic neurocognitive impairment and mild neurocognitive disorder.
- Despite peripheral blood and cerebrospinal fluid viral suppression, cognitive impairment has been demonstrated to occur and progress for reasons that are unclear at present.
- This article provides a review of the current theories behind the development of HAND, clinical and pathologic findings, recent developments, and future research opportunities.

INTRODUCTION

In the era of combination antiretroviral therapy (cART), the diagnostic and management issue of HIV-associated neurocognitive disorders (HANDs) has arisen. Traditionally, severe HAND, known as HIV-associated dementia (HAD), was seen in those with untreated HIV infection and had a guarded prognosis.[1] The introduction of antiretroviral therapy (ART) has provided longevity and viral control to many of those living with the disease, in turn revealing an overall increase in prevalence of the less severe forms of HAND: asymptomatic neurocognitive impairment (ANI) and mild

[a] Department of Neurology, University of New South Wales, University of Notre Dame, Sydney, Australia; [b] Department of Neurology, HIV Medicine, Neurosciences Program, Peter Duncan Neurosciences Unit, St Vincent's Hospital, St Vincent's Centre for Applied Medical Research, University of New South Wales, University of Notre Dame, Level 4 Xavier Building, Victoria Street, Darlinghurst, Sydney, Australia
* Corresponding author.
E-mail address: B.Brew@UNSW.edu.au

Neurol Clin 36 (2018) 751–765
https://doi.org/10.1016/j.ncl.2018.07.002   **neurologic.theclinics.com**

neurocognitive disorder (MND).[1–4] Despite peripheral blood and cerebrospinal fluid (CSF) viral suppression, cognitive impairment has been demonstrated to occur and progress[5] for reasons that are unclear at present. This article reviews the current theories behind the development of HAND, clinical and pathologic findings, recent developments, and future research opportunities.

CLASSIFICATION

Introduced in 2007, the Frascati criteria are internationally accepted as a method of classifying HANDs, stratifying patients into 3 distinct groups (**Fig. 1**).[6,7]

ANI is the term used for those who have MND that does not affect their activities of daily living and general function.[6–8] Mild neurocognitive impairment necessitates abnormal results in at least 2 cognitive domains with performance more than 1 SD below the mean of a matched HIV-negative group, whereas moderate to severe impairment is demonstrated with scores more than 2 SDs below the mean.[6]

EPIDEMIOLOGY

During the pre-ART era, rates of diagnosis of HAD ranged between 10% and 20%; however, the CHARTER and MACS studies demonstrated a reduction in HAD in the ART era, with rates of 2% to 3% indicating a beneficial effect of cART on the more severe form of cognitive impairment associated with HIV.[1,9,10] Mild to moderate rates of impairment, however, have not changed significantly, as the authors' early study showed,[11] and which was confirmed in the CHARTER study (CNS HIV Antiretroviral Therapy Effects Research). Indeed, 44% of the CHARTER study participants met diagnostic criteria for ANI and MND, similar to statistics from the pre-ART era,[9] implying less protective benefit in this cohort. The MACS study (Multicentre AIDS Cohort Study) excluded many possible confounders and found a frequency of ANI and MND of 24% over a 6-year period; however, a different demographic profile may have contributed to these results.[1] A major risk factor for the diagnosis of HAND is a history of a low CD4 count nadir[9,12]; however, this does not seem to influence progression of disease.[1] Other risk factors include low educational level and anemia. Acquiring the disease through sexual contact rather than intravenous drug use has been advanced as a potential risk factor; however, this is likely related to selection bias due to higher mortality rates in the latter group (intravenous drug users)[13]; intravenous drug use is associated with more severe cognitive impairment likely through several mechanisms. In general, cognition is

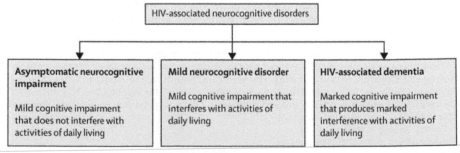

Fig. 1. The Frascati criteria for HIV-associated neurocognitive disorders. (*From* Nightingale S, Winston A, Letendre S, et al. Controversies in HIV-associated neurocognitive disorders. Lancet Neurol 2014;13(11):1139–51; with permission.)

stable, a small amount improve a small proportion of those affected; however, decline rates have been reported to be between 13% and 17%.[1,9,12] The MACS study did not demonstrate any associated between risk of HAND progression and age, duration of infection, type of cART, or hepatitis C coinfection, although these results are open to controversy. The only positive risk factor identified for stage progression was hypercholesterolemia, which possibly indicates cerebrovascular pathology as a contributor to HAND or the relative lack of central nervous system (CNS) efficacy of protease inhibitor therapy, which is associated with hypercholesterolaemia.[1]

PATHOPHYSIOLOGY

A wide range of direct and indirect pathologic mechanisms have been described as contributing to neuronal damage and subsequent cognitive decline in HIV, as demonstrated in **Fig. 2**. During the initial stages of infection, the virus enters the brain via migrating myeloid and lymphoid cells and in some but not all patients it establishes infection in perivascular macrophages, microglia, and astrocytes.[4,8,14,15] Traditionally, it was believed that HIV encephalitis and subsequent high levels of CNS inflammation were a driving factor behind the cognitive changes seen with HAND; however, in the cART era with adequate viral suppression, it may be changes in neurovascular biology that are contributing more to these cognitive changes.[16] Some of the main pathophysiological mechanisms believed to contribute to the development of HAND in the cART era are severe initial immunosuppression infected CNS monocytes and macrophages acting as a viral reservoir,[17] low-grade chronic CNS inflammation from both viral factors and host immune factors,[14,18,19] neuroreceptor tropism, possibly ARV neurotoxicity,[20] and comorbid conditions.[8] These factors are discussed later.

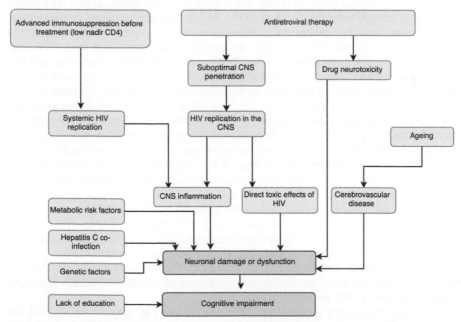

Fig. 2. Suggested pathologic mechanisms for cognitive decline in HIV. (*Adapted from* Nightingale S, Winston A, Letendre S, et al. Controversies in HIV-associated neurocognitive disorders. Lancet Neurol 2014;13(11):1139–51; with permission.)

In regard to mechanisms behind the progression of HAND, the main risk factors associated are longer duration of infection, older age, low CD4[+] count nadir, and ongoing viral replication in serum and in the CNS.[8,21] Metabolic risk factors likely enhance the cognitive decline seen with HAND. It is well known that vascular disease is common in those with HIV,[22] which in itself is a risk factor for cognitive impairment. Other factors that may affect progressive cognitive decline with HAND include anemia, impaired renal function, substance abuse, and type 2 diabetes mellitus.[23,24]

Advanced Immunosuppression Prior to Combination Antiretroviral Therapy Treatment

Historically, cART was introduced after diagnosis of HIV-related immunosuppression or a low CD4 T-cell count. Many studies have demonstrated advanced immunosuppression conferring a greater risk for cognitive impairment,[8,25–27] which may be explained by almost unchecked viral replication in the CNS.[5] Since the START study (Strategic Timing of Antiretroviral Treatment), guidelines now recommend commencing ART immediately after diagnosis of HIV rather than after impaired immune function or a low CD4[+] cell count has developed.[28] Hopefully, the early introduction of treatment will decrease rates of all subtypes of HAND, although the neurologic substudy of START did not find any difference neuropsychologically between immediate versus delayed cART, possibly because of limited follow-up.[29]

Central Nervous System Viral Reservoir

During early stages of the disease, monocytes and macrophages are infected and probably become viral reservoirs because they do not undergo apoptosis due to viral cytopathy or immune surveillance.[30] Many anatomic sites throughout the body have been identified as sanctuaries for viral reservoirs; hence, complete eradication has proved difficult with current therapies that target the virus during active replication. These sites include peripheral resting CD4[+] T cells, gut-associated lymphoid tissue, bone marrow, and the genital tract. There is good but indirect evidence that HIV can be present in the brain despite an undetectable peripheral and CSF viral load.[17,31] There are several reasons the CNS is a viral reservoir, including variable penetration of cART into the CNS (thereby making it a sanctuary), variable efficacy of cART in brain cells as opposed to lymphocytes, noncytolitic infection of very long-lived cells (of the order of many years) such as microglia and astrocytes, and cART inability to inhibit transcription of nonstructural HIV proteins. Although not demonstrated in humans, simian immunodeficiency virus–infected macaques with complete peripheral viral suppression harbored latently infected macrophages with the ability for viral replication in regions of the brain that had no detectable viral RNA.[32,33] Epigenetic factors and inherent viral mutations found only in the CSF also may promote viral latency.[26,30,34]

At some point, the virus seems to become autonomous in the CSF, independent of activity in the periphery, termed *CSF viral escape*.[26,35] This can occur even in those on ART with long-term serum viral control and adequate CD4[+] counts. In particular, most cART regimens containing protease inhibitors have been demonstrated to have inadequate activity for CNS viral suppression.[36] A low CD4[+] count nadir can predispose patients to CNS viral escape, which may not be able to be completely suppressed with the introduction of CNS-penetrating ART.[25]

Circulating monocytes expressing CD16 are believed to migrate throughout the body, acting as a viral reservoir.[37] CD16[+] monocytes are increased in the periphery in uncontrolled viremia, and high levels of peripheral CD16[+] monocytes are associated with cognitive impairment, more so than CSF viral load or proportion of

HIV-infected cells in the CNS.[21,37] CD163 is a scavenger receptor found on monocytes and macrophages with higher expression on CD16$^+$ monocytes. The receptor is shed as sCD163 after activation or damage of each monocyte; hence, sCD163 levels have been found higher in those with HIV.[21,37] A correlation has also been found between CSF sCD14 and sCD163 with CNS inflammatory biomarkers, indicating ongoing monocyte and macrophage activation is likely contributing to neuronal injury.[38] Considering this, it is not surprising that higher sCD14 and sCD163 levels have been associated with worse cognitive performance.[39]

Central Nervous System Inflammation

Sustained low-level and latent infection of the meninges, and likely the brain, may cause continuous CNS inflammation due to direct and indirect toxicity from viral proteins, such as Nef, Tat, vpr, rev, and the envelope protein gp120. In those with viral suppression and, therefore, none or little whole virus production, Nef, Tat, rev and vpr, seem important whereas in those without viral suppression it is the envelope protein gp120 that is probably most important (**Fig. 3**).[18,40] These proteins activate CSF anti-inflammatory macrophages via cytokines to alter their phenotype to become proinflammatory.[18,34] Nef can promote T-cell activation and viral replication and atherosclerosis.[41] Chronic low-level expression of Tat in mice was associated with reduced brain volume and neuronal damage with advanced age.[15] Tat causes neuronal death in multiple ways—through activation of tumor necrosis factor α, dysregulation of cellular calcium homeostasis, excitotoxicity through N-methyl-D-aspartate receptor activation, mitochondrial hyperpolarization, up-regulation of p53, and alteration of microRNA expression.[42] A gp120 mice model has demonstrated ongoing activation of innate immunity, loss of synapses, disturbed nerve cell growth, and astrocytosis.[43]

Neopterin is a pteridine produced by cells of the monocyte and macrophage lineage when activated by proinflammatory stimuli, which itself induces downstream expression of proinflammatory cytokines and mediators.[14] Higher CSF levels have been found to correlate with HAND severity in ART-naïve individuals[44]; however, this prediction cannot be made in those treated with ART who are virally suppressed. CSF neopterin levels decline with ART but are persistently higher than HIV-seronegative people, indicating ongoing inflammation despite control of whole virus production,

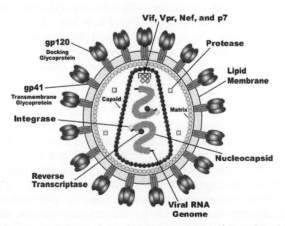

Fig. 3. HIV virion structure. (*From* Inform P. HIV Structure and Function. 2016. Available at: https://www.projectinform.org/glossary/hiv-structure-function/. Accessed November, 2017.)

further supporting the theory of HIV or possibly a dysregulated immune system acting autonomously in the CNS at least in some patients.[14]

Along with higher levels of CSF inflammation, it has been shown that with HIV infection there is a loss of neuroprotective proteins in the CSF, which in turn correlated with higher levels of cognitive impairment.[19] Ongoing inflammation and dysregulation of defense mechanisms is likely to cause ongoing cytokine release and cellular damage in a self-perpetuating manner, resulting in neuronal death.[4,21] This theory of chronic CNS inflammation may be a reason behind the lack of a strong relationship between CSF HIV RNA levels and cognitive impairment, that is, immune dysregulation rather than direct virus-related cellular damage causing irreversible neuronal loss.[8] There are emerging data from several groups, however, that sustained very low-level (using single-copy assays) HIV RNA in the CSF or nonstructural components of the virus, such as Tat, may be driving HAND.

Receptor Neurotropism

CCR5 is one of the HIV coreceptors required to bind CD4, for HIV entry into host cells. CCR5 has been identified as the most important coreceptor for microglia and CNS macrophage infection. HIV strains detected in the CSF and brain almost exclusively use the CCR5 coreceptor, with decreased dependence on CD4 for cellular entry.[30,34] Some neural cells, including astrocytes, express the other important coreceptor CXCR4 but it is often coexpressed with CCR5. Neural cells express CCR5 ligands in response to infection and inflammation, which in turn increases the migration of T cells into the CNS, amplifying the CNS immune response.[21] Maraviroc is an oral CCR5 inhibitor, currently used in cART. It and has been shown to suppress monocyte migration, lower the HIV burden in $CD14^+$ monocytes, and possibly alter the coreceptor signaling. Two studies, one of which was randomized, have demonstrated improvement in cognitive performance and a decrease in plasma sCD163 levels with maraviroc-intensified ART regimes.[37,45]

Antiretroviral Therapy Neurotoxicity

Several studies have raised the possibility of ARV neurotoxicity. These have ranged from in vitro to suggestive in vivo publications.[46] The issue is still controversial except for data relating to efavirenz.[47] Even in this instance, however, it has been emphasized that such toxicity likely only occurs in a small proportion of patients taking efavirenz. Nucleoside analogs have been associated with mitochondrial damage although again this does not occur in all patients and at a clinical level has only been associated with the development of neuropathy from didanosine and dideoxycytidine. Protease inhibitors have been potentially linked to neurotoxicity through their effect on the P-glycoprotein transporter systems, particularly in relation to brain clearance of amyloid fragments and other putative toxins.[48]

Comorbidities

It is commonly known that cerebrovascular disease contributes to cognitive decline, and those with HIV are predisposed because both HIV infection per se and the use of ARVs can induce severe metabolic complications and widespread premature vascular disease.[8,41,49,50] Coinfection with hepatitis C has also been shown to make people at a higher risk of cognitive impairment, even after adjustment for level of education and history of intravenous drug use[51] and such impairment responds to therapy.[52] Hepatic fibrosis may also contribute to poor cognitive scores, with the proposed theory relating to ammonia clearance and astrocyte dysfunction.[53] There is ongoing controversy as to whether HIV interacts with neurodegenerative diseases, such as

Alzheimer and Parkinson.[54] The nature of the interaction could be through acceleration and/or facilitation of the disease in someone predisposed. Until recently, there was a similar controversy as to whether HIV accelerated aging of the brain. The data from the MACS study, however, have convincingly shown that this is the case.[55,56]

CLINICAL FINDINGS

The typical features seen in HAND are those of a subcortical type of cognitive impairment with psychomotor slowing, delay in information processing, and difficulties with executive functioning and memory recall.[57,58] There also may be extrapyramidal features, depending on the extent of basal ganglia dysfunction. If there is progression from ANI to MND, there will be some disturbance to activities of daily living and routines. As the disorder progresses, these subcortical distinguishing features are lost and the impairment becomes more generalized with both subcortical and cortical features.[58] HANDs developing in the context of viral suppression may be different. There is some evidence that there are more cortical features, possibly as a consequence of the influence of comorbidities as patients live longer.[59]

SCREENING AND DIAGNOSIS

An ethical dilemma arises when discussing screening for HANDs in those who are asymptomatic because there are currently limited therapeutic interventions. Nonetheless, there is a strong relationship between medication adherence and cognitive impairment. Thus, the identification of HAND patients should at least focus efforts to improve adherence lest a virtual cycle be established whereby cognitive impairment leads to poor cART adherence, which in turn leads to the development of ARV resistance with further cognitive impairment and further compromised adherence. Additionally, there is some evidence albeit controversial that intensification of cART with the addition of another ARV with good CNS penetration may improve cognitive impairment in the context of viral suppression.[37,45] Finally, there is some evidence for the use of ARVs that have better CNS penetration.[60] There is currently no formally accepted international guideline regarding screening, and routine screening is not widely adopted.[8] The British HIV Association recommends screening within the first 3 months of diagnosis and subsequent annual screening; however, it does not clarify which screening tool to use.[27] The European AIDS Clinical Society has a clear algorithm for screening in those who self-report cognitive problems with a 3-question assessment, exclusion of depression, and subsequent formal neuropsychological testing.[61] The Australasian Society for HIV, Viral Hepatitis and Sexual Health Medicine recommends referral for neuropsychological testing but does not provide clear guidelines about timing of screening.[62] Formal neuropsychological testing remains the gold standard for formal diagnosis of HAND, with the exclusion of psychiatric and/or neurodegenerative disorders.[63]

Screening Tools

The HIV Dementia Scale (HDS) is a commonly used screening tool that assesses eye movements, motor skills, learning, and attention. It has been found most useful in identifying HAD; however, it is much less helpful in detecting symptoms of the milder forms of HAND.[57,64] There is some evidence, however, that a higher cutoff score of 14 instead of 10 can be more sensitive in detecting milder forms of HAND.[65] The International HIV Dementia Scale evaluates memory and psychomotor skills; it is a globally validated tool that allows clinicians to easily assess patients and can be used in younger age groups. Unfortunately, it also lacks accuracy as a screening tool for ANI and MND.[57,64] The Mini-Mental State Examination, traditionally used in Alzheimer dementia, has minimal use in screening for HANDs.[57] Studies have shown the Montreal Cognitive Assessment can be used as a screening tool with high sensitivity but poor specificity. A score of 26 or less indicates need for formal neuropsychological testing.[58,66]

Cogstate is a more recently developed computerized screening tool that focuses on sustained attention, information processing speed, verbal learning, and verbal memory. The results were impressive compared with formal neuropsychological testing—sensitivity of 76% and specificity of 82% over all stages of HAND and sensitivity of 100% and specificity of 98% when evaluating MND and HAD combined.[63] This tool may be useful for identifying the more advanced cases of HAND, allowing for prompt specialist referral.

NEUROIMAGING

A preferred neuroimaging modality has yet to be agreed on in the setting of HAND, although there is a wealth of data on the utility of magnetic resonance spectroscopy as an ancillary aid to the diagnosis of HAND and its response to therapy.[67] Typical MRI findings include cortical and subcortical atrophy as well as diffuse white matter lesions, which have been associated with CSF viral escape, especially in those taking ART.[58,68] A recent study revealed higher levels of age-associated changes to brain structure in those with peripheral viral suppression compared with the HIV-negative population, implying that chronic HIV infection may cause abnormal brain aging.[69] MRI measures of brain volume are beginning to provide insight into the cognitive deficits seen with HAND,[70] especially ANI.[71] MRI diffusion tensor imaging has also been used in a research setting to demonstrate CNS inflammation in those who are neurologically asymptomatic, hence a possibility of use as a diagnostic tool in the future.[72] Similarly, resting state MRI is proving useful in early studies.[73]

BIOMARKERS

Although currently in use in some centers for predicting or monitoring disease, future biomarkers may be useful to help target treatment. As discussed previously, CSF sCD163, circulating CD16[+] monocytes, and neopterin are detected at higher levels during CNS inflammation so can be useful biomarkers of disease; however, their use may be less robust in the context of effective ART.[21] Neurofilament light chain protein is a marker of CNS axonal damage, which may be able to predict those who are at risk of developing HANDs; however, this is less clear with the introduction of ART.[38,74] Levels have been found significantly elevated in those with HAD in comparison with ANI and MND but only in those with CD4[+] nadirs less than 200.[38] It may also be elevated in the CSF in who are cognitively asymptomatic and have a suppressed peripheral viral load, again supporting the idea of the virus acting autonomously in the CNS.[26]

As a biomarker for monocyte activation, high CSF sCD14 levels confer an increased risk of all-cause mortality and correlate with worse neurocognitive performance, suggesting this could be a useful biomarker. Its usefulness may be limited, however, because sCD14 levels did not correlate between HAND subtypes.[75–77]

CSF HIV RNA levels were more useful in the pre-ART era; however, decreasing levels can still be correlated with improvements in cognition in those who are not virally suppressed.[21] As discussed previously, the single-copy assay for HIV RNA in the CSF has promising early data for HANDs. microRNAs are noncoding RNA molecules that regulate gene expression, which may have a role in the pathogenesis of HANDs and have been shown useful as biomarkers. Nonetheless, further research to substantiate current findings is needed.[78] Other biomarkers under investigation include interleukins, BCL11B, monocyte chemoattractant protein-1, matrix metalloproteinases, and interferon gamma.[79–82]

TREATMENT

To date, there is no specific treatment of HANDs. As discussed previously, the introduction of ART has had a significant effect on the incidence of HAD; however, it has not had an impact on the development and continued presence of milder forms of HAND.[26] Alteration in the ART regimen to ARVs with putative better CNS penetration has not been found to improve cognitive function,[4,83] although there are difficulties in trial design, such as appropriate power and stability of HAND, that undermine these findings.[21,60] The weight of evidence from all studies tends to favor a more penetrating CNS ART regimen.[59] In response to the detection of CSF HIV RNA and its detrimental effect on cognition, the CNS penetration effectiveness (CPE) score was developed to rank drugs regarding their penetration and efficacy in the CNS. **Table 1** outlines CPE scores of common ARVs, with a score of 4 indicating higher CNS effectiveness and a score of 1 indicating below-average effectiveness.[8,58]

Changing to a more CNS-intensive ART regimen might lower the risk for HAND stage progression and has been shown to improve learning and memory in those with HAD[58]; however, there is currently only suggestive evidence regarding overall clinical benefit, and some groups do not promote the use of the CPE score.[8,27,60] The varied cognitive testing results with high CPE score ART regimens may indicate that CSF drug concentrations have several explanations, including issues relating to the scoring methodology per se.[21]

As discussed previously, a majority of HIV strains found in the CSF are CCR5 tropic, hence the theory behind maraviroc-boosted regimens. Maraviroc has been found to have good CSF penetration, low rates of resistance, and the ability to inhibit viral replication and has inherent CSF anti-inflammatory properties. Boosted regimens have also shown improved cognitive performance.[37,45] This provides hope for a possible enhanced treatment regimen for those diagnosed with HAND.

Many other pharmacotherapies have been trialed in HANDs, including selegiline, serotonin reuptake inhibitors, lithium, and sodium valproate; however, a clinical benefit has failed to be described.[26]

A strong link has been demonstrated between the length of duration with undetectable viral load and improved cognitive performance,[5] indicating that in some circumstances more importance should be on tailoring an ART regimen that each patient can

Table 1
Total central nervous system penetration effectiveness score is the sum of individual drug scores on the antiretroviral therapy regimen

	4	3	2	1
Nucleoside reverse transcriptase inhibitors	Zidovudine	Abavavir Emtricitabine	Lamivudine Stavudine	Tenofovir
Non-nucleoside reverse transcriptase inhibitors	Nevirapine	Delavirdine Efavirenz	Etravirine	
Protease inhibitors	Indinavir*	Darunavir* Lopinavir*	Atazanavir*	Ritonavir Nelfinavir
Cell fusion and entry inhibitors		Maraviroc		
Integrase inhibitors		Raltegravir		

Adapted from Nightingale S, Winston A, Letendre S, et al. Controversies in HIV-associated neurocognitive disorders. Lancet Neurol 2014;13(11):1139–51; with permission.

both tolerate and afford. Cognitive rehabilitation also may be of value for those with cognitive impairment[84]; however, it is unclear whether this will provide long-term benefit or decrease the risk of stage advancement.

THE FUTURE

Ongoing research into biomarkers and treatment targets may provide insight into the pathophysiology behind HANDs, especially when they occur in the context of viral suppression and hopefully will provide either a preventative treatment or a cure. This will require a treatment that can completely eradicate the CNS viral reservoir with significant issues around penetration of the therapy into the brain, efficacy, and safety. On a more general note, the following are treatments that currently are under investigation: intranasal insulin, interleukin antagonists, Tat monoclonal antibodies, and antisense oligonucleotides.[21,85] It is also necessary for clear international guidelines to be established and for 1 screening tool to be recommended.

For the current generation of people living with HIV, perhaps the more important element to be examined is how early initiation of therapy will affect rates of HANDs.

REFERENCES

1. Sacktor N, Skolasky RL, Seaberg E, et al. Prevalence of HIV-associated neurocognitive disorders in the Multicenter AIDS Cohort Study. Neurology 2016; 86(4):334–40.
2. Gonzalez-Perez MP, Peters PJ, O'Connell O, et al. Identification of emerging macrophage-Tropic HIV-1 R5 variants in brain tissue of AIDS patients without severe neurological complications. J Virol 2017;91(20).
3. Hogan C, Wilkins E. Neurological complications in HIV. Clin Med (Lond) 2011; 11(6):571–5.
4. Tan IL, McArthur JC. HIV-associated neurological disorders: a guide to pharmacotherapy. CNS Drugs 2012;26(2):123–34.
5. Rubin LH, Maki PM, Springer G, et al. Cognitive trajectories over 4 years among HIV-infected women with optimal viral suppression. Neurology 2017;89(15): 1594–603.
6. Antinori A, Arendt G, Becker JT, et al. Updated research nosology for HIV-associated neurocognitive disorders. Neurology 2007;69(18):1789–99.
7. Gandhi NS, Moxley RT, Creighton J, et al. Comparison of scales to evaluate the progression of HIV-associated neurocognitive disorder. HIV Ther 2010;4(3): 371–9.
8. Nightingale S, Winston A, Letendre S, et al. Controversies in HIV-associated neurocognitive disorders. Lancet Neurol 2014;13(11):1139–51.
9. Heaton RK, Clifford DB, Franklin DR Jr, et al. HIV-associated neurocognitive disorders persist in the era of potent antiretroviral therapy: CHARTER Study. Neurology 2010;75(23):2087–96.
10. Dore GJ, Correll PK, Li Y, et al. Changes to AIDS dementia complex in the era of highly active antiretroviral therapy. AIDS 1999;13(10):1249–53.
11. Cysique LA, Maruff P, Brew BJ. Prevalence and pattern of neuropsychological impairment in human immunodeficiency virus-infected/acquired immunodeficiency syndrome (HIV/AIDS) patients across pre- and post-highly active antiretroviral therapy eras: a combined study of two cohorts. J Neurovirol 2004;10(6): 350–7.
12. Cysique LA, Maruff P, Brew BJ. Variable benefit in neuropsychological function in HIV-infected HAART-treated patients. Neurology 2006;66(9):1447–50.

13. De Ronchi D, Faranca I, Berardi D, et al. Risk factors for cognitive impairment in HIV-1-infected persons with different risk behaviors. Arch Neurol 2002;59(5): 812–8.

14. Hagberg L, Cinque P, Gisslen M, et al. Cerebrospinal fluid neopterin: an informative biomarker of central nervous system immune activation in HIV-1 infection. AIDS Res Ther 2010;7:15.

15. Dickens AM, Yoo SW, Chin AC, et al. Chronic low-level expression of HIV-1 Tat promotes a neurodegenerative phenotype with aging. Sci Rep 2017;7(1):7748.

16. Gelman BB. Neuropathology of HAND with suppressive antiretroviral therapy: encephalitis and neurodegeneration reconsidered. Curr HIV/AIDS Rep 2015;12(2): 272–9.

17. Dahl V, Peterson J, Fuchs D, et al. Low levels of HIV-1 RNA detected in the cerebrospinal fluid after up to 10 years of suppressive therapy are associated with local immune activation. AIDS 2014;28(15):2251–8.

18. Chihara T, Hashimoto M, Osman A, et al. HIV-1 proteins preferentially activate anti-inflammatory M2-type macrophages. J Immunol 2012;188(8):3620–7.

19. Meeker RB, Poulton W, Markovic-Plese S, et al. Protein changes in CSF of HIV-infected patients: evidence for loss of neuroprotection. J Neurovirol 2011;17(3): 258–73.

20. Heaton RK, Franklin DR, Ellis RJ, et al. HIV-associated neurocognitive disorders before and during the era of combination antiretroviral therapy: differences in rates, nature, and predictors. J Neurovirol 2011;17(1):3–16.

21. Carroll A, Brew B. HIV-associated neurocognitive disorders: recent advances in pathogenesis, biomarkers, and treatment. F1000Res 2017;6:312.

22. Su T, Wit FW, Caan MW, et al. White matter hyperintensities in relation to cognition in HIV-infected men with sustained suppressed viral load on combination antiretroviral therapy. AIDS 2016;30(15):2329–39.

23. Kallianpur AR, Wang Q, Jia P, et al. Anemia and red blood cell indices predict HIV-associated neurocognitive impairment in the highly active antiretroviral therapy era. J Infect Dis 2016;213(7):1065–73.

24. Schouten J, Su T, Wit FW, et al. Determinants of reduced cognitive performance in HIV-1-infected middle-aged men on combination antiretroviral therapy. AIDS 2016;30(7):1027–38.

25. Peluso MJ, Ferretti F, Peterson J, et al. Cerebrospinal fluid HIV escape associated with progressive neurologic dysfunction in patients on antiretroviral therapy with well controlled plasma viral load. AIDS 2012;26(14):1765–74.

26. Zayyad Z, Spudich S. Neuropathogenesis of HIV: from initial neuroinvasion to HIV-associated neurocognitive disorder (HAND). Curr HIV/AIDS Rep 2015; 12(1):16–24.

27. Association, B.H., British HIV Association guidelines for the routine investigation and monitoring of adult HIV-1-positive individuals 2016, N.H. Service, Editor. 2016.

28. Lundgren JD, Babiker AG, Gordin F, et al. Initiation of antiretroviral therapy in early asymptomatic HIV infection. N Engl J Med 2015;373(9):795–807.

29. Wright EJ, Grund B, Cysique LA, et al. Factors associated with neurocognitive test performance at baseline: a substudy of the INSIGHT Strategic Timing of AntiRetroviral Treatment (START) trial. HIV Med 2015;16(Suppl 1):97–108.

30. Gray L, Roche M, Churchill MJ, et al. Tissue-specific sequence alterations in the human immunodeficiency virus type 1 envelope favoring CCR5 usage contribute to persistence of dual-tropic virus in the brain. J Virol 2009;83(11):5430–41.

31. Nightingale S, Michael BD, Fisher M, et al. CSF/plasma HIV-1 RNA discordance even at low levels is associated with up-regulation of host inflammatory mediators in CSF. Cytokine 2016;83:139–46.

32. Avalos CR, Abreu CM, Queen SE, et al. Brain macrophages in simian immunodeficiency virus-infected, antiretroviral-suppressed macaques: a functional latent reservoir. MBio 2017;8(4).

33. Avalos CR, Price SL, Forsyth ER, et al. Quantitation of productively infected monocytes and macrophages of simian immunodeficiency virus-infected macaques. J Virol 2016;90(12):5643–56.

34. Gray LR, Brew BJ, Churchill MJ. Strategies to target HIV-1 in the central nervous system. Curr Opin HIV AIDS 2016;11(4):371–5.

35. Chen MF, Gill AJ, Kolson DL. Neuropathogenesis of HIV-associated neurocognitive disorders: roles for immune activation, HIV blipping and viral tropism. Curr Opin HIV AIDS 2014;9(6):559–64.

36. Joseph J, Cinque P, Colosi D, et al. Highlights of the global HIV-1 CSF escape consortium meeting, 9 June 2016, Bethesda, MD, USA. J Virus Erad 2016;2(4): 243–50.

37. Ndhlovu LC, Umaki T, Chew GM, et al. Treatment intensification with maraviroc (CCR5 antagonist) leads to declines in CD16-expressing monocytes in cART-suppressed chronic HIV-infected subjects and is associated with improvements in neurocognitive test performance: implications for HIV-associated neurocognitive disease (HAND). J Neurovirol 2014;20(6):571–82.

38. McGuire JL, Gill AJ, Douglas SD, et al. Central and peripheral markers of neurodegeneration and monocyte activation in HIV-associated neurocognitive disorders. J Neurovirol 2015;21(4):439–48.

39. Imp BM, Rubin LH, Tien PC, et al. Monocyte activation Is associated with worse cognitive performance in HIV-infected women with virologic suppression. J Infect Dis 2017;215(1):114–21.

40. Anderson AM, Fennema-Notestine C, Umlauf A, et al. CSF biomarkers of monocyte activation and chemotaxis correlate with magnetic resonance spectroscopy metabolites during chronic HIV disease. J Neurovirol 2015;21(5):559–67.

41. Wang T, Yi R, Green LA, et al. Increased cardiovascular disease risk in the HIV-positive population on ART: potential role of HIV-Nef and Tat. Cardiovasc Pathol 2015;24(5):279–82.

42. Chang JR, Mukerjee R, Bagashev A, et al. HIV-1 Tat protein promotes neuronal dysfunction through disruption of microRNAs. J Biol Chem 2011;286(47): 41125–34.

43. Thaney VE, Sanchez AB, Fields JA, et al. Transgenic mice expressing HIV-1 envelope protein gp120 in the brain as an animal model in neuroAIDS research. J Neurovirol 2018;24(2):156–67.

44. Brew BJ, Dunbar N, Pemberton L, et al. Predictive markers of AIDS dementia complex: CD4 cell count and cerebrospinal fluid concentrations of beta 2-microglobulin and neopterin. J Infect Dis 1996;174(2):294–8.

45. Gates TM, Cysique LA, Siefried KJ, et al. Maraviroc-intensified combined antiretroviral therapy improves cognition in virally suppressed HIV-associated neurocognitive disorder. Aids 2016;30(4):591–600.

46. Underwood J, Robertson KR, Winston A. Could antiretroviral neurotoxicity play a role in the pathogenesis of cognitive impairment in treated HIV disease? AIDS 2015;29(3):253–61.

47. Sandkovsky U, Podany AT, Fletcher CV, et al. Impact of efavirenz pharmacokinetics and pharmacogenomics on neuropsychological performance in older HIV-infected patients. J Antimicrob Chemother 2017;72(1):200–4.

48. Treisman GJ, Soudry O. Neuropsychiatric effects of HIV antiviral medications. Drug Saf 2016;39(10):945–57.

49. Samaras K, Wand H, Law M, et al. Prevalence of metabolic syndrome in HIV-infected patients receiving highly active antiretroviral therapy using International Diabetes Foundation and Adult Treatment Panel III criteria: associations with insulin resistance, disturbed body fat compartmentalization, elevated C-reactive protein, and [corrected] hypoadiponectinemia. Diabetes Care 2007;30(1):113–9.

50. Wright EJ, Grund B, Robertson K, et al. Cardiovascular risk factors associated with lower baseline cognitive performance in HIV-positive persons. Neurology 2010;75(10):864–73.

51. Ciccarelli N, Fabbiani M, Grima P, et al. Comparison of cognitive performance in HIV or HCV mono-infected and HIV-HCV co-infected patients. Infection 2013; 41(6):1103–9.

52. Thein HH, Maruff P, Krahn MD, et al. Improved cognitive function as a consequence of hepatitis C virus treatment. HIV Med 2007;8(8):520–8.

53. Valcour VG, Rubin LH, Obasi MU, et al. Liver fibrosis linked to cognitive performance in HIV and hepatitis C. J Acquir Immune Defic Syndr 2016;72(3):266–73.

54. Brew BJ, Crowe SM, Landay A, et al. Neurodegeneration and ageing in the HAART era. J Neuroimmune Pharmacol 2009;4(2):163–74.

55. Goodkin K, Miller EN, Cox C, et al. Effect of ageing on neurocognitive function by stage of HIV infection: evidence from the Multicenter AIDS Cohort Study. Lancet HIV 2017;4(9):e411–22.

56. Brew BJ, Cysique L. Does HIV prematurely age the brain? Lancet HIV 2017;4(9): e380–1.

57. Valcour V, Paul R, Chiao S, et al. Screening for cognitive impairment in human immunodeficiency virus. Clin Infect Dis 2011;53(8):836–42.

58. Watkins CC, Treisman GJ. Cognitive impairment in patients with AIDS – prevalence and severity. HIV/AIDS (Auckl) 2015;7:35–47.

59. Cysique LA, Moffat K, Moore DM, et al. HIV, vascular and aging injuries in the brain of clinically stable HIV-infected adults: a (1)H MRS study. PLoS One 2013;8(4):e61738.

60. Cysique LA, Waters EK, Brew BJ. Central nervous system antiretroviral efficacy in HIV infection: a qualitative and quantitative review and implications for future research. BMC Neurol 2011;11:148.

61. Society, E.A.C., EACS Guidelines 8.0. 2015.

62. Australian Society for HIV, V.H.a.S.H.M. General Practitioners and HIV. 2017. Available at: http://hivmanagement.ashm.org.au/index.php/populations-and-situations/gps-and-hiv#summary. Accessed Nov 8, 2017.

63. Bloch M, Kamminga J, Jayewardene A, et al. A screening strategy for HIV-associated neurocognitive disorders that accurately identifies patients requiring neurological review. Clin Infect Dis 2016;63(5):687–93.

64. Haddow LJ, Floyd S, Copas A, et al. A systematic review of the screening accuracy of the HIV Dementia Scale and International HIV Dementia Scale. PLoS One 2013;8(4):e61826.

65. Kamminga J, Lal L, Wright EJ, et al. Monitoring HIV-associated neurocognitive disorder using screenings: a critical review including guidelines for clinical and research use. Curr HIV/AIDS Rep 2017;14(3):83–92.

66. Hasbun R, Eraso J, Ramireddy S, et al. Screening for neurocognitive impairment in HIV individuals: the utility of the montreal cognitive assessment test. J AIDS Clin Res 2012;3(10):186.

67. Chang LS, DK. The neurology of HIV infection - handbook of clinical neurology. In: Brew B, editor. Elsevier Press.

68. Kugathasan R, Collier DA, Haddow LJ, et al. Diffuse white matter signal abnormalities on magnetic resonance imaging are associated with human immunodeficiency virus type 1 viral escape in the central nervous system among patients with neurological symptoms. Clin Infect Dis 2017;64(8):1059–65.

69. Cole JH, Underwood J, Caan MW, et al. Increased brain-predicted aging in treated HIV disease. Neurology 2017;88(14):1349–57.

70. Heaps JM, Sithinamsuwan P, Paul R, et al. Association between brain volumes and HAND in cART-naive HIV+ individuals from Thailand. J Neurovirol 2015; 21(2):105–12.

71. Nichols M, Gates T, Soares J, et al. HIV and brain atrophic signature in asymptomatic neurocognitive imapairment. in CROI Boston. Boston, MA, March 4–7, 2018.

72. Zhu T, Zhong J, Hu R, et al. Patterns of white matter injury in hiv infection after partial immune reconstitution: a DTI tract-based spatial statistics study. J Neurovirol 2013;19(1):10–23.

73. Chaganti JR, Heinecke A, Gates TM, et al. Functional connectivity in virally suppressed patients with HIV-associated neurocognitive disorder: a resting-state analysis. AJNR Am J Neuroradiol 2017;38(8):1623–9.

74. Gisslen M, Hagberg L, Brew BJ, et al. Elevated cerebrospinal fluid neurofilament light protein concentrations predict the development of AIDS dementia complex. J Infect Dis 2007;195(12):1774–8.

75. Kamat A, Lyons JL, Misra V, et al. Monocyte activation markers in cerebrospinal fluid associated with impaired neurocognitive testing in advanced HIV infection. J Acquir Immune Defic Syndr 2012;60(3):234–43.

76. Sandler NG, Wand H, Roque A, et al. Plasma levels of soluble CD14 independently predict mortality in HIV infection. J Infect Dis 2011;203(6):780–90.

77. Lyons JL, Uno H, Ancuta P, et al. Plasma sCD14 is a biomarker associated with impaired neurocognitive test performance in attention and learning domains in HIV infection. J Acquir Immune Defic Syndr 2011;57(5):371–9.

78. Asahchop EL, Akinwumi SM, Branton WG, et al. Plasma microRNA profiling predicts HIV-associated neurocognitive disorder. AIDS 2016;30(13):2021–31.

79. Agsalda-Garcia MA, Sithinamsuwan P, Valcour VG, et al. Brief report: CD14+ enriched peripheral cells secrete cytokines unique to HIV-associated neurocognitive disorders. J Acquir Immune Defic Syndr 2017;74(4):454–8.

80. Abassi M, Morawski BM, Nakigozi G, et al. Cerebrospinal fluid biomarkers and HIV-associated neurocognitive disorders in HIV-infected individuals in Rakai, Uganda. J Neurovirol 2017;23(3):369–75.

81. Ellero J, Lubomski M, Brew B. Interventions for neurocognitive dysfunction. Curr HIV/AIDS Rep 2017;14(1):8–16.

82. Cassol E, Misra V, Morgello S, et al. Applications and limitations of inflammatory biomarkers for studies on neurocognitive impairment in HIV infection. J Neuroimmune Pharmacol 2013;8(5):1087–97.

83. Ellis RJ, Letendre S, Vaida F, et al. Randomized trial of central nervous system–targeted antiretrovirals for HIV-associated neurocognitive disorder. Clin Infect Dis 2014;58(7):1015–22.

84. Hakkers CS, Kraaijenhof JM, van Oers-Hazelzet EB, et al. HIV and cognitive impairment in clinical practice: the evaluation of a stepwise screening protocol in relation to clinical outcomes and management. AIDS Patient Care STDS 2017;31(9):363–9.
85. Bora A, Ubaida Mohien C, Chaerkady R, et al. Identification of putative biomarkers for HIV-associated neurocognitive impairment in the CSF of HIV-infected patients under cART therapy determined by mass spectrometry. J Neurovirol 2014;20(5):457–65.

Zika Virus and Neurologic Disease

Savina Reid, BS[a], Kathryn Rimmer, MD[a], Kiran Thakur, MD[b],*

KEYWORDS

- Zika virus • Neurologic manifestations of Zika virus • Congenital Zika syndrome
- Guillain-Barré syndrome

KEY POINTS

- Although Guillain-Barré syndrome (GBS) is the most frequent Zika-associated neurologic manifestation among adolescents and adults, additional neurologic manifestations have been identified, including myelitis, encephalitis, and sensory neuropathy.
- ZIKV has been identified to disrupt proliferation and migration of neural progenitor cells.
- Long-term management of CZS requires a comprehensive combination of supportive services throughout early development. Early childhood stimulation and rehabilitation programs coupled with psychosocial support are imperative for optimal outcomes.
- Debate remains regarding the neurovirulence of Asian and African ZIKV strains and whether this may have contributed to the severity of the most recent outbreak.
- Although there are more than 40 vaccine candidates in the pipeline, a vaccine will likely not be available for at least 2 years. It is also not known if ZIKV infections lead to lifelong immunity, although the significant decline in cases over the last several months suggests that there is herd immunity.

INTRODUCTION

Zika virus (ZIKV), an arthropod-borne virus, is a single-stranded, positive-sense RNA virus that belongs to the Flaviviridae family, which includes Dengue (DENV), yellow fever (YFV), St. Louis encephalitis, Japanese encephalitis, and West Nile viruses (WNV).[1,2] This emerging infectious disease most recently caused a widespread epidemic throughout the Americas and prompted the World Health Organization

Author Contributions: K. Thakur, Drafting and revising the article for intellectual content. K. Rimmer, Drafting the article for intellectual content. S. Reid, Drafting the article for intellectual content.

Author Disclosures: S. Reid reports no disclosures; Dr K. Rimmer reports no disclosures; Dr K. Thakur is an external consultant for the World Health Organization.

[a] Department of Neurology, Columbia University Medical Center, Milstein Hospital, 177 Fort Washington Avenue, 8GS-300, New York, NY 10032, USA; [b] Division of Critical Care and Hospitalist Neurology, Department of Neurology, Columbia University Medical Center, Milstein Hospital, 177 Fort Washington Avenue, 8GS-300, New York, NY 10032, USA
* Corresponding author.
E-mail address: ktt2115@cumc.columbia.edu

(WHO) to declare ZIKV a Public Health Emergency of International Concern from February 2016 to November 2016.[1,3,4] According to the most recent WHO ZIKV situation report published in March 2017, a total of 84 countries, territories, or subnational areas had evidence of vector-borne ZIKV transmission.[5] Compared with the peak incidence of ZIKV from November 2015 to February 2016, the number of suspected and confirmed ZIKV cases has recently declined (http://www.paho.org/hq/index.php?option=com_content&view=article&id=11599%3Aregional-zika-epidemiological-update-americas).[6] Many experts attribute the recent decrease in ZIKV cases to the development of a widespread immunity across populations in previous epidemic regions, although it remains unknown whether lifelong immunity exists.[7] Individuals from nonepidemic regions traveling to ZIKV endemic regions and those who are not immune remain at high risk. Although most cases are mild or go undetected, rare severe neurologic effects including congenital ZIKV syndrome (CZS) in neonates and Guillain-Barré syndrome (GBS) in adolescents and adults have been identified.[8,9] The serious neurologic complications associated with ZIKV prompted the declaration of the public health emergency of international concern and are the focus of this review.

EPIDEMIOLOGY

ZIKV was first identified in a febrile sentinel Rhesus monkey in Uganda's Zika forest in 1947, and the first documented human illness caused by ZIKV was reported in Africa in 1952.[3,10] Thereafter, only a dozen additional cases were reported in equatorial Africa and Asia until 2007 when an outbreak occurred on Yap island in Micronesia.[11] Sporadic cases were subsequently found in various Southeast Asian countries, including Thailand, Cambodia, Malaysia, Indonesia, and the Philippines in the late 2000s to early 2010s, at which time no known neurologic manifestations were reported.[3] A second major epidemic, leading to more than 19,000 symptomatic infections, occurred in the French Polynesian archipelago in 2013 and 2014.[1,4] It is suspected that the lack of community-acquired immunity and a large population of mosquito vectors contributed to the widespread outbreak.[3] The ZIKV strain isolated during this outbreak was similar to the Asian lineage strains from Yap Island in 2007 and Cambodia in 2010.[12,13] The concern for a link between ZIKV infection and neurologic complications was first identified in the French Polynesia outbreak, where a significant increase in GBS cases was seen compared with the previous 4 years. In addition, a retrospective analysis found supportive evidence of the potential association between ZIKV infection during pregnancy and microcephaly.[1,2,14–16] The increases in microcephaly and GBS cases were temporally and geographically related to the increase in ZIKV, shedding light on the magnitude of the infection and its potential severe consequences. Outbreaks subsequently followed in other Pacific islands, including the Cook Islands, New Caledonia, and Chile's Easter Island.[10,17] In January 2015, there were reports of an increase in acute febrile illness cases in northeast Brazil accompanied by rash, muscle pain, joint pain, and headache. In 25 patients sampled, all tested negative for Chikungunya (CHIKV), rubella, and measles, whereas 11 were also negative for DENV.[17] It is important to note that CHIKV and DENV are endemic to these regions, are carried by the same vector as ZIKV, and present symptoms that are similar to ZIKV.

The first case of autochthonous transmission of ZIKV in Brazil was reported by a laboratory in Paraná, Brazil on specimens received in March 2015 for patients who initially presented with a "dengue-like syndrome."[18] In April 2015, a preliminary report from a laboratory in the Brazilian state of Bahia heralded the detection of ZIKV in samples, but confirmatory tests were still pending.[17] The WHO confirmed the first case of ZIKV in

May 2015, although the virus was likely introduced more than 12 months before, potentially via the World Cup in 2014.[2,4,18–20] By July 2015, ZIKV transmission was reported in 12 Brazilian states.[17] Colombia confirmed ZIKV cases in October 2015 followed by Suriname, El Salvador, Guatemala, Paraguay, and Venezuela in November 2015.[17] Over the next 2 months leading into the beginning of 2016, 18 additional countries in the Americas and the Caribbean reported cases of ZIKV infection.[17] In February 2016, ZIKV was announced a Public Health Emergency of International Concern by the WHO because of significant reported increases in microcephaly and other neurologic disorders identified in Brazil, and previously in French Polynesia.[17] Overall, transmission spread throughout South and Central America as well as the Caribbean, affecting 48 countries and territories from March 2015 to March 2017.[1,3]

Effective monitoring of ZIKV was enforced because of the concern for sexual transmission, congenital birth defects, and other neurologic manifestations, which led to ZIKV detection outside of the Americas and Caribbean. Cape Verde, an island off the coast of West Africa, reported their first outbreak of ZIKV, caused by the Asian strain, in October 2015. Later analysis revealed that it was most likely imported to Africa from Brazil.[10,21] There was a large concern that ZIKV may spread to the African continent during the most recent outbreak, although there is a lack of evidence currently that neurovirulent strains have emerged in the region. Although ZIKV did not reach the African continent, it did reach the continental United States. According to the Centers for Disease Control and Prevention (CDC), the first known outbreak of ZIKV caused by local mosquito-borne transmission occurred between June 30, 2016 and August 5, 2016 in Florida.[22] Of the 29 individuals who displayed diagnostic evidence of recent ZIKV infection in the affected areas, 4 infections were attributed to likely local mosquito-borne transmission.[22] In the US territories during the 2015 to 2017 time period, there were 37,103 symptomatic ZIKV cases reported (not including congenital disease cases), 611 (2%) of which occurred in 2017.[23,24] During the same time period, there have been 5613 symptomatic ZIKV cases reported in the United States (not including congenital disease cases), 385 (7%) of which occurred between January 1, 2017 and December 20, 2017.[23,24] In 2017, 4 (1%) of these cases were acquired via sexual transmission; 3 (1%) were acquired through presumed local mosquito-borne transmission, and 378 (98%) cases occurred in travelers returning from endemic areas.[23] Two cases of locally transmitted ZIKV by mosquitoes have been reported in the southernmost counties of Texas in 2017.[25] Most recently in November 2017, a single case of presumed local transmission of ZIKV was reported in Miami-Dade County, Florida after an individual, who had not traveled to active ZIKV transmission areas nor had a sexual partner with recent travel history, tested positive for ZIKV.[26] Despite this single case report, there is no current evidence of ongoing, active transmission of ZIKV in Florida at this time.[26]

TRANSMISSION

Transmission occurs primarily through vector routes, predominantly *Aedes aegypti* mosquitoes, which are also largely responsible for transmitting DENV, CHIKV, and YFV.[1,4] Although bites can be acquired throughout the day and night, most tend to occur in the early morning, late afternoon, and early evening.[27] Individuals who live in tropical or subtropical areas, where *Aedes* mosquito vectors are located, are at increased risk for ZIKV.[4] A recent study investigated potential ZIKV transmission via *Aedes albopictus* mosquitoes and revealed that although *A albopictus* had a higher susceptibility to ZIKV infection, *A aegypti* had higher transmission efficiency.[28] Because *A albopictus* mosquitoes are capable ZIKV vectors, they should be closely monitored because this raises potential concern that they may be able to transmit the virus more effectively in the future through adaptive events.[28] Prevention, treatment, and surveillance of *Aedes* vectors are imperative for optimal disease control. One report highlighted how active community prevention participation in Cuba helped to sustain control of vector-borne diseases, including DENV and ZIKV through treatment with pesticides, which decreased the number of infected female carrier mosquitoes.[29] Along with the primary modes of preventing mosquito transmission (ie, insecticides and breeding site removal), other methods include introduction of *Wolbachia* bacteria and transgenic mosquitoes.[30] Further treatment and prevention measures are discussed later in the "Prevention, Treatment, and Vaccine Development" section.

In addition to vector-borne transmission, maternal-fetal transmission occurs when pregnant mothers infected with ZIKV pass the infection on to their fetus, which may lead to CZS, which is discussed in detail later in the section on "Congenital Zika Syndrome." Unlike other Flaviviridae viruses, sexual transmission has also been documented and has contributed to ZIKV's outbreak potential. Although the first man-to-woman transmission occurred in 2008, the first reported case of woman-to-man sexual transmission occurred in July 2016 in New York City.[31,32] Sexual transmission may occur via vaginal, anal, and oral routes even if individuals are asymptomatic.[33] Between January and April 2016, 9 reported cases of man-to-woman sexual transmission occurred in the United States as a result of recent male travel to outbreak regions.[34] All male travelers had laboratory evidence of a recent ZIKV or unspecified flavivirus infection, whereas all female nontravelers had laboratory-confirmed ZIKV infection.[34] Although not yet documented in the United States, ZIKV has also been transmitted via blood transfusions in multiple cases in Brazil, and laboratory exposure of ZIKV has occurred.[33,35,36] Although ZIKV has been detected in breast milk up to 9 days after delivery, no reports have linked ZIKV infections to breastfeeding.[37] Transmission through organ transplantation is theoretically possible; however, there have been no reported cases to date.[37-39]

NEUROLOGIC MANIFESTATIONS
Adolescent and Adult Neurologic Manifestations

Although rare, various severe neurologic complications are associated with ZIKV infection in adolescents and adults. GBS, an acute autoimmune polyneuropathy, has been the most common neurologic complication associated with ZIKV in those age groups.[8,9,40,41] The first report of GBS associated with ZIKV occurred during the French Polynesia outbreak in November 2013.[42] In a case-control study, 42 cases were identified, a significant increase from the number of annual GBS cases compared with previous years.[43,44] Thirty-seven (88%) patients had a recent history of viral syndrome in a median of 6 days (interquartile range [IQR] 4–10) before neurologic onset with all patients no longer viremic at the time of admission. Most had electrophysiological findings compatible with acute motor axonal neuropathy (AMAN), although incomplete electrophysiological testing was performed.[43] Interestingly, 95% of GBS patients were found to have preexisting DENV immunity. Antibodies against DENV serotypes 1 and 3 were detected during that time. Past DENV history, however, did not significantly differ from either of the 2 control groups (group 1: individuals presenting with a nonfebrile illness; group 2: reverse-transcription polymerase chain reaction [RT-PCR] -confirmed ZIKV, but no neurologic complications; 89% and 83%, respectively).[43]

A study performed in Rio de Janeiro, Brazil between December 5, 2015 and March 18, 2016 found an increased incidence of GBS from approximately 0.6 GBS cases per month in 2013 to 2014 to 5.4 cases per month.[45] In a case series involving

7 geographic locations (Bahia State, Colombia, the Dominican Republic, El Salvador, Honduras, Suriname, and Venezuela) between April 1, 2015 and March 31, 2016, 1474 cases of GBS were reported among 164,237 confirmed or suspected ZIKV infections.[46] Data were analyzed on ZIKV and GBS incidence, and a strong association between GBS incidence was found with 2.0 to 9.8 times higher incidence compared with pre-ZIKA time periods.[46] Across Colombia, approximately 90 GBS cases were documented per month during the peak of ZIKV outbreak, an increase from the mean 20 cases per month from 2009 to 2015.[47] In Puerto Rico, it was predicted that the annual incidence of GBS would be 3.2 to 5.1 times the baseline incidence in 2016 and that long-term care needs would be 3 to 5 times those of the years before ZIKV circulation.[48] Between January 1 and July 31, 2016, 56 suspected GBS cases were identified in Puerto Rico and 34 (61%) had evidence of ZIKV or flavivirus infection (10 confirmed, 16 presumptive ZIKV, 8 presumptive flavivirus infection). All patients were hospitalized and treated with intravenous immunoglobulin.[49] The median age was 55 years; 20 (59%) of patients were women, and out of the 32 GBS patients whose charts were completely reviewed, the most common symptoms included hyporeflexia or areflexia (97%), leg weakness (97%), leg paresthesia (75%), arm weakness (75%), facial weakness (63%), arm numbness (59%), and dysphagia (59%).[49] Twenty-one patients (62%) required intensive care unit (ICU) care; 12 (35%) were required mechanical ventilation, and one succumbed to septic shock.[49]

Both acute inflammatory demyelinating polyneuropathy (AIDP) and AMAN subtypes have been identified in ZIKV-infected individuals, although AMAN has been identified less frequently.[43,47,50,51] Seventy-eight percent (36/46) of GBS patients in a Colombian cohort who received nerve-conduction and electromyography studies from January to March 2016 were found to have AIDP subtype.[47] Thirty-eight patients (56%) were men, and the median time from acute ZIKV symptom onset to GBS symptom onset was 7 days (IQR, 3–10).[47] Sixty-six patients (97%) experienced limb weakness, 56 (82%) presented with ascending paralysis, 52 (76%) experienced paresthesias, and 22 (32%) had facial palsy.[47] When investigating the severity of illness, 40 (59%) required ICU stays, 21 (31%) required mechanical ventilation, 21 (31%) had autonomic dysfunction, and 3 (4%) died of respiratory failure/sepsis.[47] In a separate case-control study in Barranquilla, Colombia during October 2015 to April 2016, 47 GBS cases were confirmed with a median age of 49 years (range, 10–83), and 25 (53%) were women.[52] Thirty-six (77%) had antecedent illness in the 2 months before the onset of neurologic symptoms with a median of 6 days (range, 0–55) from the time of antecedent illness onset to onset of neurologic symptoms.[52] Of the 13 patients who received electrodiagnostic testing, 10 (77%) were consistent with AIDP, 1 (8%) was consistent with AMAN, and 2 (15%) were undefined electrophysiologically.[52] Thirty-two (68%) received intensive care, 11 (23%) required mechanical ventilation, 32 (88%) were discharged home, and 2 (6%) died before discharge.[52] Across the larger studies investigating GBS cases in conjunction with ZIKV, approximately 63% of patients visited the ICU, about 30% were mechanically ventilated, and the mortality rate was about 5%.[47,49,52] In contrast to the case-control study in French Polynesia, but consistent with studies in Colombia, AIDP was found in the 5 GBS patients who underwent electrophysiological testing.[49] Although AMAN has been identified less frequently, a descriptive case series in Cúcuta, Colombia of 19 GBS patients admitted to various ICUs from December 2015 to March 2016 revealed that all patients had AMAN subtype and the median time to neurologic findings following the first viral symptoms was 10 days (IQR, 5–12; range, 2–60).[53]

Complementing the French Polynesian case-control study is a study performed in Salvador, Brazil during 2015 that found a strong correlation between GBS and an acute exanthematous illness outbreak (AEI) with ZIKV noted as the likeliest underlying cause.[54] Of 17,503 AEI cases, 51 patients were hospitalized with GBS or GBS variants (eg, Miller Fisher syndrome), yielding approximately 1.74 hospitalized GBS cases per 100,000 people during 2015.[54] The peak incidence of GBS occurred 5 to 9 weeks after the peak AEI incidence, which is longer than in other studies.[43,54] Other variants of GBS have been described, including a 35-year-old man in Haiti who presented with the GBS variant facial diplegia with acral paresthesias and later developed the features of Miller Fisher syndrome.[55] Although the patient's ataxia improved, he still required the use of a cane 3 weeks after discharge, and there was only minimal improvement of his bilateral facial weakness.[55] As of March 10, 2017, the latest situation report published by the WHO, 23 countries/territories reported GBS potentially associated with ZIKV infection.[5]

Urine studies for ZIKV may be particularly helpful in detecting ZIKV-associated GBS cases. In a case report in January 2016 from Martinique, urine PCR was used to definitively diagnosis GBS associated ZIKV.[56] Although all RT-PCR tests performed on plasma and cerebrospinal fluid (CSF) were negative for ZIKV, the first patient had a positive ZIKV in urine via RT-PCR 15 days after the onset of neurologic symptom onset, whereas ZIKV was detected in the urine of the second patient via RT-PCR on days 5, 15, and 21 after the development of neurologic symptoms.[56] Similarly, in a study performed in Colombia, of the 17/68 (25%) patients who tested positive for ZIKV, most of the positive results were detected in urine samples (16), whereas there were also 3 positive CSF samples and 1 positive serum sample.[47]

In addition to GBS and its variants, other neurologic manifestations associated with ZIKV infections have been identified, including myelitis, encephalitis, meningoencephalitis, acute disseminated encephalomyelitis (ADEM), sensory polyneuropathy, and optic neuropathy.[9,57–59] ZIKV-associated encephalitis cases have been reported with a neurologic onset varying from 1 to 8 days.[40] In addition, 3 adult cases of ZIKV-associated ADEM and 9 ZIKV-associated myelitis cases have been reported.[40] Various case reports have revealed a range of neurologic manifestations, including an 81-year-old with meningoencephalitis, a 15-year-old from Guadeloupe with acute myelitis, one young adult and one elderly individual who suffered from encephalopathy, an adolescent who suffered cognitive impairment and neuropsychiatric symptoms following ZIKV infection, and an 18-year-old with encephalomyelitis.[60–63] In a recently published single-center observational study in Brazil, ZIKV infection was associated with an increase in the incidence of a diverse spectrum of serious neurologic syndromes. Of the 35 patients (88%) who had molecular and/or serologic evidence of recent ZIKV infection in the serum and/or CSF, 27 had GBS (18 demyelinating, 8 axonal, and 1 Miller Fisher syndrome), 5 had encephalitis (3 with concomitant acute neuromuscular disease), 2 had transverse myelitis, and 1 had chronic inflammatory demyelinating polyneuropathy.

Congenital Zika Syndrome

CZS results from vertical transmission of ZIKV from an infected woman to the fetus during pregnancy. According to the CDC, CZS is categorized by 5 features (**Box 1**), and neuroimaging examples of severe CZS can be found in **Fig. 1**.[64] Other abnormalities of CZS reported by the CDC are displayed in **Box 2**.[64] Children who are impacted by CZS may experience severe neurodevelopmental delay, epilepsy, blindness, hearing loss, and hypotonia.[8,65]

An increase in reported microcephaly cases in Brazil during October 2015 initially raised concern of a potential link between maternal ZIKV and congenital ZIKV.[8] Subsequently, scientific evidence has linked ZIKV with microcephaly (see the section

---

Box 1
Congenital Zika syndrome (Centers for Disease Control and Prevention)

Five features of congenital Zika syndrome

1. Severe microcephaly in which the skull has partially collapsed

2. Decreased brain tissue with a specific pattern of brain damage, including subcortical calcifications

3. Damage to the back of the eye, including macular scarring and focal pigmentary retinal mottling

4. Congenital contractures, such as clubfoot or arthrogryposis

5. Hypertonia restricting body movement soon after birth

From Congenital Zika syndrome & other birth defects. 2017. Available at: https://www.cdc.gov/zika/hc-providers/infants-children/zika-syndrome-birth-defects.html. Accessed November 10, 2017.

"Neuropathogenesis"). Twenty-seven countries/territories in the Americas have reported confirmed cases of CZS since 2015.[6] A large case series of 602 ZIKV cases in Brazil between November 19, 2015 and February 27, 2016 and of 899 newborns without suspicion of ZIKV found that the ZIKV cases had smaller head circumference and higher first-week mortality.[66] A postmortem case series of 7 RT-PCR–confirmed cases in neonates from Ceará, Brazil reported that all had microcephaly, ventriculomegaly, dystrophic calcifications, and severe cortical neuronal depletion; 6 additionally had arthrogryposis.[67] Importantly, some CZS cases have presented with normal head circumference, which indicates that additional screening measures for CZS are necessary because microcephaly alone is insufficient to detect all affected newborns.[8,68–70] For example, in a retrospective Brazilian study of 13 neonates with laboratory-confirmed ZIKV, all were born without microcephaly, although later neuroimaging revealed brain abnormalities, including decreased brain volume, ventriculomegaly, subcortical calcifications, and cortical malformations in all (**Fig. 2**).[71] Subsequently, slower rates of head growth occurring in 11 of the infants was confirmed as early as 5 months after birth and was accompanied by neurologic dysfunctions (ie, hypertonia, hemiparesis, dyskinesia/dystonia, dysphagia, epilepsy, persistence of primitive reflexes).[71] In addition, a recent report demonstrates how CZS can present with a spectrum of changes, including microcephaly at birth, postnatal microcephaly, or no microcephaly.[72] A retrospective analysis of 77 infants revealed that 19 (24.7%) had evidence of CZS, 16 (20.8%) had microcephaly, and 3 (3.9%) did not.[72] All 3 in the latter group were recognized as having brain impairment a few months after birth and were found to have asymmetric polymicrogyria, predominantly in the frontal lobes; calcifications restricted to the leukocortical region, mild ventricular enlargement, and delayed myelination.[72] Another study that supports the need for improved CZS detection measures was a review of major radiological studies in which the most common abnormalities among 66 fetuses with suspected or confirmed ZIKV were ventriculomegaly (n = 21, 33%), microcephaly (n = 15–17, 24%), and intracranial calcifications (n = 17, 27%).[66] Two novel abnormalities found on neonatal brain MRIs of infants with CZS include enhancement of multiple cranial nerves and chronic ischemic cerebral infarction.[73] A separate contemporaneous case report described a 10-month-old boy who presented with an acute ZIKV infection that was also associated with cerebral infarction.[74] Further investigation is needed to establish the link between ZIKV and strokes in infants. CZS has also recently been associated with hydrocephalus.[64,75–77] The initial report included 21 CZS cases with

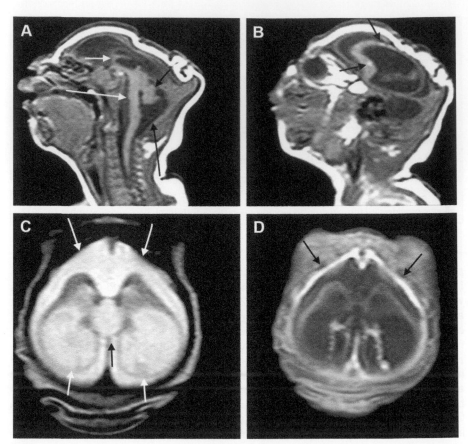

Fig. 1. Images of microcephaly associated with ZIKV infection. Severe microcephaly. Sagittal T1-weighted image (*A*) shows a profound craniofacial disproportion, noticeably hypogenetic corpus callosum (*short white arrow*), and brainstem (*long white arrow*) and cerebellum hypoplasia (*short black arrow*). In addition, the cisterna magna is enlarged (*long black arrow*). Observe the small dystrophic calcifications hyperintense on T1-weighted image (*B*) in the frontal lobe (*black arrows*) and extremely simplified gyral pattern. Axial T2-weighted image (*C*) shows severe ventriculomegaly, mainly at the posterior horn and ventricular atrium (*short white arrows*). Note the bulging walls of the ventricle, the upward dilated third ventricle (*black arrow*), and enlargement of the subarachnoid space (*long white arrows*). Axial T1-weighted image fat-suppression postcontrast (*D*) shows thickness and enhancement of frontal pachymeninges (*black arrows*). These last findings (*C, D*) may indicate a blockage in the CSF pathways and/or reduced absorption of CSF owing to impairment of the meninges or injury of arachnoid granulations. (*From* de Fatima Vasco Aragao M, van der Linden V, Brainer-Lima AM, et al. Clinical features and neuroimaging (CT and MRI) findings in presumed Zika virus related congenital infection and microcephaly: retrospective case series study. BMJ 2016;353:i1901; with permission.)

ventricular enlargement between November 2015 and July 2017, 6 (28.6%) of which required ventriculoperitoneal shunting due to progressive ventricular enlargement complicated by seizures. Postoperative improvements were seen in all cases.[75]

Ocular and hearing abnormalities have also been associated with ZIKV (see **Box 2**). In a recent prospective case series from Cúcuta, Colombia and Maracaibo, Venezuela, of 43 infants evaluated in ophthalmology centers with presumed CZS all

---

Box 2
Other birth defects of congenital Zika syndrome (Centers for Disease Control and Prevention)

Other abnormalities associated with congenital Zika syndrome:
  Brain atrophy and asymmetry
  Abnormally formed or absent brain structures
  Hydrocephalus
  Neuronal migration disorders
  Excessive and redundant scalp skin

Reported neurologic findings
  Hyperreflexia
  Irritability
  Tremors
  Seizures
  Brainstem dysfunction
  Dysphagia

Reported eye abnormalities:
  Focal pigmentary mottling and chorioretinal atrophy in the macula
  Optic nerve hypoplasia
  Cupping
  Atrophy
  Other retinal lesions
  Iris colobomas
  Congenital glaucoma
  Microphthalmia
  Lens subluxation
  Cataracts
  Intraocular calcifications

From Congenital Zika syndrome & other birth defects. 2017. Available at: https://www.cdc.gov/zika/hc-providers/infants-children/zika-syndrome-birth-defects.html. Accessed November 10, 2017.

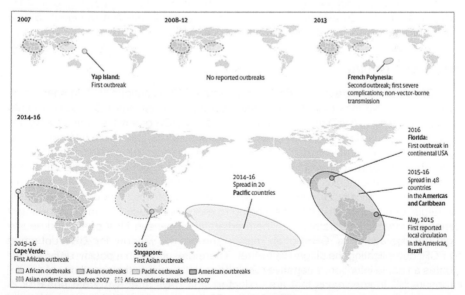

Fig. 2. ZIKV outbreaks 2007 to 2016. (*From* Baud D, Gubler DJ, Schaub B, et al. An update on Zika virus infection. Lancet 2017;390(10107):2101; with permission.)

infants presented with bilateral ocular findings, such as focal macular pigment mottling, lacunar maculopathy, chorioretinal scarring, congenital glaucoma, optic nerve hypoplasia, and other optic disc abnormalities.[78] Although glaucoma is a rare manifestation associated with CZS, the first report of ZIKV-associated glaucoma occurred in an infant 95 days after birth despite no detected signs of glaucoma in the ophthalmologic examination 3 days after birth.[79] In a case series that examined 29 infants with presumed ZIKV exposure in Salvador, Brazil, 10 children (34.5%) experienced ocular abnormalities, including focal pigment mottling of the retina and chorioretinal atrophy, optic nerve abnormalities, bilateral iris coloboma, and lens subluxation.[80] The mechanism behind the ocular abnormalities may be directly induced by ZIKV or may be secondary to cerebral manifestations of CZS (see "Neuropathogenesis").[80–82] A retrospective evaluation of 70 infants with microcephaly and laboratory evidence of ZIKV revealed 5 (7%) with sensorineural hearing loss (3 bilateral, 2 unilateral), although when eliminating an infant who received amikacin before the hearing test, the percentage of ocular abnormalities was 6%.[83]

Between 2015 and December 2017 in the United States and its territories, there were 244 live-born infants with Zika-associated birth defects and 17 pregnancy losses with Zika-associated birth defects.[84] As of December 21, 2017, there were 3715 confirmed congenital ZIKV infections throughout the Americas, 79% (2952) of which were from Brazil.[85] The incidence of reported cases of microcephaly in Brazil dropped from 41.3/10,000 live births before July 2016 to 17.0/10,000 live births after July 2016.[86] Although evidence shows an increased risk of CZS during the first trimester of pregnancy, there remains a risk in the second and third trimesters. One study showed that the earlier a rash occurred during pregnancy, the smaller the mean head circumferences at birth, supporting the claim that there is an increased risk of CZS during the first trimester.[66] Similarly, the CDC reported that approximately 9/60 (15%, 95% confidence interval = 8%–26%) of confirmed ZIKV infections during the first trimester led to ZIKV-related birth defects.[87,88] In this same report, the incidence for other trimesters was not calculated due to small numbers.[88] A report in the US territories found that among pregnant women with confirmed ZIKV infection, 8% of fetuses and infants had evidence of CZS with exposure in the first trimester, 5% in the second trimester, and 4% in the third trimester.[89,90]

DIAGNOSTIC TESTING

RT-PCR is used to detect ZIKV RNA during acute ZIKV infections.[91–94] In specimens that are collected less than 14 days after symptom onset, the CDC recommends nucleic acid testing (NAT) on serum and urine (ie, RT-PCR or any test that detects genetic material of an infecting pathogen).[95] Urine specimens can be useful because reports have demonstrated a relatively long detection time. ZIKV RNA is detected in urine up to 39 days (approximately 6 weeks) after symptom onset, although it has been detected in a man as late as 91 days.[96,97] Because patients with ZIKV may present asymptomatically or with mild symptoms (ie, fever, maculopapular rash, arthralgia, or conjunctivitis), it is challenging to ensure diagnostic testing is conducted during the viremic time frame.[98,99] The median time between ZIKV onset and neurologic manifestations (ie, GBS) often misses the narrow window for ZIKV detection by PCR, complicating the diagnosis further. Therefore, although a positive RT-PCR indicates an acute infection, a negative result does not eliminate the possibility of a ZIKV exposure.[8,91] In specimens that are collected ≥14 days after symptom onset or in specimens that are negative by RT-PCR, the CDC recommends ZIKV immunoglobulin M (IgM) serology testing followed by a plaque reduction neutralization test (PRNT) if the IgM result is nonnegative (ie, positive, equivocal, presumptive positive, or possible positive).[95] ZIKV PRNT $\geq$10 and DENV PRNT <10 indicate a ZIKV infection but do not distinguish between an active or a prior infection.[95] Although PRNT is highly specific, the test is only performed by a limited number of laboratories across the world because it is expensive, labor intensive, and requires materials not widely accessible to all areas impacted by ZIKV and other flaviviruses.[8,92]

In addition to serum and urine, ZIKV RNA has been detected in other bodily fluids, including whole blood, saliva, semen, vaginal secretions, breast milk, and CSF.[40] ZIKV RNA has been detected in whole blood longer than in serum.[8] ZIKV RNA has been detected in semen up to 188 days after onset of symptoms, although it is still unclear how long one may be infectious.[100] Viral shedding of ZIKV RNA has been detected for up to 14 days in vaginal secretions.[101] In addition, CSF can be used to test for ZIKV IgM.[102]

For pregnant women with a possible exposure to ZIKV and who present with ZIKV symptoms, ZIKV NAT on serum and urine should be performed in addition to ZIKV IgM serology.[102,103] Because ZIKV IgM antibodies can persist past 12 weeks after infection, these results alone are unable to distinguish between an infection that occurred before or during pregnancy.[104] For detailed information about test interpretations, visit https://www.cdc.gov/zika/pdfs/testing_algorithm.pdf.[103]

A major challenge associated with the current diagnostic techniques includes the high cross-reactivity with other flaviviruses due to structural and genetic similarities, including DENV and CHIKV, as well as coinfections in individuals given that many flaviviruses circulate simultaneously throughout various geographic locations.[92,99] DENV and ZIKV, in particular, share many amino acid sequence similarities in the main targets for antibody responses, including the envelope, premembrane proteins, and the nonstructural protein NS1, which makes interpretation of antibody-based testing challenging.[94]

For pregnant women who have evidence of a possible ZIKV infection, prenatal ultrasound is recommended every 3 to 4 weeks to evaluate fetal anatomy.[104] Although ZIKV has also been detected in amniotic fluid using ultrasound-guided transabdominal amniocentesis, the data on its utility and optimal performance time are limited and should be considered on a case-by-case basis.[105] The sensitivity and specificity of RNA testing of amniotic fluid are not currently established at this time, and it is unclear whether infants who test positive for congenital ZIKV via amniotic fluid will present with abnormalities at or after birth.[106] A negative ZIKV RNA result from amniotic fluid does not eliminate the possibility of congenital ZIKV because research has suggested that the detectable viremic time period may be transient.[107]

The complications caused by past exposures, asymptomatic or mild symptom presentation, cross-reactivity between flaviviruses, transient viremic time period in various biological samples, uncertainties involved in prenatal testing and monitoring, and limited resources in various geographic settings make ZIKV diagnosis challenging. Future research is needed to help address those challenges.

NEUROPATHOGENESIS
Viral Lineages and Neurovirulence

Phylogenetic studies have revealed that there are 2 ZIKV lineages, African and Asian, and that the latter was responsible for the 2007 and 2013 Pacific Islands outbreaks as well as the most recent outbreak throughout the Americas.[2,108,109] ZIKV analyzed from the Yap Island provided phylogenetic evidence that the Yap Island outbreak originated in Southeast Asia.[32] Between the African and epidemic Asian strains of ZIKV, most genetic changes were observed in the NS5 proteins (involved in blockade of type 1 interferon signaling and formation of replication complex of flavivirus genome), NS4, and E (envelope).[41] Nonstructural proteins NS1, NS2B, and NS4A have been identified to contribute to virulence via immune evasion effects.[41] E protein glycosylation at Arg-154 is also seen in epidemic Asian strains but not the African wild type, and it may be involved in assembly and infectivity of flaviviruses.[41]

Debate remains about whether newer strains have evolved to cause neurotropic infections. It is unclear whether the African ZIKV is as capable of the Asian lineage in causing severe neurologic complications in fetuses, neonates, and adults.[8,110] Some research suggests that more neurovirulent strains of ZIKV have evolved via new mutations, while a recent report using organotypic brain slice cultures generated from embryonic mice of various ages reports that all lineages of ZIKV appear to be neurotropic and that even the older strains from 1947 can affect developing brains.[41,111]

A recent study found evidence of antibody-dependent enhancement (ADE) in mice that had antibodies from a previous DENV or WNV infection and experienced more severe manifestations of ZIKV.[112,113] Mice that had been injected with DENV or WNV-convalescent plasma experienced increased morbidity (ie, fever and viral loads in the spinal cord and testes), increased ZIKV antibodies in their testes and spinal cords, and increased mortality compared with controls. Those findings support the hypothesis that ADE may have contributed to the severity of the most recent ZIKV outbreak due to geographic cocirculation of other flaviviruses, including DENV.[113] However, some researchers have expressed concern that the findings of this may not mimic human pathogenesis.[112]

Pathogenesis of Congenital ZIKV Syndrome

Various studies provide evidence that ZIKV disrupts proliferation and migration of neural progenitor cells (NPCs).[110,114–116] The consequent cell death of NPCs prematurely arrests the development of the fetal brain. Studies have shown that ZIKV crosses the placental barrier to infect the developing fetus.[110] One study revealed that when human NPCs and neuronal cells were infected with the Brazilian strain of ZIKV (ZIKV[BR]), there were more viral copies in NPCs and neuronal cells compared with the wild-type African strain (ZIKV[AF]).[114] Both ZIKV[BR]- and ZIKV[AF]-infected NPC cultures showed signs of cell death after 96 hours postinfection.[114] In addition, offspring of pregnant SJL mice (a strain that is immunocompetent but more susceptible to viral infections and has known immune irregularities) infected with ZIKV[BR] had cortical malformations and thinner cortical layers, analogous to findings of microcephaly in humans.[114] The brain tissue from those offspring also had evidence of viral RNA and neuronal cell death. Further PCR analysis reveals that in those affected offspring, genes related to autophagy and apoptosis were upregulated.[114] In another study consisting of 5 postmortem evaluations of fetal and neonatal cases of CZS, all mothers had symptoms of fever and rash in the first trimester and ZIKV was confirmed in the central nervous system tissue of offspring.[115] On autopsy, histopathological changes were seen in brain and placental tissue but not in other organs. On gross examination of the brain, there were malformations including lissencephaly, alobar holoprosencephaly, and cerebellar hypoplasia.[115] ZIKV antigen was isolated in the placenta, specifically in the chorionic villi.[115] One study demonstrates that ZIKV RNA binds to Musashi-I (MSI1), a translational regulator protein found in neural precursors, retina, and testis that is required for neurodevelopment. This prevents interaction between MSI1 and its target RNAs *MCHP1* and *NUMB*, thereby resulting in defective migration and cell-cycle disruption in the NPCs.[116]

Pathogenesis of Guillain-Barré Syndrome

Hypotheses on the pathogenesis of ZIKV-associated GBS include direct neuropathogenic mechanisms, a hyperacute immune response, immune dysregulation, and molecular mimicry against neural antigens.[8,117] Given the short time period between ZIKV symptoms and GBS onset found in several studies, it is likely that a parainfectious process involving immune-mediated inflammation of neural tissue is involved.[41,51] Molecular mimicry in which infectious molecules resemble membrane molecules in neural tissue as seen in other cases of GBS triggered by infections such as *Campylobacter jejuni* likely also play a pathogenic role in ZIKV-associated GBS.[41] This "mistaken immune attack" may arise because the surface of ZIKV contains polysaccharides that resemble glycoconjugates of the human nerve tissues. There is dual recognition, by a single B- or T-cell receptor, of a microbe's structure and an antigen of the host. ADE of ZIKV infection may also play a role given an observation that patients who developed GBS had higher titers of cross-reacting IgM or IgG antibodies to flavivirus antigens, including DENV infection, although this is confounded by the high degree of cross-reactivity seen in antibody-based testing for flaviviruses.[41]

Prevention, Treatment, and Vaccine Development

Prevention measures

The key measure to interrupt the transmission of ZIKV is through control of the *Aedes* mosquito vector density through mechanisms including proper cleaning and maintenance of water supplies and storage systems, adequate solid waste management systems, and alterations in human behavior and residence systems (**Table 1**).[118] Another vector control strategy is to genetically modify mosquitoes, giving rise to the population of mosquitoes whose offspring are not able to survive.[119] Another strategy that

Table 1	
Prevention recommendation	
Strategy	**Action**
Control vector design	• Diligent management and control of environmental factors • Eliminate or reduce vector breeding sites in common areas • Conduct mass sanitation campaigns to educate the public • Ensure mosquitoes are removed within the predetermined radius of critical places like schools, hospitals, transport terminals, using risk stratification paradigms • In areas with viral activity, use mosquito adulticidal sprays to interrupt ZIKA transmission • Ensure proper monitoring and follow-up during integrated actions for vector control
Preventative measure	Individual protection • Encourage individuals to use bed nets • Appropriate clothing to cover exposed skin • Use repellents Household/residential protection • Encourage installation and use of wire-mesh screens on doors and windows • Once per week emptying, cleaning, turning over, and disposal of containers that can hold water inside or outside the houses to reduce any mosquito breeding sites

From Sikka V, Chattu V, Popli R, et al. The emergence of ZIKA as a global health security threat: a review and a consensus statement of the INDUSEM Joint Working Group. J Glob Infect Dis 2016;8:3; with permission.

has been shown to reduce the mosquito-to-human transmission events, particularly with DENV, involves the introduction of *Wolbachia* bacteria into the mosquito population, reducing the transmission of virus to humans from mosquito.[120] Because of the unique traits of *Wolbachia* that cause cytoplasmic incompatibility, the bacteria are useful as a promoter of genetic drive within a population. *Wolbachia*-infected females are able to produce offspring with uninfected and infected males; however, uninfected females are only able to produce viable offspring with uninfected males. Thus, infected females have a frequency-dependent reproductive advantage.

With regards to personal protection, individuals should avoid contact with mosquitoes in areas endemic for ZIKV (see **Table 1**). Individuals living in and traveling to ZIKV-affected regions should refer to the CDC Web site for further guidance on prevention measures (https://www.cdc.gov/zika/prevention/protect-yourself-and-others.html). It is important to advise those living in endemic regions and travelers to ZIKV-affected areas to practice safe sex or abstinence for at least 6 months from exposure and to not donate blood for at least 1 month after returning to reduce the risk of potential transmission.[121] In addition, pregnant women with potential risk of exposure to ZIKV should have fetuses evaluated and monitored closely for CZS. For further information, it is recommended that travelers and pregnant women visit the following CDC Web site for the most up-to-date recommendations: https://www.cdc.gov/zika/pregnancy/protect-yourself.html.[122–124]

Treatment

ZIKV disease is usually mild and requires no specific treatment. People sick with acute ZIKV infection should remain adequately hydrated and treat pain and fever with acetaminophen.[8,125] By use of large screening strategies, several compounds have been found to have in vitro activity against ZIKV, but there are no antiviral drugs that have shown activity against the virus in vivo.[8] Management recommendations for GBS and myelitis as a result of ZIKV include immunomodulatory therapy and supportive care, as per guidelines for management of these respective syndromes triggered by other causes.[126] Long-term management of CZS requires a comprehensive combination of supportive services throughout early development. Early childhood stimulation and rehabilitation programs coupled with psychosocial support are imperative for optimal outcomes. For further guidance on the management ZIKV neurologic complications, including CZS, refer to the WHO Zika Toolkit (http://www.who.int/mental_health/neurology/zika_toolkit/en/).[126]

Vaccine development

A safe, effective, and rapidly scalable vaccine against ZIKV is needed. A recent study describes a purified formalin-inactivated Zika virus vaccine candidate that showed protection in mice and nonhuman primates against viremia after ZIKV infection.[127] Although there are more than 40 vaccine candidates in the pipeline, a vaccine will likely not be available for at least 2 years. It is also not known if ZIKV infections lead to life-long immunity, although the significant decline in cases over the last several months suggests that herd immunity exists in endemic regions.

SUMMARY

Although most cases of ZIKV are mild or not detected, rare severe neurologic effects have been identified, including but not limited to GBS and CZS. Over the last year, scientific evidence has established a causal link between ZIKV and neurologic manifestations, including congenital birth defects. Diagnostic and treatment challenges remain due to cross-reactivity between flaviviruses, the transient viremic time period, uncertainties involved in prenatal testing and monitoring, and limited resources for supportive care in various geographic settings. Longitudinal studies are needed to evaluate the long-term effects of ZIKV infection, including the long-term risks in infants exposed to ZIKV in utero. Whether alterations of the Asian strain have led to increased neurovirulence remains under debate. Although herd immunity is suspected, it is unknown at this time whether ZIKV infections lead to lifelong immunity. Thus, prevention efforts, including reduction in mosquito vector transmission and sexual transmission, are required as well as ongoing international efforts for vaccine development.

REFERENCES

1. Epelboin S, Dulioust E, Epelboin L, et al. Zika virus and reproduction: facts, questions and current management. Hum Reprod Update 2017;23(6):629–45.
2. White MK, Wollebo HS, Beckham JD, et al. Zika virus: an emergent neuropathological agent. Ann Neurol 2016;80(4):479–89.
3. Song B-H, Yun S-I, Woolley M, et al. Zika virus: history, epidemiology, transmission, and clinical presentation. J Neuroimmunol 2017;308:50–64.
4. Deseda CC. Epidemiology of Zika. Curr Opin Pediatr 2017;29(1):97–101.
5. Situation report ZIKA virus microcephaly Guillain-Barré syndrome. 2017. Available at: http://apps.who.int/iris/bitstream/10665/254714/1/zikasitrep10Mar17-eng.pdf?ua=1. Accessed March 10, 2017.
6. Regional Zika epidemiological update (Americas). 2017. Available at: http://www.paho.org/hq/index.php?option=com_content&view=article&id=11599%3Aregional-zika-epidemiological-update-americas. Accessed August 25, 2017.
7. Cohen J. Where has all the Zika gone? Science 2017;357(6352):631–2.
8. Baud D, Gubler DJ, Schaub B, et al. An update on Zika virus infection. Lancet 2017;390(10107):2099–109.
9. Assessment and management of Guillain-Barre syndrome in the context of Zika virus infection, interim guidance update. 2016. Available at: http://apps.who.int/iris/bitstream/10665/204474/1/WHO_ZIKV_MOC_16.4_eng.pdf?ua=1. Accessed November 5, 2017.
10. The history of Zika virus. 2017. Available at: http://www.who.int/emergencies/zika-virus/history/en/. Accessed November 29, 2017.
11. Duffy MR, Chen T-H, Hancock WT, et al. Zika virus outbreak on Yap Island, federated states of Micronesia. N Engl J Med 2009;360(24):2536–43.
12. Lim S-K, Lim JK, Yoon I-K. An update on zika virus in asia. Infect Chemother 2017;49(2):91–100.
13. Cao-Lormeau V-M, Roche C, Teissier A, et al. Zika virus, French polynesia, South pacific, 2013. Emerg Infect Dis 2014;20(6):1085.
14. Watrin L, Ghawché F, Larre P, et al. Guillain-Barré syndrome (42 Cases) occurring during a Zika virus outbreak in French Polynesia. Medicine (Baltimore) 2016;95(14):e3257.
15. Guillain-Barré syndrome – France - French Polynesia. 2016. Available at: http://www.who.int/csr/don/7-march-2016-gbs-french-polynesia/en/. Accessed November 1, 2017.
16. Cauchemez S, Besnard M, Bompard P, et al. Association between Zika virus and microcephaly in French Polynesia, 2013–15: a retrospective study. Lancet 2016;387(10033):2125–32.

17. Timeline of emergence of Zika virus in the Americas. Pan American Health Organization/World Health Organization. 2016. Available at: http://www.paho.org/hq/index.php?option=com_content&view=article&id=11959%3Atimeline-of-emergence-of-zika-virus-in-the-americas&catid=8424%3Acontents&Itemid=41711&lang=en. Accessed November 5, 2017.

18. Zanluca C, Melo VCAD, Mosimann ALP, et al. First report of autochthonous transmission of Zika virus in Brazil. Mem Inst Oswaldo Cruz 2015;110(4):569–72.

19. Meaney-Delman D, Rasmussen SA, Staples JE, et al. Zika virus and pregnancy: what obstetric health care providers need to know. Obstet Gynecol 2016;127(4): 642–8.

20. Metsky HC, Matranga CB, Wohl S, et al. Zika virus evolution and spread in the Americas. Nature 2017;546(7658):411–5.

21. [press release]WHO confirms Zika virus strain imported from the Americas to Cabo Verde. World Health Organization; 2016.

22. Likos A, Griffin I, Bingham AM, et al. Local mosquito-borne transmission of Zika Virus - Miami-Dade and Broward Counties, Florida, June-August 2016. MMWR Morb Mortal Wkly Rep 2016;65(38):1032–8.

23. 2017 case counts in the US. 2017. Available at: https://www.cdc.gov/zika/reporting/2017-case-counts.html. Accessed October 25, 2017.

24. Zika cases in the United States. 2017. Available at: https://www.cdc.gov/zika/reporting/case-counts.html. Accessed October 25, 2017.

25. Zika virus. 2017. Available at: https://www.dshs.texas.gov/news/updates.shtm. Accessed October 25, 2017.

26. Single case of locally transmitted Zika identified in Miami-Dade County. 2017. Available at: http://www.floridahealth.gov/newsroom/2017/11/111717-zika-update.html. Accessed October 25, 2017.

27. Zika virus fact sheet. 2016. Available at: http://www.who.int/mediacentre/factsheets/zika/en/. Accessed October 23, 2017.

28. Ciota AT, Bialosuknia SM, Zink SD, et al. Effects of Zika virus strain and Aedes mosquito species on vector competence. Emerg Infect Dis 2017;23(7):1110.

29. Castro M, Pérez D, Guzman MG, et al. Why did Zika not explode in Cuba? The role of active community participation to sustain control of Vector-Borne diseases. Am J Trop Med Hyg 2017;97(2):311–2.

30. Epelboin Y, Talaga S, Epelboin L, et al. Zika virus: an updated review of competent or naturally infected mosquitoes. PLoS Negl Trop Dis 2017;11(11): e0005933.

31. First female-to-male sexual transmission of Zika virus infection reported in New York City. 2016. Available at: https://www.cdc.gov/media/releases/2016/s0715-zika-female-to-male.html. Accessed November 1, 2017.

32. Zika: the origin and spread of a mosquito-borne virus. 2016. Available at: http://www.who.int/bulletin/online_first/16-171082/en/. Accessed November 2, 2017.

33. Zika virus transmission. 2017. Available at: https://www.cdc.gov/zika/transmission/index.html. Accessed November 2, 2017.

34. Russell K, Hills SL, Oster AM, et al. Male-to-female sexual transmission of Zika virus—United States, January–April 2016. Clin Infect Dis 2016;64(2):211–3.

35. Musso D, Nhan T, Robin E, et al. Potential for Zika virus transmission through blood transfusion demonstrated during an outbreak in French Polynesia, November 2013 to February 2014. Euro Surveill 2014;19(14):20761.

36. Motta IJ, Spencer BR, Cordeiro da Silva SG, et al. Evidence for transmission of Zika virus by platelet transfusion. N Engl J Med 2016;375(11):1101–3.

37. Sotelo JR, Sotelo AB, Sotelo FJ, et al. Persistence of Zika virus in breast milk after infection in late stage of pregnancy. Emerg Infect Dis 2017;23(5):854.
38. Guidance on Zika virus. Available at: https://optn.transplant.hrsa.gov/news/guidance-on-zika-virus/. Accessed November 2, 2017.
39. Zika in infants & children. 2017. Available at: https://www.cdc.gov/pregnancy/zika/testing-follow-up/zika-in-infants-children.html. Accessed November 1, 2017.
40. De Broucker T, Mailles A, Stahl J-P. Neurological presentation of Zika virus infection beyond the perinatal period. Curr Infect Dis Rep 2017;19(10):35.
41. Morris G, Barichello T, Stubbs B, et al. Zika virus as an emerging neuropathogen: mechanisms of neurovirulence and neuro-immune interactions. Mol Neurobiol 2018;55(5):4160–84.
42. Oehler E, Watrin L, Larre P, et al. Zika virus infection complicated by Guillain-Barre syndrome–case report, French Polynesia, December 2013. Euro Surveill 2014;19(9):20720.
43. Cao-Lormeau V-M, Blake A, Mons S, et al. Guillain-Barré Syndrome outbreak associated with Zika virus infection in French Polynesia: a case-control study. Lancet 2016;387(10027):1531–9.
44. Prevention ECfD, Control. Rapid risk assessment: Zika virus infection outbreak, French Polynesia. Stockholm (Sweden): European Centre for Disease Prevention and Control; 2014.
45. Ferreira da Silva IR, Frontera JA, Moreira do Nascimento OJ. News from the battlefront: Zika virus–associated Guillain-Barré syndrome in Brazil. Neurology 2016;87(15):e180–1.
46. Dos Santos T, Rodriguez A, Almiron M, et al. Zika virus and the Guillain–Barré syndrome—case series from seven countries. N Engl J Med 2016;375(16):1598–601.
47. Parra B, Lizarazo J, Jiménez-Arango JA, et al. Guillain–Barré syndrome associated with Zika virus infection in Colombia. N Engl J Med 2016;375(16):1513–23.
48. Dirlikov E, Kniss K, Major C, et al. Guillain-Barré syndrome and healthcare needs during Zika virus transmission, Puerto Rico, 2016. Emerg Infect Dis 2017;23(1):134.
49. Dirlikov E, Major CG, Mayshack M, et al. Guillain-Barré syndrome during ongoing Zika virus transmission - Puerto Rico, January 1-July 31, 2016. MMWR Morb Mortal Wkly Rep 2016;65(34):910–4.
50. Willison HJ, Jacobs BC, Van Doorn PA. Guillain-Barré syndrome. Lancet 2016; 388(10045):717–27.
51. Muñoz LS, Parra B, Pardo CA, Neuroviruses Emerging in the Americas Study. Neurological implications of Zika virus infection in adults. J Infect Dis 2017; 216(suppl_10):S897–905.
52. Salinas JL, Walteros DM, Styczynski A, et al. Zika virus disease-associated Guillain-Barré syndrome—Barranquilla, Colombia 2015–2016. J Neurol Sci 2017; 381:272–7.
53. Arias A, Torres-Tobar L, Hernández G, et al. Guillain-Barré syndrome in patients with a recent history of Zika in Cucuta, Colombia: a descriptive case series of 19 patients from December 2015 to March 2016. J Crit Care 2017;37:19–23.
54. Paploski IA, Prates APP, Cardoso CW, et al. Time lags between exanthematous illness attributed to Zika virus, Guillain-Barré syndrome, and microcephaly, Salvador, Brazil. Emerg Infect Dis 2016;22(8):1438.
55. Kassavetis P, Joseph J-MB, Francois R, et al. Zika virus–associated Guillain-Barré syndrome variant in Haiti. Neurology 2016;87(3):336–7.

56. Rozé B, Najioullah F, Fergé J-L, et al. Zika virus detection in urine from patients with Guillain-Barré syndrome on Martinique, January 2016. Euro Surveill 2016; 21(9):30154.

57. Sebastián UU, Ricardo AVA, Alvarez BC, et al. Zika virus-induced neurological critical illness in Latin America: severe Guillain-Barre Syndrome and encephalitis. J Crit Care 2017;42:275–81.

58. Ferreira MLB, de Brito CAA, Moreira ÁJP, et al. Guillain–Barré syndrome, acute disseminated encephalomyelitis and encephalitis associated with Zika virus infection in brazil: detection of viral RNA and isolation of virus during late infection. Am J Trop Med Hyg 2017;97(5):1405–9.

59. Medina MT, Medina-Montoya M. New spectrum of the neurologic consequences of Zika. J Neurol Sci 2017;383:214–5.

60. Carteaux G, Maquart M, Bedet A, et al. Zika virus associated with meningoencephalitis. N Engl J Med 2016;374(16):1595–6.

61. Mécharles S, Herrmann C, Poullain P, et al. Acute myelitis due to Zika virus infection. Lancet 2016;387(10026):1481.

62. Roth W, Tyshkov C, Thakur K, et al. Encephalomyelitis following definitive zika virus infection. Neurol Neuroimmunol Neuroinflamm 2017;4(4):e349.

63. Rozé B, Najioullah F, Signate A, et al. Zika virus detection in cerebrospinal fluid from two patients with encephalopathy, Martinique, February 2016. Euro Surveill 2016;21(16).

64. Congenital Zika syndrome & other birth defects. 2017. Available at: https://www.cdc.gov/zika/hc-providers/infants-children/zika-syndrome-birth-defects.html. Accessed Novemeber 10, 2017.

65. Adebanjo T, Godfred-Cato S, Viens L, et al. Update: interim guidance for the diagnosis, evaluation, and management of infants with possible congenital Zika virus infection - United States, October 2017. MMWR Morb Mortal Wkly Rep 2017;66(41):1089–99.

66. Vouga M, Baud D. Imaging of congenital Zika virus infection: the route to identification of prognostic factors. Prenat Diagn 2016;36(9):799–811.

67. Sousa AQ, Cavalcante DIM, Franco LM, et al. Postmortem findings for 7 neonates with congenital Zika virus infection. Emerg Infect Dis 2017;23(7):1164–7.

68. Eppes C, Rac M, Dunn J, et al. Testing for Zika virus infection in pregnancy: key concepts to deal with an emerging epidemic. Am J Obstet Gynecol 2017; 216(3):209–25.

69. França GV, Schuler-Faccini L, Oliveira WK, et al. Congenital Zika virus syndrome in Brazil: a case series of the first 1501 livebirths with complete investigation. Lancet 2016;388(10047):891–7.

70. Heukelbach J, Werneck GL. Surveillance of Zika virus infection and microcephaly in Brazil. Lancet 2016;388(10047):846–7.

71. van der Linden V, Pessoa A, Dobyns W, et al. Description of 13 infants born during October 2015-January 2016 with congenital Zika virus infection without microcephaly at birth - Brazil. MMWR Morb Mortal Wkly Rep 2016;65(47): 1343–8.

72. Aragao M, Holanda A, Brainer-Lima A, et al. Nonmicrocephalic infants with congenital Zika syndrome suspected only after neuroimaging evaluation compared with those with microcephaly at birth and postnatally: how large is the Zika virus "iceberg"? AJNR Am J Neuroradiol 2017;38(7):1427–34.

73. Mulkey SB, Vezina G, Bulas DI, et al. Neuroimaging findings in normocephalic newborns with intrauterine Zika virus exposure. Pediatr Neurol 2018;78:75–8.

74. Landais A, Césaire A, Fernandez M, et al. ZIKA vasculitis: a new cause of stroke in children? J Neurol Sci 2017;383:211–3.
75. Jucá E, Pessoa A, Ribeiro E, et al. Hydrocephalus associated to congenital Zika syndrome: does shunting improve clinical features? Childs Nerv Syst 2018; 34(1):101–6.
76. Joob B, Wiwanitkit V. Hydrocephalus associated to congenital Zika syndrome and shunting. Childs Nerv Syst 2018;34(2):183.
77. Jucá E, Pessoa A, Cavalcanti LP. Reply to the letter by Joob and Wiwanitkit regarding our article on congenital Zika syndrome and hydrocephalus. Childs Nerv Syst 2018;34(2):185–6.
78. Yepez JB, Murati FA, Pettito M, et al. Ophthalmic manifestations of congenital Zika syndrome in Colombia and Venezuela. JAMA Ophthalmol 2017;135(5):440–5.
79. de Paula Freitas B, Ko AI, Khouri R, et al. Glaucoma and congenital Zika syndrome. Ophthalmology 2017;124(3):407–8.
80. de Paula Freitas B, de Oliveira Dias JR, Prazeres J, et al. Ocular findings in infants with microcephaly associated with presumed Zika virus congenital infection in Salvador, Brazil. JAMA Ophthalmol 2016;134(5):529–35.
81. Moshfeghi DM, de Miranda HA, Costa MC. Zika virus, microcephaly, and ocular findings. JAMA Ophthalmol 2016;134(8):945.
82. Belfort R, de Paula Freitas B, de Oliveira Dias JR. Zika virus, microcephaly, and ocular findings—reply. JAMA Ophthalmol 2016;134(8):946–7.
83. Leal MC, Muniz LF, Ferreira TS, et al. Hearing loss in infants with microcephaly and evidence of congenital Zika virus infection - Brazil, November 2015-May 2016. MMWR Morb Mortal Wkly Rep 2016;65(34):917–9.
84. Outcomes of pregnancies with laboratory evidence of possible Zika virus infection, 2015-2017. 2017. Available at: https://www.cdc.gov/pregnancy/zika/data/pregnancy-outcomes.html. Accessed November 5, 2017.
85. Zika cumulative cases. 2017. Available at: http://www.paho.org/hq/index.php?option=com_content&view=article&id=12390%3Azika-cumulative-cases&catid=8424%3Acontents&Itemid=42090&lang=en. Accessed November 4, 2017.
86. de Magalhães-Barbosa MC, Prata-Barbosa A, Robaina JR, et al. New trends of the microcephaly and Zika virus outbreak in Brazil, July 2016–December 2016. Travel Med Infect Dis 2017;16:52–7.
87. About 1 in 10 U.S. pregnant women with confirmed Zika infection had a fetus or baby with birth defects in 2016. 2017. Available at: https://www.cdc.gov/media/releases/2017/p0404-zika-pregnancy.html. Accessed November 5, 2017.
88. Ital signs: update on Zika virus–Associated birth defects and evaluation of all U.S. infants with congenital Zika virus exposure — U.S. Zika Pregnancy Registry, 2016. 2017. Available at: https://www.cdc.gov/mmwr/volumes/66/wr/mm6613e1.htm. Accessed November 6, 2017.
89. Update: interim guidance for health care providers caring for pregnant women with possible Zika virus exposure — United States (Including U.S. Territories), July 2017. 2017. Available at: https://www.cdc.gov/mmwr/volumes/66/wr/mm6629e1.htm. Accessed November 1, 2017.
90. CDC analysis of data from US territories finds serious birth defects in about 1 in 12 fetuses or infants of pregnant women with Zika infection in the first trimester. 2017. Available at: https://www.cdc.gov/media/releases/2017/p0608-zika-data-first-trimester.html. Accessed November 2, 2017.
91. Lum FM, Lin C, Susova OY, et al. A sensitive method for detecting Zika virus antigen in patients' whole-blood specimens as an alternative diagnostic approach. J Infect Dis 2017;216(2):182–90.

92. Chua A, Prat I, Nuebling CM, et al. Update on Zika diagnostic tests and WHO's related activities. PLoS Negl Trop Dis 2017;11(2):e0005269.

93. Rapid molecular detection of Zika virus in acute-phase urine samples using the recombinase polymerase amplification assay. 2017. Available at: http://currents. plos.org/outbreaks/article/rapid-molecular-detection-of-zika-virus-in-urine-using-the-recombinase-polymerase-amplification-assay/. Accessed November 8, 2017.

94. Priyamvada L, Hudson W, Ahmed R, et al. Humoral cross-reactivity between Zika and dengue viruses: implications for protection and pathology. Emerg Microbes Infec 2017;6(5):e33.

95. ZIKA virus testing guidance: symptomatic non-pregnant individuals with possible Zika virus exposure. Available at: https://www.cdc.gov/zika/pdfs/testing-algorithm-symptomatic-nonpregnant.pdf. Accessed November 15, 2017.

96. Paz-Bailey G, Rosenberg ES, Doyle K, et al. Persistence of Zika virus in body fluids - Preliminary report. N Engl J Med 2017. [Epub ahead of print].

97. Nicastri E, Castilletti C, Liuzzi G, et al. Persistent detection of Zika virus RNA in semen for six months after symptom onset in a traveller returning from Haiti to Italy, February 2016. Euro Surveill 2016;21(32).

98. Zhang B, Pinsky BA, Ananta JS, et al. Diagnosis of Zika virus infection on a nanotechnology platform. Nat Med 2017;23(5):548–50.

99. Lee AJ, Bhattacharya R, Scheuermann RH, et al. Identification of diagnostic peptide regions that distinguish Zika virus from related mosquito-borne Flaviviruses. PLoS One 2017;12(5):e0178199.

100. Clinical guidance for healthcare providers for prevention of sexual transmission of Zika virus. 2017. Available at: https://www.cdc.gov/zika/hc-providers/clinical-guidance/sexualtransmission.html. Accessed November 12, 2017.

101. Murray KO, Gorchakov R, Carlson AR, et al. Prolonged detection of Zika virus in vaginal secretions and whole blood. Emerg Infect Dis 2017;23(1):99.

102. Diagnostic tests for Zika virus. 2017. Available at: https://www.cdc.gov/zika/hc-providers/types-of-tests.html. Accessed November 10, 2017.

103. Testing guidance. 2017. Available at: https://www.cdc.gov/zika/hc-providers/testing-guidance.html. Accessed November 15, 2017.

104. Oduyebo T, Polen KD, Walke HT, et al. Update: interim guidance for health care providers caring for pregnant women with possible Zika virus exposure - United States (Including U.S. Territories), July 2017. MMWR Morb Mortal Wkly Rep 2017;66(29):781–93.

105. Calvet G, Aguiar RS, Melo ASO, et al. Detection and sequencing of Zika virus from amniotic fluid of fetuses with microcephaly in Brazil: a case study. Lancet Infect Dis 2016;16(6):653–60.

106. Testing & diagnosis. Available at: https://www.cdc.gov/zika/hc-providers/pregnant-women/testing-and-diagnosis.html. Accessed November 10, 2017.

107. Schaub B, Vouga M, Najioullah F, et al. Analysis of blood from Zika virus-infected fetuses: a prospective case series. Lancet Infect Dis 2017;17(5):520–7.

108. Liu Y, Liu J, Du S, et al. Evolutionary enhancement of Zika virus infectivity in Aedes aegypti mosquitoes. Nature 2017;545(7655):482–6.

109. Faria NR, da Silva Azevedo RDS, Kraemer MU, et al. Zika virus in the Americas: early epidemiological and genetic findings. Science 2016;352(6283):345–9.

110. Simonin Y, van Riel D, Van de Perre P, et al. Differential virulence between Asian and African lineages of Zika virus. PLoS Negl Trop Dis 2017;11(9): e0005821.

111. Rosenfeld AB, Doobin DJ, Warren AL, et al. Replication of early and recent Zika virus isolates throughout mouse brain development. Proc Natl Acad Sci U S A 2017;114(46):12273–8.
112. Cohen J. Dengue may bring out the worst in Zika. American Association for the Advancement of Science; 2017.
113. Bardina SV, Bunduc P, Tripathi S, et al. Enhancement of Zika virus pathogenesis by preexisting antiflavivirus immunity. Science 2017;356(6334):175–80.
114. Cugola FR, Fernandes IR, Russo FB, et al. The Brazilian Zika virus strain causes birth defects in experimental models. Nature 2016;534(7606):267–71.
115. Martines RB, Bhatnagar J, de Oliveira Ramos AM, et al. Pathology of congenital Zika syndrome in Brazil: a case series. Lancet 2016;388(10047):898–904.
116. Chavali PL, Stojic L, Meredith LW, et al. Neurodevelopmental protein Musashi-1 interacts with the Zika genome and promotes viral replication. Science 2017; 357(6346):83–8.
117. Uncini A, Shahrizaila N, Kuwabara S. Zika virus infection and Guillain-Barré syndrome: a review focused on clinical and electrophysiological subtypes. J Neurol Neurosurg Psychiatry 2017;88(3):266–71.
118. Sikka V, Chattu V, Popli R, et al. The emergence of ZIKA as a global health security threat: a review and a consensus statement of the INDUSEM Joint working Group. J Glob Infect Dis 2016;8:3.
119. Rather IA, Kumar S, Bajpai VK, et al. Prevention and control strategies to counter ZIKA epidemic. Front Microbiol 2017;8:305.
120. Nguyen T, Nguyen H, Nguyen T, et al. Field evaluation of the establishment potential of wmelpop Wolbachia in Australia and Vietnam for dengue control. Parasit Vectors 2015;8:563.
121. Zika virus. World Health Organization. 2017. Available at: http://www.who.int/mediacentre/factsheets/zika/en/. Accessed December 20, 2017.
122. Mailand MT, Frederiksen JL. Vaccines and multiple sclerosis: a systematic review. J Neurol 2017;264(6):1035–50.
123. Pregnant women. Center for Disease Control and Prevention. 2017. Available at: https://www.cdc.gov/zika/pregnancy/protect-yourself.html. Accessed December 20, 2017.
124. Diagnostic tests for Zika virus. 2017. Available at: https://www.cdc.gov/zika/hc-providers/types-of-tests.html. Accessed December 30, 2017.
125. Updated guidance for US Laboratories testing for Zika virus infection July 24, 2017. Centers for Disease Control and Prevention. 2017. Available at: https://www.cdc.gov/zika/pdfs/laboratory-guidance-zika.pdf. Accessed December 1, 2017.
126. Diagnostic tests for Zika virus. 2017. Available at: https://www.cdc.gov/zika/hc-providers/types-of-tests.html. Accessed December 20, 2017.
127. Modjarrad K, Lin L, George SL, et al. Preliminary aggregate safety and immunogenicity results from three trials of a purified inactivated Zika virus vaccine candidate: phase 1, randomised, double-blind, placebo-controlled clinical trials. Lancet 2018;391(10120):563–71.

Infectious Myelopathies

Mayra Montavo, MD[a], Tracey A. Cho, MD[b],*

KEYWORDS

- Viral myelitis • Bacterial myelitis • Myeloradiculitis • Acute flaccid paralysis

KEY POINTS

- Myelopathies can be caused by viral, bacterial, parasitic, and fungal infections, each of them causing distinct classic syndromes including radiculomyelitis, transverse myelitis, acute flaccid paralysis, and compressive lesions.
- The increase of immunosuppressed patients especially due to human immunodeficiency virus coinfection has led to the resurgence of pathogens that were previously rarely seen.
- Some pathogens are ubiquitous throughout the world, but many are encountered in specific geographic areas. Knowledge about travel to and immigration from endemic areas is key information when evaluating infectious myelopathies.
- Preventive measures and advanced imaging and laboratory techniques have improved both diagnostic and management strategies resulting in improved outcomes.

INTRODUCTION

Infectious diseases are an important cause of spinal cord dysfunction (**Box 1**). Infectious pathogens can affect the cord directly or can trigger autoimmune reactions, which may result in damage to cord structures. Myelopathy is a term used to describe spinal cord dysfunction, whereas myelitis refers to inflammation of the cord. Myelopathy due to infection may present with distinct syndromes, including acute flaccid paralysis (AFP), acute transverse myelitis, cord compression, myeloradiculitis, and chronic spastic paralysis. AFP results from infection of the anterior horns of the central gray matter. Transverse myelitis is a segmental spinal cord injury caused by acute inflammation resulting in transverse injury to the motor and sensory pathways below the lesion. Microbes may infect structures adjacent to the spinal cord that can result in mass effect with subsequent cord compression. Finally, some infectious organisms can affect the nerve roots along with the cord, resulting in myeloradiculitis. Certain retroviruses can result in a slowly progressive painless myelopathy affecting mainly the lateral white matter corticospinal tracts leading to chronic spastic paralysis (**Fig. 1**).

No disclosures.
[a] Department of Neurology, Brown University, Rhode Island Hospital, 222 Richmond Street, Providence, RI 02903, USA; [b] Department of Neurology, University of Iowa Hospitals and Clinics, 200 Hawkins Drive, Iowa City, Iowa 52242, USA
* Corresponding author.
E-mail address: tracey-cho@uiowa.edu

Box 1
Classification of infectious myelopathies according to etiology

A. Viral

DNA viruses
  Herpesvirus
    Human herpes virus 1 (HHV1)
    Human herpes virus 2 (HHV2)
    Varicella zoster virus (HHV 3)
    Epstein-Barr virus (HHV 4)
    Cytomegalovirus (HHV 5)
    Human herpes virus 6 (HHV 6)
    Human herpes virus 7 (HHV 7)

RNA viruses
  Flaviridae
    West Nile, Japanese encephalitis
    Tick-borne encephalitis virus
    Dengue virus
    Hepatitis C virus
    Zika virus
  Alphaviridae
    Chicungunya virus
  Orthomyxoviridae
    Influenza virus
  Paramyxoviridae
    Mumps virus
    Measles virus
  Picornaviridae
    Polio virus 1, 2, and 3
    Enterovirus 71
    Enterovirus 68
    Coxsackieviruses
    Echoviruses
    Hepataitis A virus
  Retroviridae
    Human immunodeficiency virus (HIV)
    Human T-cell lymphotropic virus (HTLV)
  Rhabdoviridae
    Rabies virus

B. Bacterial

Pyogenic bacteria
  Gram positive
    Staphylococcus spp
    Streptococcus spp
    Propionibacterium acnes
  Gram negative
    Proteus spp
    Salmonella spp
    Enterobacter spp
    Serratia spp
    Pseudomonas aeruginosa

Spirochaetes
  Treponema pallidum
  Borrelia burgdorferi

Miscellaneous
  Mycobacterium tuberculosis
  Mycoplasma pneumonia

Brucella spp
Bartonella henselae

C. Parasitic

Schistosoma mansoni

Schistosoma haematobium

Taenia solium

Toxoplasma gondii

Echinococcus granulosum

Gnathostoma spinigerum

Toxocara canis

D. Fungal

Cryptococcus neoformans

Actinomyces

Aspergillus

Coccidioides immitis

Nocardia

Candida

Blastomyces dermatitidis

Histoplasma capsulatum

Physicians must be familiar with the clinical syndromes and geographic distribution of pathogens, and host immune status. Prompt recognition and early treatment of infectious myelitis can improve outcomes. The purpose of this review was to describe the most common pathogens causing infections of the spinal cord, their mode of infection, diagnosis, and recommended treatment practices.

Bacterial Epidural Abscess

Pyogenic bacteria can infiltrate the epidural space and result in spinal epidural abscess. The epidural space is the area between the dura mater and the vertebral wall. Below the foramen magnum there is a true space containing fat that is well supplied with arteries and veins. Because of this anatomy, epidural abscesses are usually located posteriorly and in the thoracic and lumbar region, because that is where the epidural space is largest.[1,2]

Approximately 30% of epidural abscesses will arise from contiguous infection, such as vertebral osteomyelitis or discitis, psoas, perinephric, paraspinal, or retropharyngeal abscesses. Another mechanism is via local invasion, which may arise from penetrating injuries, surgery, or spinal procedures. Finally, hematogenous spread from a systemic infection also can lead to an epidural abscess.[1] Risk factors for epidural abscess include intravenous (IV) drug use, diabetes mellitus, alcohol abuse, cancer, renal failure requiring hemodialysis, and trauma or instrumentation.[2]

Myelopathy due to epidural abscess is caused by 4 mechanisms: direct compression of the cord, interruption of arterial blood flow causing ischemia, thrombosis and thrombophlebitis of nearby veins, and contiguous inflammatory response. *Staphylococcus aureus* is the most common bacteria involved, followed by *Streptococcus* species.[1] Coagulase-negative *Staphylococcus* and *Propionibacterium acnes* are

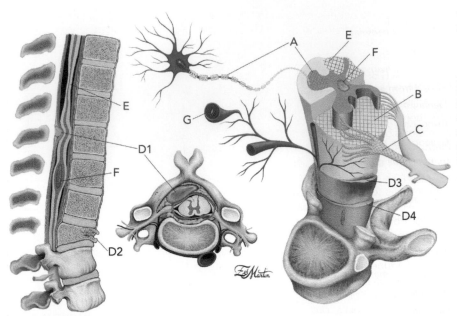

Fig. 1. Infectious myelopathies and characteristic syndromes according to anatomic location. A, AFP, or "anterior horn syndrome": Flaviviruses (WNV, Japanese encephalitis virus, tick-borne encephalitis viruses); Picornaviruses (poliovirus, enterovirus, coxsackievirus). B, C Transverse myelitis/radiculomyelitis: Herpesviruses (HSV, VZV, CMV), TB, syphilis, Lyme, schistosomiasis, *Cryptococcus*. D, Space-occupying lesions: D1, Epidural abscess (pyogenic bacteria, TB, syphilis); D2, Vertebral osteomyelitis (pyogenic bacteria, TB, syphilis, *Coccidioides, Blastomyces*); D3, Arachnoiditis (TB, syphilis, neurocysticercosis); D4, Pachymeningitis (syphilis, TB). E, Chronic spastic paraparesis resulting in cord atrophy depicted in sagittal image: Retroviruses (HTLV, HIV). F, Syringomyelia: TB, syphilis. G, Vasculitis affecting small vessels: TB, syphilis, VZV, *Aspergillus*.

associated with osteomyelitis following spinal surgery. *Escherichia coli* is the most common Enterobacter, but others, such as *Proteus, Salmonella, Enterobacter, Serratia,* and *Pseudomonas,* also have been implicated.[1]

The most common initial symptom of osteomyelitis is back pain, and the presence of fever can vary.[3] C-reactive protein is elevated in virtually every patient and should guide the clinician to promptly obtain an MRI, which is the most sensitive noninvasive diagnostic test. Lumbar puncture is contraindicated due to risk of inoculation of bacteria into the subarachnoid space. This is particularly important given that the cord damage by an epidural abscess results from compression, not direct infection. A spinal epidural abscess is a surgical emergency. Decompressive surgery and drainage of the abscess, coupled with parental antibiotic therapy, is the optimal management. Neurologic deterioration can occur rapidly, making a prompt diagnosis imperative. The severity of neurologic impairment is the most reliable predictor of mortality, which can be high even with proper treatment.[1,4]

Bacterial Spinal Cord Abscess

Compared with epidural abscess, intramedullary spinal cord abscess is rare. The most common risk factors are dermal sinuses (especially in children), concomitant infection, and a compromised immune system. MRI shows gadolinium ring enhancement in the spinal cord in 64% of patients. Management, as with epidural abscess, includes anti-biotics and surgical drainage; despite proper treatment, outcomes are poor.[5]

Tuberculous Spinal Infection

Tuberculosis (TB) is the ninth leading cause of death worldwide and the leading cause of death from a single infectious agent, ranking above human immunodeficiency virus (HIV)/AIDS. Tuberculosis is an infection caused by *Mycobacterium tuberculosis*. In 2016, there were 6.3 million new cases of TB globally, with a 3% mortality.[6] Meningeal tuberculosis occurs in 1% to 6% of cases.[7–9] There are several different ways in which tuberculosis can cause myelopathy. In tuberculous meningitis, inflammatory exudates can result in several spinal complications, including radiculomyelitis (tuberculous arachnoiditis), intradural extramedullary tuberculoma, intramedullary tuberculoma, acute myelitis (demyelination and axonal injury), longitudinally extensive transverse myelitis, vertebral tuberculosis (Pott disease), syringomyelia, and rarely tuberculous abscess. Pott disease with vertebral collapse causing spinal cord compression and tuberculous arachnoiditis resulting in myeloradiculitis are the most frequent spinal cord complications. TB may spread to the spinal cord through several mechanisms: rupture of a tuberculous lesion in the spinal meninges, downward extension of intra-cranial exudates to spinal subarachnoid space, and extension from adjacent vertebra to the meninges. Spinal blood vessels can be involved via necrotizing granulomas or inflammatory vasculitis processes, and can lead to thrombosis and spinal cord ischemia.[10]

Cerebrospinal fluid (CSF) examination typically shows lymphocytic pleocytosis, decreased glucose, and elevated protein, with tuberculous meningitis and the associated syndromes. Protein elevation may be remarkably high in the case of spinal block of CSF flow (up to 2–6 g/dL). Bacteriologic confirmation is performed by smear exam-ination for acid-fast bacteria, like Ziehl-Neelsen staining, mycobacterial culture, or polymerase chain reaction (PCR) analysis for mycobacterial DNA. It is recommended to sample large volumes and use the last tube for microbiology to increase test sensitivity.

MRI is a helpful diagnostic tool for spinal tuberculosis. It can help with differential diagnosis and to establish the extent of disease.[11] Tuberculous myelitis presents with cord edema, hyperintensity on T2, isointense or hypointense on T1, and segmental enhancement on postcontrast images (**Fig. 2**). Radiculomyelitis presents with linear or nodular enhancement coating the nerve roots and spinal cord. Tubercu-lous granulomas (tuberculomas) are T1 hypointense, T2 hyperintense, and have T1 postcontrast solid or rim-enhancing pattern. The center of the lesion may be either solid due to caseous necrosis or cystic with liquefactive necrosis, the latter also may cause restricted diffusion.[12] Tuberculous abscesses are similar in radiographic appearance to pyogenic brain abscesses. They are larger in comparison with tubercu-lomas, with central hypointensity on T2 due to mycobacteria-filled pus and liquefac-tion of tissue, and may be solitary or multiloculated. Pott disease is characterized by T1 hypointensity, T2 hyperintensity, and contrast enhancement of the vertebral bone, and can result in vertebral body collapse with mechanical cord compression. Syringomyelia is isointense to CSF and does not enhance.[13,14]

The cornerstone treatment for spinal tuberculosis is antimicrobial therapy with a combination of 4 first-line drugs: isoniazid, rifampicin, streptomycin, and pyrazinamide for 2 months continued by 7 to 10 months of a 2-drug regimen (isoniazid and rifampin). Corticosteroids reduce mortality in patients with tuberculous meningitis[15]; however, the role of corticosteroids in spinal cord tuberculosis has not been established. A para-doxic reaction may occur, in which a patient who is receiving appropriate antibiotic

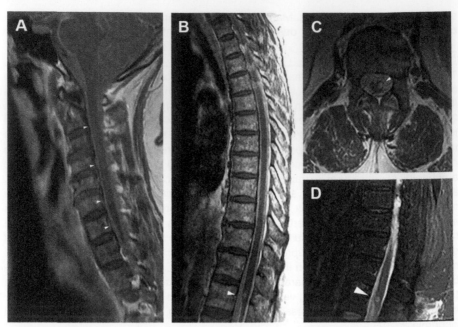

Fig. 2. Tuberculous myelitis: Sagittal T1-weighted postcontrast MRI (*A*) depicting nodular leptomeningeal enhancement in the cervical spine (*white arrowheads*). Sagittal T1-weighted postcontrast (*B*), axial T2-weighted (*C*), sagittal short tau inversion recovery (*D*), MRI demonstrate an intramedullary lesion at the level of the conus medullaris (*white arrowheads*).

therapy develops clinical or radiological worsening. This is thought to result from an exaggerated cell-mediated immune response against mycobacterial antigens. Corticosteroids used temporarily may be beneficial in this scenario, but other immunomodulatory drugs have been used in severe paradoxic reactions with varying efficacy.[16] Severe cases, including paraplegia, severe vertebral body collapse, cord compression, and medical failure, may require adjunctive surgical treatment.[10,17]

Lyme-Associated Spinal Disease

Lyme disease is caused by the spirochete *Borrelia burgdorferi,* and is the most common vector-borne disease in the northern hemisphere. It is endemic in North America, Europe, and Asia. The endemic area mirrors the distribution of the disease vector, small ticks of the genus *Ixodes.*[1] Neurologic involvement is reported in 5% to 20% of cases. The most common neurologic manifestations are cranial nerve palsies (especially cranial nerve 7), lymphocytic meningitis, and painful radiculopathy. More commonly in Europe, Lyme disease presents as painful meningoradiculitis known as Bannwarth syndrome,[18] which was the most common manifestation in one European case series.[19] Myelopathy is a rare manifestation of Lyme disease. In patients affected with early neuroborreliosis, 4% had spinal cord involvement. Myelitis often presents at the same level as painful meningoradiculitis.[19] Rarely it can present as isolated transverse myelitis.[20]

Lyme neuroborreliosis should be suspected in any patient exposed to an endemic area who presents with the classic neurologic manifestations (especially facial palsy). When these symptoms are preceded by erythema migrans, Lyme arthritis, or acrodermatitis chronica atrophicans (in Europe), the diagnosis is straightforward. Serologic evaluation is made with a screening enzyme-linked immunosorbent assay followed by confirmatory Western blot. In a patient presenting with a common neurologic syndrome in an endemic area, systemic serologic evidence of Lyme disease is often enough to make a presumptive diagnosis and begin treatment. CSF typically shows lymphocytic pleocytosis, elevated protein, and increased immunoglobulin (Ig) G index. Elevated CSF antibody index (quantitative comparison of serum to CSF Lyme-specific antibody levels) can give further support for Lyme neuroborreliosis, but is not 100% sensitive. CSF levels of the chemokine CXCL13 might be useful as a complementary diagnostic tool for early Lyme neuroborreliosis when antibody index is negative; however, CSF CXCL13 may also be elevated in other infections, multiple sclerosis, and central nervous system (CNS) lymphoma.[21] PCR from CSF samples is insensitive and not widely validated, and thus has no role in the diagnosis of neuroborreliosis.[1] Treatment with ceftriaxone 2 g IV daily for 10 to 28 days is recommended for patients with meningitis, myelitis, and meningoradiculitis. Oral antibiotics, such as doxycycline, are recommended for isolated cranial nerve palsy.[1,22]

Neurosyphilis of the Spinal Cord

Syphilis is caused by the spirochete Treponema pallidum, subspecies pallidum. After the introduction of penicillin in the 1940s, the number of cases dramatically decreased. Despite this, the rates of neurosyphilis have increased in the HIV era. Syphilis can affect the spinal cord in different ways. Meningovascular syphilis consists of endarteritis of vessels anywhere in the CNS, leading to thrombosis and infarction. In the spinal cord, it usually affects small radicular vessels but can also affect the anterior spinal artery and less commonly the posterior spinal arteries leading to infarction or hemorrhage. A better known manifestation is tabes dorsalis, which consists of degeneration of the dorsal roots and posterior column of the spinal cord. The classic symptoms include lancinating pains, ataxic gait, paresthesias, and bladder dysfunction. Classic signs include Argyll Robertson pupils, diminished reflexes, impaired vibration and proprioception, impaired pain and temperature with development of Charcot joints, and extraocular muscle palsies.[23,24] Rarely, syphilis can result in meningomyelitis.[25] It can also affect the spinal cord by compression due to space-occupying lesions, such as spinal cord gummas, hypertrophic pachymeningitis, aortic aneurysm, and a Charcot vertebra with compression. Other rare manifestations of neurosyphilis are syringomyelia and anterior horn cell syndrome.[24,26]

If neurosyphilis is suspected, the first step is to establish systemic infection through serum treponemal antibody. If negative, neurosyphilis is excluded. In patients with neurosyphilis, CSF studies reveal lymphocytic pleocytosis and mildly elevated protein. For patients coinfected with HIV, some investigators use a white blood cell cutoff in CSF greater than 20 cells/μL to avoid confusion with the mild pleocytosis that can be seen in chronic HIV infection. CSF-VDRL is considered diagnostic for neurosyphilis but has incomplete sensitivity. CSF fluorescent treponemal antibody test can be used to exclude a diagnosis of neurosyphilis, but false positives are common due to contamination from serum.[27]

First-line therapy involves penicillin G 4 g IV every 4 hours for 10 to 14 days. In cases of myelitis, patients can be pretreated with steroids to avoid the paradoxic worsening symptoms due to lysis of spirochetes seen in Jarisch-Herxheimer reaction.[14]

Other Bacterial Infections of the Spine

Other bacteria may occasionally affect the spinal cord. Brucella species can affect the spine through several mechanisms, such as infections of vertebral bodies, intervertebral discs, epidural space, meninges, subarachnoid space, and the spinal cord itself (myelitis).[28] *Mycoplasma pneumonia*[29] and *Bartonella henselae*[30] have also been associated with transverse myelitis, mainly as a parainfectious immune reaction rather than direct infection of the CNS.

DNA Viruses

Herpesviruses

The herpes viruses are ubiquitous with worldwide distribution. When affecting the spinal cord, they characteristically cause a transverse myelitis syndrome (see **Fig. 1**). Herpes simplex virus (HSV) 1 and 2 and varicella zoster virus (VZV) are the most common human neurotropic viruses. They establish latent infection in the trigeminal and dorsal root ganglia, which persists throughout the entire life of the host. During latency, the pathogen can reactivate, resume replication, and cause recurrent disease.

HSV is the most common cause of sporadic viral encephalitis worldwide and causes substantial morbidity and mortality. Less commonly, HSV may also affect the spinal cord, typically manifesting as partial or complete transverse myelitis. HSV-1 is acquired by oral mucosa infection.[31,32] HSV-2 is acquired by genital mucosa infection and may cause a reactivation myelitis in adults. HSV-2 myelitis can present as a mild syndrome with excellent recovery, but it can also present as a recurrent disease or as acute necrotizing myelitis, especially in immunocompromised hosts.[33–36] HSV-2 can reactivate in sacral spinal ganglia, causing lumbosacral polyradiculitis and CSF pleocytosis (Elsberg syndrome).[37,38] CSF usually reveals lymphocytic pleocytosis but polymorphonuclear cells may dominate early in the disease.[39] Detection of viral DNA by PCR is the gold standard method for diagnosing HSV infection of the CNS.[40] MRI shows T2 hyperintensities with cord edema and contrast enhancement of cord and roots.[41,42]

VZV most commonly causes varicella (chicken pox) in children and zoster in adults. Myelitis is a rare complication but it may occur even in immunocompetent patients. Patients may present with impaired sensation at a level compatible with the segment in which VZV reactivation occurs. Potentially, myelitis is due to spread from dorsal root ganglia to the spinal cord.[31] Most patients have dermatomal zoster preceding the myelitis by a few days to 3 weeks, which gives clue to the diagnosis. However, patients can develop myelitis with no prior rash. CSF DNA PCR assays are a method of rapid detection, but in contrast to HSV infections, the sensitivity for VZV myelitis is not well defined and is likely less sensitive than HSV PCR. CSF IgM and IgG antibodies can help improve sensitivity.[43] MRI may show spinal cord T2 hyperintense signal, cord enhancement, and nerve root enhancement (**Fig. 3**). Treatment for both HSV and VZV myelitis is extrapolated from HSV encephalitis: acyclovir 10 mg/kg IV every 8 hours for 14 to 21 days. In milder cases, patients may transition to oral acyclovir or valacyclovir to complete the treatment course. For severe cases with cord swelling and severe deficit, corticosteroids are sometimes used in addition to antiviral therapy.[36]

Cytomegalovirus is an important cause of myelitis in immune-compromised patients, especially those with advanced HIV (CD4 count <100 cells/μL). It can cause lumbosacral polyradiculitis or myeloradiculitis.[44] It is rare in immunocompetent patients but it has been described in case reports. Treatment includes ganciclovir with or without foscarnet depending on severity.[45] Epstein-Barr virus,[46] human herpesvirus (HHV)6,[47] and HHV7[48] have all been associated with inflammatory myelitis thought to occur through a parainfectious mechanism.

RNA Viruses

Flaviviruses and enteroviruses may infect the spinal cord gray matter, typically presenting as AFP, affecting the anterior horn cells, also called poliomyelitis syndrome

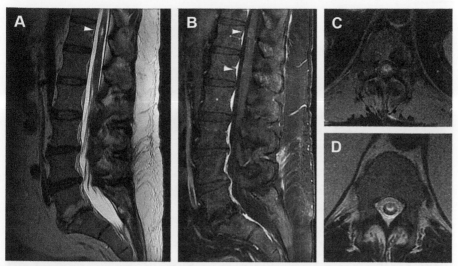

Fig. 3. Varicella zoster radiculomyelitis. Sagittal T2-weighted (*A*) MRI showing intrinsic cord hyperintense T2 signal (*arrowhead*), sagittal T1-weighted postcontrast (*B*) showing patchy cord enhancement (*arrowheads*), axial T2-weighted (*C*) showing cord enhancement, and axial T1-weighted postcontrast (*D*) MRI showing intramedullary hyperintense T2 signal.

(see **Fig. 1**). Epidemiologically this is now referred to as acute flaccid myelitis. This syndrome is characterized by flaccid, asymmetric, patchy weakness without sensory loss that is classically preceded by a minor febrile illness and begins within 1 week of infection.[36]

Flaviviruses

West Nile Virus (WNV) is widely distributed in Africa, Europe, Australia, and Asia. Since 1999, it has caused outbreaks in North and South America, accounting for 20,000 cases of symptomatic infection in the United States,[49] although 80% of infections are asymptomatic. West Nile may present with invasive neurologic disease in 1% of infected patients. Most commonly, neuroinvasive disease causes meningitis or encephalitis; 10% of those with neuroinvasive disease will have AFP.[50]

When WNV invades the anterior horn cells of the spinal cord, it may cause an asymmetric AFP, with absent deep tendon reflexes, bowel or bladder dysfunction, and respiratory dysfunction, but preserved sensation.[50] Mortality can be as high as 50%.[49] Early CSF findings in WNV neuroinvasive disease include in half a neutrophilic pleocytosis (>200 nucleated cells/μL), followed by a shift to lymphocytic predominance. Because IgM antibodies are too large to cross the blood-CSF barrier, elevated IgM titers from CSF is diagnostic in the appropriate setting, although their appearance in CSF may be delayed up to 14 days after onset of neurologic symptoms. Alternatively, acute and convalescent serum antibodies showing an increase in titers is also supportive of the diagnosis, but takes several weeks. Notably, serum IgM antibodies can last up to a year, so positive results outside the acute setting must be interpreted with caution.[50] MRI of spinal cord is usually normal, although it may show T2 hyperintensities in the anterior horns or cauda equina/nerve root enhancement (**Fig. 4**).[51] In this subgroup of patients, the level of abnormal spinal MRI findings corresponds with the degree of paralysis.[52] In addition to the anterior horn involvement, WNV can also involve adjacent white matter, causing a transverse myelitis, but this is

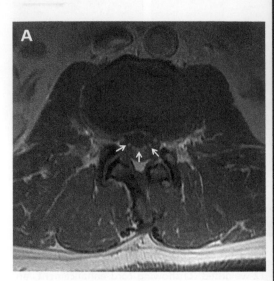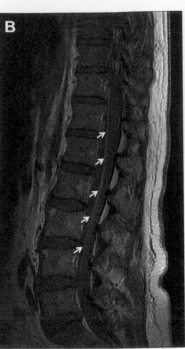

Fig. 4. West Nile radiculomyelitis. Axial (*A*) and sagittal (*B*) T1-weighted postcontrast MRI of the cauda equina shows abnormal enhancement of nerve roots (*arrows*).

rare.[53] There is currently no specific treatment for flavivirus infections. Intravenous immunoglobulin (IVIG) containing high titers of WNV antibody, ribavirin, and interferon have shown therapeutic activity in vitro but not in vivo.[54] Vector control using spray and water treatments, individual repellent, and protective clothing are important for prevention.[36]

Japanese encephalitis virus is the most important cause of viral encephalitis in eastern and southern Asia. It can also present with AFP. Diagnosis is made based on IgM antibodies in CSF. Treatment is supportive. The inactivated Japanese encephalitis vaccine is widely available in several Asian countries, and routine immunization has significantly lowered the prevalence of the disease.[55] Vaccination is not recommended for all travelers to endemic areas because of side effects, but it is recommended for those planning to spend long periods of time in rural areas.[56]

Tick-born encephalitis virus is prevalent in Europe, Russia, and Asia. The virus affects the anterior horn of the cervical spinal cord, causing a flaccid paralysis affecting the arms and shoulder muscles. In 5% of cases, this can result in paralysis of respiratory muscles, requiring ventilator support. Bulbar syndrome also has been described as a result of this virus, as well as cranial nerve involvement.[57] Diagnosis is made with IgM antibodies in CSF. Management is supportive. Plasma exchange and steroids have been tried with variable results.[57] A vaccine is available with an estimated protection rate of 95%, as seen in Austrian population studies.[58]

Other flaviviruses that have been associated with myelopathy include St. Louis encephalitis virus (StLE virus), Dengue virus,[59] hepatitis C virus,[60] and Zika virus.[61] StLE virus causes AFP, but the clinical picture in the others may be more of an inflammatory myelitis rather than AFP. It is believed to be an immune-mediated response against spinal cord, and has a favorable response to corticosteroids or other immunomodulatory therapy.

Picornaviruses

Picornaviruses are common worldwide. Although they typically result in a respiratory or gastrointestinal disease, they can also target the CNS due to neurotropism. There are 3 routes through which picornavirus may enter the CNS. Virus can infect the peripheral nerve and invade the CNS via retrograde axonal transport. In viremia, the virus can enter the CNS hetamogenously through a disrupted blood brain barrier, and it can also infect migrating cells and enter the CNS through a "Trojan-Horse" invasion.[62]

Poliovirus (PV) is the classic etiology of AFP caused by neurotropic invasion of anterior horn cells, but it has been nearly eradicated due to global vaccination efforts. Since 1988, polio cases have decreased by more than 99%. Currently only 3 countries in the world still have polio (Pakistan, Afghanistan, and Nigeria). Although polio is no longer endemic in the United States, there is a protocol for patients who present with unexplained AFP in the right clinical setting to rule out this infection.[63]

Enterovirus 71 (EV71) infection was first identified during a small outbreak in California in 1969. Since then, several epidemics have occurred around the world, most prominently in the Asia-Pacific region. Patients infected with EV71 generally present with hand-foot-and-mouth disease, but neurologic complications including aseptic meningitis, encephalitis, and AFP range from 5.8% in Brazil[64] to 9.0% in the United States[65] to 30.0% in Taiwan.[62] *Enterovirus D68 (EVD68)* is another picornavirus associated with acute AFP arising as a rare manifestation during outbreaks of upper respiratory tract infections.[66]

PV, EV71, and EV68 present with AFP primarily in young children. EV71 has been associated with myoclonus, tremor, ataxia, and herpangina, which is not commonly seen in poliovirus. EV71 has been associated with good recovery, especially if the disease is unilateral, although mortality can reach up to 8%.[62] As with flaviviruses, MRI in patients with AFP suspected of picornavirus infection may show anterior horn lesions, which generally correlate with the severity of clinical manifestations.[67]

EV71 and EV68 are usually isolated from stool and respiratory tract specimens, but CSF and blood specimens also should be obtained. CSF often shows pleocytosis and elevated protein.[68] Treatment with IVIG, plasmapheresis, corticosteroids, and antiviral agents have shown no benefit.[69] Currently there are 2 Chinese food and drug administration–approved vaccines for EV-A71, and efforts are under way to develop a multivalent vaccine that targets EV-A71 and coxsackie virus A16 (CV-A16).

Other enteroviruses can cause infectious myelopathies: coxsackie virus causes AFP[70] as well as transverse myelitis.[71,72] Echoviruses[73] and hepatitis A virus[74] have also been associated with transverse myelitis.

Retroviruses

Two retroviruses in particular, HIV and human T-cell lymphotropic virus (HTLV-1), typically present with a distinct syndrome called chronic spastic paraparesis. These viruses affect the posterior and lateral columns in a slow chronic fashion over many years, resulting in this distinct syndrome characterized by symmetric spastic paraparesis, hyperreflexia, impaired proprioception, and urinary incontinency, usually resulting in atrophy, especially in the thoracic spine (see **Fig. 1**).

Human T-cell lymphotropic virus-1 (HTLV-1) was the first described human retrovirus, which was detected in a patient with cutaneous lymphoma. It is the causative agent of HTLV-associated myelopathy or tropical spastic paraparesis (HAM/TSP). It is estimated that 5 to 10 million people are infected worldwide, but the true prevalence may be even higher.[75] HTLV-1 is endemic to Central and South America, the Caribbean islands, the Middle East, central Australia, Japan, and sub-Saharan Africa. HTLV-1 is transmitted by breastfeeding, sexual contact, and blood transfusions. Incidence is higher in women due to more efficient male-to-female sexual transmission. Once infected, the lifetime risk of developing HAM/TSP varies from 0.25% to 4.0% in infected individuals.[76,77] HAM/TSP pathogenesis begins with an initial inflammatory phase with perivascular lymphocytic infiltration, most frequently in the upper thoracic spinal cord. After months or years, this process results in loss of spinal volume, frequently apparent on MRI. The clinical syndrome is characterized by subacute-chronic-onset lower extremity weakness, low back pain, hyperreflexia, spastic gait, and loss of vibration and proprioception in keeping with posterolateral column syndrome. A sensory level is rarely present. In advanced disease, constipation, urinary frequency, nocturia, urgency, and erectile dysfunction (in men) are also common. Diagnosis is made by detection of HTLV-1 antibodies in serum and CSF, confirmed by Western blot analysis or a positive PCR for HTLV-1 in blood and/or CSF. Proviral load (PCR assay of viral DNA within peripheral blood mononuclear cells) is the strongest predictor of developing HAM/TSP. In patients with atypical or incomplete clinical features, the HTLV-1 proviral load can provide the key for diagnosis. In fact, HTLV-1 proviral load and inflammatory response have been reported to have a 100% positive predictive value and 98% negative predictive value.[76] CSF protein and lymphocytes can be normal or mildly increased. CXCL10, CXCL9, and neopterin have been proposed as biomarkers,[78] although these are used primarily in research settings.

Depending of the stage of the disease, the spinal cord can be swollen, normal, or atrophic. In early stages, MRI may show intrinsic cord T2 hyperintensity, which is associated with rapidly progressive disease. As the disease progresses, the radiological findings correlate with the neurodegenerative process resulting in atrophy of the spinal cord.

Management of HAM/TSP is mostly symptomatic, as there is no proven effective treatment to stop or reverse the myelopathy. It is widely believed that the therapeutic window in HAM/TSP lies within the first few years of presentation when the symptoms are due to inflammation rather than subsequent neurodegeneration. Corticosteroids are the first-line treatment early in disease.[49] Motor disability has been shown to improve, but this is usually not sustained. Other agents, such as interferon-alfa,[79] cyclosporine A,[80] methotrexate,[81] and pentoxifylline,[82] have been used with variable success. Prosultiamine[83] and pentosan polysulfate sodium[84] have shown some promise in small open trials. A monoclonal antibody against CCR4, mogamulizumab, has shown some promise in an early-phase trial in Japan, but requires a larger phase 3 study.[85]

HIV has infected an estimated 65 million people since it was first identified in the early 1980s. Currently there are 36.7 million people living with HIV in the world and 1 million living with HIV in the United States.[86,87] HIV enters the CNS early in the course of infection. In addition to microglia and macrophage infection, there is a sustained inflammatory reaction that persists even after virus replication is under control.[88,89]

HIV-associated vacuolar myelopathy affects 10% of untreated patients with AIDS. Its incidence has markedly decreased now that antiretroviral therapy (ART) is established throughout the world. This posterolateral column syndrome is characterized by symmetric spastic paraparesis, hyperreflexia, impaired proprioception, and urinary incontinency. Unfortunately, once the syndrome is established, there is limited reversal of symptoms with ART and management is mainly symptomatic.[87] Neuropathological specimens reveal axonal injury with macrophage infiltration localized in the lateral and dorsal columns of the thoracic cord, which are thought to represent intramyelinic edema that can look similar to subacute combined degeneration secondary to vitamin B12 deficiency. Despite this similarity, B12 repletion does not reverse vacuolar myelopathy. A small pilot study showed improvement of strength with IVIG, but further investigation is required to confirm these results.[90] HIV-associated vacuolar myelopathy is a diagnosis of exclusion and it should be questioned especially if the presentation is acute, painful, there is upper extremity predominance, and/or CSF is inflammatory.[14]

Transverse myelitis associated with primary HIV infection, as occurs with other viruses, has also been described in case reports. This entity responds to ART and steroids.[91–93]

Parasites

Schistosomiasis affects more than 230 million people worldwide. The causative agent is the trematode parasite of the genus *Schistosoma*. The adult worms live within the venous system of the human host. They release fertilized eggs that are excreted via feces and urine or are trapped in host tissues. The eggs that remain in the host's tissue can trigger an immune-mediated granulomatous response largely characterized by lymphocytes, eosinophils, and activated macrophages. The main species that cause neurologic disease are *Schistosoma haematobium* and *Schistosoma mansoni*, which are endemic to Africa and the Middle East. *S mansoni* is present in Central and South America, Africa, and the Arabian peninsula. *Staphylococcus japonicum*, which is endemic in Asia, mainly affects the brain. Neuroschistosomiasis myelitis associated with *S mansoni* is one of the most severe clinical syndromes of infection. Eggs can migrate to the CNS from the portal venous system through the pelvic and epidural veins and cause spinal cord involvement. The mass of thousands of eggs and large granulomas surrounding the spinal cord leads to either acute myelitis or subacute myeloradiculitis, especially of the conus medullaris of the cord. Symptoms include lumbar pain, radicular pain, weakness, and bladder dysfunction.[94]

The CSF may demonstrate eosinophilic pleocytosis but eosinophilia is not universal. MRI shows T2 hyperintense signal in the conus medullaris and cauda equina, edematous cord, and patchy enhancement of the cord and nerve roots (**Fig. 5**). Intramedullary schistosomal granulomas can present as heterogeneous hyperintense lesions with no clear boundaries or as patchy nodular enhancing lesions. Atrophy of the cord can be seen in chronic cases.[95] Positive serology may be useful in travelers but has poor specificity in patients from endemic countries where seroprevalence is high. Demonstration of viable eggs in urine (*S haematobium*) or feces (*S mansoni*), or in rectal biopsy provides supportive but not direct evidence of schistosomal involvement in the CNS. This finding should be integrated with neuroimaging and clinical history. A definitive diagnosis can be done only with a tissue biopsy, which is rarely indicated due to high morbidity. Treatment includes antiparasitic therapy with praziquantel to prevent further shedding of eggs and corticosteroids to mitigate edema from the inflammatory reaction to the eggs. Surgery is reserved for severe cases with cord compression or worsening symptoms despite optimal medical management.[94,96]

Neurocysticercosis is an infection of the CNS and its meningeal covering by the larval stage of the pork tapeworm *Taenia solium*. It is endemic in most resource-poor countries where pigs are raised in close proximity to humans. Cases in industrialized countries are mainly due to immigration from endemic countries. The disease is predominantly intracranial but can cause myelopathies in 3% of infected cases.[97] Cysticerci may be located anywhere in the CNS, including brain parenchyma,

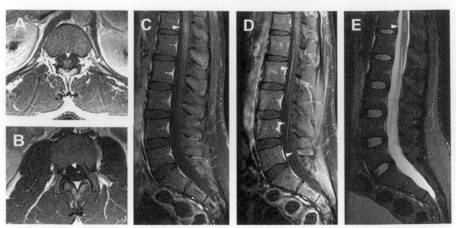

Fig. 5. Neuroschistosomiasis. Axial T12 level (*A*) and L4 level (*B*) and sagittal (*C, D*) T1-weighted postcontrast MRI showing thoracic cord (*A, C*) and nerve root (*B, D*) enhancement (*arrowheads*). Sagittal T2-weighted (*E*) MRI demonstrating T2 hyperintense intramedullary lesion (*arrowhead*).

intracranial subarachnoid space, the ventricular system, or the spinal column. The parasites can reach the spinal subarachnoid space via spread from intracranial subarachnoid space. Basal subarachnoid neurocysticercosis is associated with spinal involvement in 60% of cases, often with deposition of cysts in the lumbosacral region where they may cause radiculopathy.[98] Spinal neurocysticercosis can also present as an intramedullary lesion, but this is uncommon, with fewer than 50 cases reported in the literature.[99] Most spinal cord parenchymal cysts are located in the thoracic region, possibly because cysticerci enter the parenchyma by hematogenous dissemination through the artery of Adamkiewicz, which originates from the aorta and enters the spine between T9 and T11.

CSF may reveal high protein and eosinophilia. MRI is the best modality for imaging the spinal cord and the spinal subarachnoid space. Leptomeningeal cysts are seen on MRI as cystic lesions or areas of arachnoiditis (**Fig. 6**). Intramedullary cysticercus appears as a rounded cyst with a scolex, but can be misdiagnosed as neoplasm.[98] Treatment usually involves albendazole and corticosteroids; however, in selected cases with progressive neurologic deficits and especially with intradural extramedullary lesions, surgical decompression may be necessary.[100]

Toxoplasma can present with mass lesions in patients with advanced HIV. Usually located in the brain, toxoplasma can also be rarely found in the spinal cord. The treatment of choice is pyrimethamine (with leucovorin rescue) and sulfadiazole.[101] *Gnathostoma spiegerum*,[102] *Toxocara canis*,[103] *Angiostrongylus cantonensis*,[104] and *Echinococcus granulosum*[105,106] can also cause myelopathy but are more geographically restricted.

Fungi

Fungal infections can affect the spinal cord, usually in patients with some degree of immunosuppression. The primary syndrome is typically meningitis, with secondary injury to the spinal cord through a number of mechanisms. *Cryptococcus, Actinomyces, Aspergillus,* and *Nocardia* can present as intramedullary abscesses. *Coccidioides* and *Nocardia* can form granulomas. Most cases of fungal spinal cord

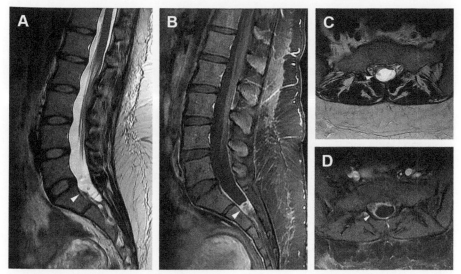

Fig. 6. Spinal neurocysticercosis. Sagittal (*A*) and axial (*C*) T2-weighted MRI demonstrating an extramedullary intradural spinal cysticercus at the level of S1 (*arrowheads*). Sagittal (*B*) and axial (*D*) T1-weighted postcontrast MRI showing an extramedullary intradural spinal cysticercus with meningeal enhancement at the level of S2 (*arrowheads*).

disease are caused by *Cryptococcus neoformans* in immunosuppressed patients, with arachnoiditis leading to myelopathy. Fungi also can cause vasculitis with resulting cord infarction. Diagnosis is typically made by identification of fungal antigens, cultures, or antibodies in CSF. Management consists of targeted antifungal medications.[36]

SUMMARY

Infections constitute a rare but often treatable cause of myelopathy. With globalization increasing the presentation of endemic infections in developed countries and expanded use of immunotherapy altering host defenses, infections will likely expand as a cause of myelopathy. Knowledge of potential infectious etiologies and their typical spinal cord syndromes can help clinicians diagnose these myelopathies efficiently and initiate early treatment.

REFERENCES

1. Scheld MW, Whitley RJ, Marra CM. Infections of the central nervous system. Philadelphia: Lippincott Williams & Wilkins; 2014.
2. Zimmerli W. Vertebral osteomyelitis. N Engl J Med 2010;362:1022–9.
3. Davis DP, Wold RM, Patel RJ, et al. The clinical presentation and impact of diagnostic delays on emergency department patients with spinal epidural abscess. J Emerg Med 2004;26:285–91.
4. Patel AR, Alton TB, Bransford RJ, et al. Spinal epidural abscesses: risk factors, medical versus surgical management, a retrospective review of 128 cases. Spine J 2014;14:326–30.
5. Lapointe S, Legault C, Altman R, et al. Intramedullary spinal cord abscess; descriptive review of the literature (P2. 015). Neurology 2016;86:P2. 015.

6. World Health Organization. Global tuberculosis report 2017. Global tuberculosis report 20172017. Available at: http://www.who.int/tb/publications/global_report/gtbr2017_main_text.pdf?ua=1.

7. Ducomble T, Tolksdorf K, Karagiannis I, et al. The burden of extrapulmonary and meningitis tuberculosis: an investigation of national surveillance data, Germany, 2002 to 2009. Euro Surveill 2013;18:20436.

8. Peto HM, Pratt RH, Harrington TA, et al. Epidemiology of extrapulmonary tuberculosis in the United States, 1993–2006. Clin Infect Dis 2009;49:1350–7.

9. Sandgren A, Hollo V, Van der Werf M. Extrapulmonary tuberculosis in the European Union and European economic area, 2002 to 2011. Euro Surveill 2013;18: 20431.

10. Garg R, Malhotra H, Gupta R. Spinal cord involvement in tuberculous meningitis. Spinal Cord 2015;53:649.

11. Khan S, Zahir MZ, Khan J, et al. Spectrum of MRI findings in spinal tuberculosis. Kaohsiung J Med Sci 2016;9:96.

12. Marais S, Roos I, Mitha A, et al. Spinal tuberculosis: clinicoradiological findings in 274 patients. Clin Infect Dis 2018. https://doi.org/10.1093/cid/ciy020.

13. Bernaerts A, Vanhoenacker F, Parizel P, et al. Tuberculosis of the central nervous system: overview of neuroradiological findings. Eur Radiol 2003;13:1876–90.

14. Cho TA, Vaitkevicius H. Infectious myelopathies. Continuum (Minneap Minn) 2012;18:1351–73.

15. Thwaites GE, Bang ND, Dung NH, et al. Dexamethasone for the treatment of tuberculous meningitis in adolescents and adults. N Engl J Med 2004;351: 1741–51.

16. Garg RK, Malhotra HS, Kumar N. Paradoxical reaction in HIV negative tuberculous meningitis. J Neurol Sci 2014;340:26–36.

17. Chandra SP, Singh A, Goyal N, et al. Analysis of changing paradigms of management in 179 patients with spinal tuberculosis over a 12-year period and proposal of a new management algorithm. World Neurosurg 2013;80:190–203.

18. Ogrinc K, Lusa L, Lotrič-Furlan S, et al. Course and outcome of early European Lyme neuroborreliosis (Bannwarth syndrome): clinical and laboratory findings. Rev Infect Dis 2016;63:346–53.

19. Hansen K, Lebech A-M. The clinical and epidemiological profile of lyme neuroborreliosis in Denmark 1985–1990: a prospective study of 187 patients with *Borrelia burgdorferi* specific intrathecal antibody productionm. Brain 1992;115: 399–423.

20. Bigi S, Aebi C, Nauer C, et al. Acute transverse myelitis in Lyme neuroborreliosis. Infection 2010;38:413–6.

21. Koedel U, Fingerle V, Pfister H-W. Lyme neuroborreliosis—epidemiology, diagnosis and management. Nat Rev Neurol 2015;11:446.

22. Halperin JJ. Nervous system Lyme disease. Infect Dis Clin North Am 2008;22: 261–74.

23. Simon RP. Neurosyphilis. Arch Neurol 1985;42:606–13.

24. Ghanem KG. Neurosyphilis: a historical perspective and review. CNS Neurosci Ther 2010;16:e157–68.

25. Kikuchi S, Shinpo K, Niino M, et al. Subacute syphilitic meningomyelitis with characteristic spinal MRI findings. J Neurol 2003;250:106–7.

26. Berger JR. Neurosyphilis and the spinal cord: then and now. J Nerv Ment Dis 2011;199:912–3.

27. Marra CM. Update on neurosyphilis. Curr Infect Dis Rep 2009;11:127–34.

28. Tali ET, Koc AM, Oner AY. Spinal brucellosis. Neuroimaging Clin N Am 2015;25: 233–45.
29. Weng W-C, Peng SS-F, Wang S-B, et al. Mycoplasma pneumoniae–associated transverse myelitis and rhabdomyolysis. Pediatr Neurol 2009;40:128–30.
30. Baylor P, Garoufi A, Karpathios T, et al. Transverse myelitis in 2 patients with *Bartonella henselae* infection (cat scratch disease). Clin Infect Dis 2007;45:e42–5.
31. Steiner I, Kennedy PG, Pachner AR. The neurotropic herpes viruses: herpes simplex and varicella-zoster. Lancet Neurol 2007;6:1015–28.
32. Irani DN. Aseptic meningitis and viral myelitis. Neurol Clin 2008;26:635–55.
33. Folpe A, Lapham LW, Smith HC. Herpes simplex myelitis as a cause of acute necrotizing myelitis syndrome. Neurology 1994;44:1955.
34. Wiley C, VanPatten P, Carpenter P, et al. Acute ascending necrotizing myelopathy caused by herpes simplex virus type 2. Neurology 1987;37:1791.
35. Iwamasa T, Yoshitake H, Sakuda H, et al. Acute ascending necrotizing myelitis in Okinawa caused by herpes simplex virus type 2. Virchows Arch A Pathol Anat Histopathol 1991;418:71–5.
36. Mihai C, Jubelt B. Infectious myelitis. Curr Neurol Neurosci Rep 2012;12: 633–41.
37. Suarez-Calvet M, Rojas-Garcia R, Querol L, et al. Polyradiculoneuropathy associated to human herpesvirus 2 in an HIV-1-infected patient (Elsberg syndrome): case report and literature review. Sex Transm Dis 2010;37:123–5.
38. Eberhardt O, Küker W, Dichgans J, et al. HSV-2 sacral radiculitis (Elsberg syndrome). Neurology 2004;63:758–9.
39. Koskiniemi M, Vaheri A, Taskinen E. Cerebrospinal fluid alterations in herpes simplex virus encephalitis. Rev Infect Dis 1984;6:608–18.
40. Sauerbrei A, Wutzler P. Laboratory diagnosis of central nervous system infections caused by herpesviruses. J Clin Virol 2002;25:45–51.
41. Nakajima H, Furutama D, Kimura F, et al. Herpes simplex virus myelitis: clinical manifestations and diagnosis by the polymerase chain reaction method. Eur Neurol 1998;39:163–7.
42. Kincaid O, Lipton HL. Viral myelitis: an update. Curr Neurol Neurosci Rep 2006; 6:469–74.
43. Nagel M, Forghani B, Mahalingam R, et al. The value of detecting anti-VZV IgG antibody in CSF to diagnose VZV vasculopathy. Neurology 2007;68:1069–73.
44. Eidelberg D, Sotrel A, Vogel H, et al. Progressive polyradiculopathy in acquired immune deficiency syndrome. Neurology 1986;36:912.
45. Fux C, Pfister S, Nohl F, et al. Cytomegalovirus-associated acute transverse myelitis in immunocompetent adults. Clin Microbiol Infect 2003;9:1187–90.
46. Caldas C, Bernicker E, Dal Nogare A, et al. Case report: transverse myelitis associated with Epstein-Barr virus infection. Am J Med Sci 1994;307:45–8.
47. Hill A, Hicks E, Coyle P. Human herpes virus 6 and central nervous system complications. Dev Med Child Neurol 1994;36:651–2.
48. Mihara T, Mutoh T, Yoshikawa T, et al. Postinfectious myeloradiculoneuropathy with cranial nerve involvements associated with human herpesvirus 7 infection. Arch Neurol 2005;62:1755–7.
49. Croda MG, de Oliveira ACP, Vergara MPP, et al. Corticosteroid therapy in TSP/HAM patients: the results from a 10 years open cohort. J Neurol Sci 2008;269: 133–7.
50. Kramer LD, Li J, Shi P-Y. West Nile virus. Lancet Neurol 2007;6:171–81.
51. Ali M, Safriel Y, Sohi J, et al. West Nile virus infection: MR imaging findings in the nervous system. AJNR Am J Neuroradiol 2005;26:289–97.

52. Li J, Loeb JA, Shy ME, et al. Asymmetric flaccid paralysis: a neuromuscular presentation of West Nile virus infection. Ann Neurol 2003;53:703–10.
53. Leis AA, Stokic DS. Neuromuscular manifestations of West Nile virus infection. Front Neurol 2012;3:37.
54. Anderson JF, Rahal JJ. Efficacy of interferon α-2b and ribavirin against West Nile virus in vitro. Emerg Infect Dis 2002;8:107.
55. Van den Hurk AF, Ritchie SA, Mackenzie JS. Ecology and geographical expansion of Japanese encephalitis virus. Annu Rev Entomol 2009;54:17–35.
56. Mackenzie JS, Gubler DJ, Petersen LR. Emerging flaviviruses: the spread and resurgence of Japanese encephalitis, West Nile and dengue viruses. Nat Med 2004;10:S98–109.
57. Lindquist L, Vapalahti O. Tick-borne encephalitis. Lancet 2008;371:1861–71.
58. Kunz C. TBE vaccination and the Austrian experience. Vaccine 2003;21:S50–5.
59. Seet RC, Lim EC, Wilder-Smith EP. Acute transverse myelitis following dengue virus infection. J Clin Virol 2006;35:310–2.
60. Stübgen J-P. Immune-mediated myelitis associated with hepatitis virus infections. J Neuroimmunol 2011;239:21–7.
61. Mécharles S, Herrmann C, Poullain P, et al. Acute myelitis due to Zika virus infection. Lancet 2016;387:1481.
62. Anastasina M, Domanska A, Palm K, et al. Human picornaviruses associated with neurological diseases and their neutralization by antibodies. J Gen Virol 2017;98:1145–58.
63. Ayscue P, Van Haren K, Sheriff H, et al. Acute flaccid paralysis with anterior myelitis—California, June 2012–June 2014. MMWR Morb Mortal Wkly Rep 2014;63:903–6.
64. Takimoto S, Waldman EA, Moreira RC, et al. Enterovirus 71 infection and acute neurological disease among children in Brazil (1988–1990). Trans R Soc Trop Med Hyg 1998;92:25–8.
65. Hayward JC, Gillespie SM, Kaplan KM, et al. Outbreak of poliomyelitis-like paralysis associated with enterovirus 71. Pediatr Infect Dis J 1989;8:611–5.
66. Messacar K, Schreiner TL, Maloney JA, et al. A cluster of acute flaccid paralysis and cranial nerve dysfunction temporally associated with an outbreak of enterovirus D68 in children in Colorado, USA. Lancet 2015;385:1662–71.
67. Chen C-Y, Chang Y-C, Huang C-C, et al. Acute flaccid paralysis in infants and young children with enterovirus 71 infection: MR imaging findings and clinical correlates. AJNR Am J Neuroradiol 2001;22:200–5.
68. Mirand A, Peigue-Lafeuille H. Acute flaccid myelitis and enteroviruses: an ongoing story. Lancet 2015;385:1601–2.
69. Wiznitzer M, Nath A. Acute flaccid myelitis and enterovirus D68: Déjà vu all over again. Neurology 2017;89(2):112–3.
70. Chaves S, Black J, Kennett M, et al. Coxsackie virus A24 infection presenting as acute flaccid paralysis. Lancet 2001;357:605.
71. Ku B, Lee K. Acute transverse myelitis caused by coxsackie virus B4 infection. J Korean Med Sci 1998;13:449–53.
72. Minami K, Tsuda Y, Maeda H, et al. Acute transverse myelitis caused by Coxsackie virus B5 infection. J Paediatr Child Health 2004;40:66–8.
73. Knebusch M, Strassburg HM, Reiners K. Acute transverse myelitis in childhood: nine cases and review of the literature. Dev Med Child Neurol 1998;40:631–9.
74. Breningstall GN, Belani KK. Acute transverse myelitis and brainstem encephalitis associated with hepatitis A infection. Pediatr Neurol 1995;12:169–71.

75. Gessain A, Cassar O. Epidemiological aspects and world distribution of HTLV-1 infection. Front Microbiol 2012;3:388.
76. Bangham CR, Araujo A, Yamano Y, et al. HTLV-1-associated myelopathy/tropical spastic paraparesis. Nat Rev Dis Primers 2015;1:15012.
77. Tanajura D, Castro N, Oliveira P, et al. Neurological manifestations in human T-cell lymphotropic virus type 1 (HTLV-1)–infected individuals without HTLV-1–associated myelopathy/tropical spastic paraparesis: a longitudinal cohort study. Clin Infect Dis 2015;61:49–56.
78. Sato T, Coler-Reilly A, Utsunomiya A, et al. CSF CXCL10, CXCL9, and neopterin as candidate prognostic biomarkers for HTLV-1-associated myelopathy/tropical spastic paraparesis. PLoS Negl Trop Dis 2013;7:e2479.
79. Yamasaki K, Kira J, Koyanagi Y, et al. Long term, high dose interferon-alpha treatment in HTLV-I-associated myelopathy/tropical spastic paraparesis: a combined clinical, virological and immunological study. J Neurol Sci 1997;147: 135–44.
80. Martin F, Castro H, Gabriel C, et al. Ciclosporin A proof of concept study in patients with active, progressive HTLV-1 associated myelopathy/tropical spastic paraparesis. PLoS Negl Trop Dis 2012;6:e1675.
81. Ahmed S, Adonis A, Hilburn S, et al. Treatment of patients with HTLV-1-associated myelopathy with methotrexate. Retrovirology 2014;11:P33.
82. Shirabe S, Nakamura T, Tsujino A, et al. Successful application of pentoxifylline in the treatment of HTLV-I associated myelopathy. J Neurol Sci 1997;151: 97–101.
83. Nakamura T, Matsuo T, Fukuda T, et al. Efficacy of prosultiamine treatment in patients with human T lymphotropic virus type I-associated myelopathy/tropical spastic paraparesis: results from an open-label clinical trial. BMC Med 2013; 11:182.
84. Nakamura T, Satoh K, Fukuda T, et al. Pentosan polysulfate treatment ameliorates motor function with increased serum soluble vascular cell adhesion molecule-1 in HTLV-1-associated neurologic disease. J Neurovirol 2014;20: 269–77.
85. Sato T, Coler-Reilly AL, Yagishita N, et al. Mogamulizumab (Anti-CCR4) in HTLV-1–associated myelopathy. N Engl J Med 2018;378:529–38.
86. Shiels MS, Engels EA. Evolving epidemiology of HIV-associated malignancies. Curr Opin HIV AIDS 2017;12:6–11.
87. Boissé L, Gill MJ, Power C. HIV infection of the central nervous system: clinical features and neuropathogenesis. Neurol Clin 2008;26:799–819.
88. Eugenin EA, Osiecki K, Lopez L, et al. CCL2/monocyte chemoattractant protein-1 mediates enhanced transmigration of human immunodeficiency virus (HIV)-infected leukocytes across the blood–brain barrier: a potential mechanism of HIV–CNS invasion and NeuroAIDS. J Neurosci 2006;26:1098–106.
89. McArthur JC, Steiner J, Sacktor N, et al. Human immunodeficiency virus-associated neurocognitive disorders: mind the gap. Ann Neurol 2010;67: 699–714.
90. Cikurel K, Schiff L, Simpson DM. Pilot study of intravenous immunoglobulin in HIV-associated myelopathy. AIDS Patient Care STDs 2009;23:75–8.
91. Andrade P, Figueiredo C, Carvalho C, et al. Transverse myelitis and acute HIV infection: a case report. BMC Infect Dis 2014;14:149.
92. Denning DW, Anderson J, Rudge P, et al. Acute myelopathy associated with primary infection with human immunodeficiency virus. Br Med J (Clin Res Ed) 1987;294:143–4.

93. Hamada Y, Watanabe K, Aoki T, et al. Primary HIV infection with acute transverse myelitis. Intern Med 2011;50:1615–7.
94. Colley DG, Bustinduy AL, Secor WE, et al. Human schistosomiasis. Lancet 2014;383:2253–64.
95. Ross AG, McManus DP, Farrar J, et al. Neuroschistosomiasis. J Neurol 2012; 259:22–32.
96. Gray DJ, Ross AG, Li Y-S, et al. Diagnosis and management of schistosomiasis. BMJ 2011;342:d2651.
97. Garcia HH, Nash TE, Del Brutto OH. Clinical symptoms, diagnosis, and treatment of neurocysticercosis. Lancet Neurol 2014;13:1202–15.
98. Agrawal R, Chauhan SS, Misra V. Focal spinal intramedullary cysticercosis. Acta Biomed 2008;79:39–41.
99. Del Brutto OH, Garcia HH. Intramedullary cysticercosis of the spinal cord: a review of patients evaluated with MRI. J Neurol Sci 2013;331:114–7.
100. Lee HJ, Kang MS, Kim KH. Intradural spinal cysticercosis: case series. The Nerve 2015;1:20–5. Available at: https://www.thenerve.net/journal/view.php?number=47.
101. Garcia-Gubern C, Fuentes CR, Colon-Rolon L, et al. Spinal cord toxoplasmosis as an unusual presentation of AIDS: case report and review of the literature. Int J Emerg Med 2010;3:439–42.
102. Katchanov J, Sawanyawisuth K, Chotmongkol V, et al. Neurognathostomiasis, a neglected parasitosis of the central nervous system. Emerg Infect Dis 2011;17:1174.
103. Jabbour RA, Kanj SS, Sawaya RA, et al. *Toxocara canis* myelitis: clinical features, magnetic resonance imaging (MRI) findings, and treatment outcome in 17 patients. Medicine 2011;90:337–43.
104. Al Hammoud R, Nayes SL, Murphy JR, et al. *Angiostrongylus cantonensis* meningitis and myelitis, Texas, USA. Emerg Infect Dis 2017;23:1037.
105. Sapkas GS, Machinis TG, Chloros GD, et al. Spinal hydatid disease, a rare but existent pathological entity: case report and review of the literature. South Med J 2006;99:178–84.
106. Işlekel S, Erçşahin Y, Zileli M, et al. Spinal hydatid disease. Spinal Cord 1998;36:166.

Acute Community-Acquired Bacterial Meningitis

Ana Helena A. Figueiredo, MD, Matthijs C. Brouwer, MD, PhD,
Diederik van de Beek, MD, PhD*

KEYWORDS

- Community-acquired bacterial meningitis • Lumbar puncture • Antimicrobial therapy
- Conjugate vaccines • Dexamethasone • Epidemiology

KEY POINTS

- Bacterial meningitis is a disease with high mortality and morbidity. The epidemiology has changed due to the introduction of conjugate vaccines.
- The clinical presentation may vary depending on age, underlying conditions, and severity of illness and lumbar puncture is the procedure of choice for the diagnosis.
- Empirical antibiotic treatment depends on local antibiotic susceptibility patterns of common pathogens.
- Use of adjunctive dexamethasone is recommended in patients with suspected or proven bacterial meningitis in high- or medium-income countries.
- About half of the individuals who survived bacterial meningitis suffer from neurologic deficits, including cognitive impairment.

INTRODUCTION

Bacterial meningitis is an impacting disease with substantial mortality and morbidity worldwide.[1] The introduction of conjugate vaccines and the improvement of treatment over the years reduced the burden of the disease, although it remains a concern in both high- and low-income countries.[2] Community-acquired bacterial meningitis is a neurologic emergency, and early diagnosis and treatment can reduce morbidity and mortality.[3] Here, the authors provide an update on the changing epidemiology

Study Funding: This study has been funded by grants from the Netherlands Organization for Health Research and Development (ZonMw; NWO-Vidi grant 2017.[016.176.308] to M.C. Brouwer, NWO-Vidi grant 2011.[016.116.358] to D. van de Beek), the Academic Medical Center (AMC Fellowship 2008 to D. van de Beek), and the European Research Council (ERC Starting Grant [261178] to D. van de Beek).
Conflicts of Interest: All authors no conflicts.
Amsterdam UMC, University of Amsterdam, Neurology, Amsterdam Neuroscience, Meibergdreef 9, Amsterdam, 1105 AZ Amsterdam, The Netherlands
* Corresponding author.
E-mail address: d.vandebeek@amc.uva.nl

Neurol Clin 36 (2018) 809–820
https://doi.org/10.1016/j.ncl.2018.06.007
0733-8619/18/© 2018 Elsevier Inc. All rights reserved.

neurologic.theclinics.com

and predisposing factors and provide a clinical approach on patients presenting with community-acquired bacterial meningitis.

EPIDEMIOLOGY

In the past 30 years, the epidemiology of bacterial meningitis has changed substantially with a shift in causative pathogens and affected age groups.[2,4] These changes were in part due to the large-scale introduction of conjugated vaccines against *Haemophilus influenzae* type b, *Streptococcus pneumoniae*, and *Neisseria meningitidis*, but also stochastic changes in *N meningitidis* resulted in a sharp decrease in incidence.[5] The major burden of disease is still in sub-Saharan Africa with incidence rates varying between 10 and 40 per 100,000 inhabitants, whereas in the United States and Europe, incidence rate varied between 0.7 and 7.1 per 100,000.[4,6,7] Currently, the predominant causative bacteria worldwide in neonatal meningitis are *Streptococcus agalactiae* (group B streptococcus) and *Escherichia coli*, whereas in children outside the neonatal age, *S pneumoniae* and *N meningitidis* cause most cases.[8] In adults, pneumococcus and meningococcus cause 85% of cases, whereas *Listeria monocytogenes* is the third most common cause, which is most commonly found in the elderly and patients with immunodeficiency, for instance, alcoholics, patients with cancer, and patients using immunosuppressive medication.[9,10] Pneumococcus is now the most common cause of community-acquired bacterial meningitis outside of the neonatal age and is found in 50% to 70% of cases.[4,11] To reduce the burden of pneumococcal disease in general, vaccines have been developed covering a limited number of the more than 90 serotypes that can cause disease in humans. Since 1983, a pneumococcal polysaccharide vaccine including 23 serotypes is available, but because polysaccharide antigens are poorly immunogenic in young children and the elderly, this vaccine had limited effect in the at-risk population.[2] In the early 2000s, a conjugated vaccine containing 7 pneumococcal serotypes (PCV7) was introduced, resulting in a decreased incidence of meningitis caused by vaccine serotypes. This decreased incidence was first observed in children, followed by a decrease in adults caused by herd immunity.[12] Regrettably, following the reduction in vaccine serotype disease, an increase in meningitis due to nonvaccine serotype was observed, reducing the efficacy of the vaccination.[12] Subsequently, 10- and 13-valent vaccines were marketed, which were projected to cover more than 70% of pneumococcal serotypes causing meningitis.[13] Following PCV13 introduction, no dramatic decline in incidence has been observed in the United States and France. The introduction did result in a shift in serotypes toward nonvaccine serotypes.[14,15] Novel approaches to prevention of pneumococcal meningitis are needed, such as a pan-serotype vaccine, because currently available vaccines are not expected to result in a further reduction in incidence.

The meningococcus is the second-most common pathogen in bacterial meningitis in children beyond the neonatal age and adults and is infamous for major outbreaks in sub-Saharan Africa.[1,16] The predominant serogroup differs per continent with serogroup B being the most common in Europe, serogroup Y most common in the United States, and the second in Europe and serogroup A the most common in Africa. Vaccination against serogroup C was started in several countries in Europe following a sharp increase in incidence.[5,17] This vaccine introduction resulted in the virtual disappearance of serogroup C meningitis in these countries.[17] Recent surges in serogroup W disease in the United Kingdom and the Netherlands were observed after which the conjugated serogroup C vaccine was replaced with the tetra-valent serogroup A,C,W,Y vaccine and incidence decreased again.[18] Substantial efforts have been made to reduce the serogroup A meningococcal meningitis incidence in the "meningitis belt," referring to sub-Saharan Africa, where most cases occur. A sharp decrease in serogroup A disease has been observed following the stepwise serogroup A conjugate vaccine introduction in these African countries.[16] The total incidence of meningococcal disease was down by 57%, and serogroup A disease almost completely disappeared.[16] An increase in serogroup W incidence in 2010 and serogroup C in 2015, however, caused a similar number of cases as seen prior during the serogroup A epidemics.[16] Continuous monitoring of meningococcal disease epidemiology and adequate response in vaccination policy are vital to reduce the burden of meningococcal disease. The Advisory Committee on Immunization Practices in the United States recommends that persons aged 16 to 23 years may receive meningococcal vaccine for short-term protection for serogroup B in situational potential exposure, which is not covered in the quadrivalent vaccine (A,C,W,Y) used for routine immunization in the United States.

Other pathogens in bacterial meningitis occurring in less than 10% of adult meningitis cases are L monocytogenes, H influenzae, and Staphylococcus aureus.[19] Listeria meningitis typically occurs in older adults with an immunocompromised state.[10] A longitudinal study of Listeria epidemiology showed the incidence in neonates and pregnant woman has decreased, potentially due to public education on food-borne infections during pregnancy.[20] Furthermore, this study showed the predominant genotype of Listeria is clonal complex 6, which has been associated with poor disease outcome. The proposed mechanism of this clonal expansion was selection of this Listeria genotype through use of industrial disinfectants.[21] H influenzae type b has virtually disappeared as an important cause of meningitis, and nowadays other serotypes and nontypeable H influenzae strains are found as incidental causes of bacterial meningitis. It has been associated with ear or sinus infection as predisposing condition and generally has a good outcome.[22] S aureus is found in approximately 2% of adult meningitis cases and is frequently associated with concomitant endocarditis.[19,23] Streptococcus suis is the major pathogen of bacterial meningitis in South-East Asia and has been associated with contact with pigs.[24]

PREDISPOSING FACTORS

Bacterial meningitis occurs more frequently in persons with defects of the immune system, both inborn and acquired, and anatomic defects of the natural barriers of the central nervous system.[25] Immunodeficiency can be due to an immature immune system in children under 2 years of age, immunosenescence in the elderly, but also comorbid conditions such as splenectomy or asplenic states, diabetes mellitus, infections with human immunodeficiency virus, alcoholism, cancer, and use of immunosuppressive drugs.[25–30] Genetic association studies have identified several genetic deficiencies increasing the susceptibility to pneumococcal and meningococcal infections.[31] Rare genetic variations were found to result in a high risk of recurrent infections due to these pathogens, whereas population-based studies showed common genetic variants in the complement system result in a moderately increased susceptibility to meningitis.[31,32] Leakage of cerebrospinal fluid (CSF), either following surgery, after trauma, or due to inborn anatomic defects, poses a high risk of meningitis, causing an easy entry to the central nervous system for bacteria from the nasopharynx. In patients with recurrent meningitis, the search for CSF leaks should involve ears, nose, and throat consultation and cranial imaging to identify bony defects.[33]

CLINICAL PRESENTATION

Early diagnosis and rapid initiation of appropriate therapy are the keys in patients with suspected community-acquired bacterial meningitis. The clinical presentation may vary depending on age, underlying conditions, and severity of illness.[1,34,35] Infants may become irritable or lethargic, may stop feeding, and are found to have a bulging fontanelle, separation of the cranial sutures, meningism, and opisthotonos, and they may develop convulsions.[11] These findings are uncommon in neonates, who sometimes present only with respiratory distress, diarrhea, or jaundice.[11] Clinical findings of meningitis in young children are often minimal, and in childhood bacterial meningitis, classical symptoms, such as headache, fever, nuchal rigidity, and altered mental status, may be less common than in younger and middle-aged adults.[19,36] Elderly patients with bacterial meningitis often present with classic symptoms of bacterial meningitis.[35] However, in a prospective study on adults with bacterial meningitis, the classic triad of signs and symptoms consisting of fever, nuchal rigidity, and altered mental status was present in only 44% of the patients.[36] Certain clinical features may predict the bacterial cause of meningitis.[37] Rashes occur more frequently in patients with meningococcal meningitis, with reported sensitivities of 63% to 80% and with specificities of 83% to 92%.[1,38,39]

THERAPEUTIC APPROACH

Dilemmas remain for physicians who need to accurately diagnose patients with bacterial meningitis and administer antibiotics and adjunctive therapies rapidly for this life-threatening disease.[3] Once an initial patient evaluation has been completed with history and physical findings, lumbar puncture is the diagnostic procedure of choice for diagnosis of bacterial meningitis.[40] The diagnostic accuracy of the findings in history and physical examinations is reviewed elsewhere.[41] Fever, stiff neck, and change in mental status are the classic triad. About 95% will have 2 of the 4 of fever, stiff neck, altered mental status, or headache. Characteristic findings in the CSF are typically used to make the diagnosis of meningitis. Classically described, the white blood cell count in bacterial meningitis is typically greater than 1000 cells/μL, whereas in viral meningitis, it is less than 300 cells/μL, although considerable overlap exists.[42]

The measurement of protein and glucose is an important aspect of CSF analysis because abnormal protein and glucose levels are typically found in bacterial disease but are relatively normal in many cases of viral meningitis.[41] However, data in the literature concerning guidelines for predicting bacterial disease are derived mainly from pediatric patients, with several multiple retrospective models using logistic equations and other mathematical modeling[43]; however, none have yet proved robust enough for widespread clinical practice.[3]

With the urgent nature of this testing to make the diagnosis of meningitis, one of the issues physicians are faced with in an emergency department setting is whether neuroimaging is required before lumbar puncture.[34] A recent study showed that lumbar puncture can be performed safely in the large majority of patients with bacterial meningitis, because it is only very rarely complicated by cerebral herniation.[44] One set of recommendations for emergency department brain computed tomographic (CT) scanning before lumbar puncture is based on a prospective study from the United States involving 301 adult patients with suspected meningitis.[45] Items associated with abnormal CT scan included age greater than 60, altered mental status, gaze or facial palsy, abnormal language or inability to answer 2 questions or follow 2 commands, immunocompromised status, history of central nervous system disease, recent seizure, visual field abnormalities, and arm or leg drift. This study showed that if none of these features were present, there was a negative predictive value of 97% for an intracranial abnormality, confirming that clinical features can be used to identify patients who are unlikely to have abnormal findings on brain CT.

The authors think it is reasonable proceed with lumbar puncture without a CT scan if the patient does not meet any of the following: patients who have new-onset seizures, an immunocompromised status, signs that are suspicious for space-occupying lesions (papilledema or focal neurologic signs, not including cranial nerve palsy), or moderate to severe impairment of consciousness.[8,40] In other patients, cranial CT can be considered a screening method for contraindications for lumbar puncture, but one should realize that the interrater reliability of this assessment is moderate only.[44]

Gram staining and culture of CSF can identify the causative pathogen in approximately 80% of the patients.[1] The sensitivity of bacterial antigen tests is limited.[1] A promising diagnostic tool in cases of suspected bacterial meningitis and negative CSF cultures is the amplification of bacterial DNA by polymerase chain reaction.[1] A recent development is the introduction of multiplex kits for pathogen detection. Although high diagnostic sensitivity and specificity have been reported, further refinements and particularly a reduction of the false-positive rates and cost-effectiveness studies are needed before these kits are recommended in the diagnosis of bacterial meningitis.[46]

DIFFERENTIAL DIAGNOSIS

The differential diagnosis of the triad of fever, headache, and stiff neck is bacterial or viral meningitis, fungal meningitis, tuberculous meningitis, drug-induced aseptic meningitis, carcinomatous or lymphomatous meningitis, aseptic meningitis associated with inflammatory diseases (systemic lupus erythematosus, sarcoidosis, Behçet disease, Sjögren syndrome), and, when temperature is only moderately elevated and onset of headache is acute, subarachnoid hemorrhage.[47] When an impaired level of consciousness, focal neurologic deficits, or new-onset seizure activity are added to the classic triad, the differential diagnosis includes viral encephalitis, venous sinus thrombosis, tick-borne bacterial infections depending on geographic area (Borrelia and Ehrlichia infections in North America and Europe, Rocky Mountain spotted fever in North America), brain abscess, and subdural empyema.[48,49]

TREATMENT
Antibiotics

A delay in antimicrobial therapy (eg, due to cranial CT or transfer to another hospital) has been associated with an increased risk for adverse clinical outcome in community-acquired bacterial meningitis.[50,51] Therefore, if imaging precedes lumbar puncture, blood cultures should be drawn and antimicrobial therapy with adjunctive dexamethasone initiated before imaging is performed.

Empirical antibiotic treatment should be based on the most common bacterial species that cause the disease according to the patient's age group, clinical setting, epidemiology, and local antibiotic susceptibility patterns of the predominant pathogens (**Table 1**).[52] Neonatal meningitis is largely caused by group B streptococci, E coli, and L monocytogenes.[20,52,53] Initial treatment, therefore, should consist of penicillin or ampicillin plus a third-generation cephalosporin, preferably cefotaxime or ceftriaxone, or penicillin or ampicillin and an aminoglycoside.[8] Empirical coverage with a third-generation cephalosporin (cefotaxime or ceftriaxone) at appropriate doses for meningitis is recommended based on a broad spectrum of activity and excellent

Table 1
Recommendations for empiric antimicrobial therapy in suspected community-acquired bacterial meningitis

Predisposing Factor	Common Bacterial Pathogens	Initial Intravenous Antibiotic Therapy
Age		
<1 mo	S agalactiae, E coli, L monocytogenes	Ampicillin plus cefotaxime or an aminoglycoside
1–3 mo	S pneumoniae, N meningitidis, S agalactiae, H influenzae, E coli, L monocytogenes	Ampicillin plus vancomycin plus ceftriaxone or cefotaxime[a]
3–23 mo	S pneumoniae, N meningitidis, S agalactiae, H influenzae, E coli	Vancomycin plus ceftriaxone or cefotaxime[a]
2–50 y	N meningitidis, S pneumoniae	Vancomycin plus ceftriaxone or cefotaxime[a]
>50 y	N meningitidis, S pneumoniae, L monocytogenes, aerobic gram-negative bacilli	Vancomycin plus ceftriaxone or cefotaxime plus ampicillin[b]
With risk factor present[c]	S. pneumoniae, L monocytogenes, H influenzae	Vancomycin plus ceftriaxone or cefotaxime plus ampicillin[b]

[a] In areas with very low penicillin-resistance rates, monotherapy penicillin may be considered.
[b] In areas with very low penicillin-resistance and cephalosporin-resistance rates, combination treatment of amoxicillin and third-generation cephalosporin may be considered.
[c] Alcoholism, altered immune status.
Adapted from van de Beek D, Brouwer MC, Thwaites GE, et al. Advances in treatment of bacterial meningitis. Lancet 2012;380(9854):1694; with permission.

penetration into the CSF during inflammatory conditions.[52] Because of the worldwide emergence of multi-drug-resistant strains of S pneumoniae, vancomycin is added to the initial empirical antimicrobial regimen in adult patients.[8,54] In addition, in patients aged greater than 50 years, treatment with ampicillin should be added to the above antibiotic regimen for additional coverage of L monocytogenes, which is more prevalent among this age group.[10] Although no clinical data on the efficacy of rifampin in patients with pneumococcal meningitis are available, some experts would recommend the use of rifampicin, based on its susceptibility, in combination with a third-generation cephalosporin, with or without vancomycin, in patients with pneumococcal meningitis caused by bacterial strains that, on the basis of local epidemiology, are likely to be highly resistant to penicillin or cephalosporins.

Adjunctive Dexamethasone Therapy

Experimental animal models have shown that dexamethasone inhibits the production of tumor necrosis factor-α and interleukin-1, reverses development of brain edema, and limits the increase in CSF lactate and leukocyte concentrations.[55] Since publication of the experimental studies, several controlled randomized clinical trials have been performed to determine whether adjunctive steroid therapy is beneficial in children with bacterial meningitis. Initial results showed that the main beneficial effect of dexamethasone was to reduce the risk of hearing loss in children with H influenzae type b meningitis.[56] Additional data extended the likely benefit to children with pneumococcal meningitis.[57] Subsequent large randomized controlled trials in Malawian and South American children did not show benefit of this adjunctive therapy.[58,59] A Cochrane meta-analysis showed that adjunctive dexamethasone treatment did not influence overall mortality but did decrease hearing loss in surviving children with bacterial meningitis. In low-income countries, no benefit of dexamethasone was established in this meta-analysis.[60]

For adults with bacterial meningitis, results of a European randomized controlled trial showed that adjunctive dexamethasone, given before or with the first dose of antimicrobial therapy, was associated with a reduced risk of unfavorable outcome and mortality.[61] The beneficial effect was most apparent in adults with pneumococcal meningitis, in whom mortality was decreased from 34% to 14%. In this subgroup, dexamethasone prevented death due to a reduction of systemic and cerebral complications.[62] A follow-up study showed that the survival benefit from adjunctive dexamethasone therapy is obtained in the acute phase of the disease and remains for years.[63]

In 2004, a meta-analysis of 5 randomized controlled trials showed that treatment with corticosteroids reduced both mortality and neurologic sequelae in adults with bacterial meningitis.[64] However, subsequent randomized controlled trials from Malawi and Vietnam did not show that dexamethasone benefited adults.[65,66] In Vietnam, dexamethasone was associated with a decreased rate of mortality for patients with microbiologically confirmed disease.[66] An individual patient data meta-analysis showed that dexamethasone treatment reduced the rate of hearing loss irrespective of antibiotic pretreatment.[67]

European Society of Clinical Microbiology and Infectious Diseases/Infections Diseases Society of America guidelines recommend the use of adjunctive dexamethasone in patients with suspected or proven bacterial meningitis, but only in high-income countries.[8,54] The advised dexamethasone regimen is 0.6 mg/kg of body weight intravenously (IV) daily for children, and 10 mg IV given every 6 hours for adults, with the first dose being preferably given before or with the first dose of antimicrobials, for 4 days.[8,54]

The implementation of adjunctive dexamethasone therapy has led to decreased rates of unfavorable outcome and death throughout Europe and the United States.[6,19,39,68] In a prospective nationwide cohort study in the Netherlands, the drug was administered in 92% of meningitis episodes, in the period 2006 to 2009. An observational study reported a decline of mortality from 30% to 20% after the introduction of adjunctive dexamethasone therapy (P = .001).[68] The decline in mortality was observed across the whole study population but was more prominent in patients who received dexamethasone.[19]

Use of adjunctive dexamethasone has been reported to predispose patients with bacterial meningitis to a new complication, delayed cerebral thrombosis.[69,70] Pathology suggests an immunologic reaction targeting cerebral blood vessels, possibly complement mediated,[70,71] with vascular inflammation, thromboembolism of large arteries, and infectious intracranial aneurysms.[72] Pneumococcal cell wall components can be observed for weeks after pneumococcal meningitis and may be a source of resurging inflammation after the initial immunosuppression by dexamethasone.[72]

OUTCOME

Reported case fatality rates vary with age, causative pathogen, and income status.[73] Meningitis caused by S pneumoniae has the highest case fatality rates: 20% to 37% for high-income countries and up to 50% for low-income countries.[73,74] Meningococcal meningitis fatality rates are much lower: between 3% and 10% for high- and low-income countries.[74] Neurologic sequelae have been estimated to occur in a substantial number of surviving patients: about half of survivors suffer from focal neurologic deficits.[73] Most frequently reported sequelae are focal neurologic deficits, hearing loss, cognitive impairment, and epilepsy. Adults with pneumococcal meningitis have the highest risk of developing focal neurologic deficits, commonly caused by cerebral infarction,[75] but can also be due to subdural empyema,[49] cerebral abscess,[76] or intracerebral bleeding.[77] Focal deficits may improve during clinical course and even after discharge, but a proportion of patients will have persisting focal neurologic deficits that often interfere in the patient's daily life. Hearing loss occurs in a high proportion of patients with pneumococcal meningitis and has been associated with coexisting otitis.[78] Children and adults recovering from bacterial meningitis are at risk for long-term cognitive deficits.[79,80] Although corticosteroids may potentiate ischemic and apoptotic injury to neurons, treatment with adjunctive dexamethasone did not increase risk for long-term cognitive impairment.[81] Costs associated with post–meningitis sequelae have an important economic impact on health care systems.[2,82]

REFERENCES

1. Brouwer MC, Tunkel AR, van de Beek D. Epidemiology, diagnosis, and antimicrobial treatment of acute bacterial meningitis. Clin Microbiol Rev 2010;23(3): 467–92.

2. McIntyre PB, O'Brien KL, Greenwood B, et al. Effect of vaccines on bacterial meningitis worldwide. Lancet 2012;380(9854):1703–11.

3. Brouwer MC, Thwaites GE, Tunkel AR, et al. Dilemmas in the diagnosis of acute community-acquired bacterial meningitis. Lancet 2012;380(9854):1684–92.

4. Brouwer MC, van de Beek D. Epidemiology of community-acquired bacterial meningitis. Curr Opin Infect Dis 2018;31(1):78–84.

5. Bijlsma MW, Bekker V, Brouwer MC, et al. Epidemiology of invasive meningococcal disease in the Netherlands, 1960-2012: an analysis of national surveillance data. Lancet Infect Dis 2014;14(9):805-12.

6. Castelblanco RL, Lee M, Hasbun R. Epidemiology of bacterial meningitis in the USA from 1997 to 2010: a population-based observational study. Lancet Infect Dis 2014;14(9):813-9.

7. Paradowska-Stankiewicz I, Piotrowska A. Meningitis and encephalitis in Poland in 2015. Przegl Epidemiol 2017;71(4):493-500.

8. van de Beek D, Cabellos C, Dzupova O, et al. ESCMID guideline: diagnosis and treatment of acute bacterial meningitis. Clin Microbiol Infect 2016;22(Suppl 3): S37-62.

9. van Ettekoven CN, van de Beek D, Brouwer MC. Update on community-acquired bacterial meningitis: guidance and challenges. Clin Microbiol Infect 2017;23(9): 601-6.

10. Koopmans MM, Brouwer MC, Bijlsma MW, et al. Listeria monocytogenes sequence type 6 and increased rate of unfavorable outcome in meningitis: epidemiologic cohort study. Clin Infect Dis 2013;57(2):247-53.

11. van de Beek D, Brouwer M, Hasbun R, et al. Community-acquired bacterial meningitis. Nat Rev Dis Primers 2016;2:16074.

12. Hsu HE, Shutt KA, Moore MR, et al. Effect of pneumococcal conjugate vaccine on pneumococcal meningitis. N Engl J Med 2009;360(3):244-56.

13. Johnson HL, Deloria-Knoll M, Levine OS, et al. Systematic evaluation of serotypes causing invasive pneumococcal disease among children under five: the pneumococcal global serotype project. PLoS Med 2010;7(10):1-13, e1000348.

14. Olarte L, Barson WJ, Barson RM, et al. Impact of the 13-valent pneumococcal conjugate vaccine on pneumococcal meningitis in US children. Clin Infect Dis 2015;61(5):767-75.

15. Alari A, Chaussade H, Domenech De Celles M, et al. Impact of pneumococcal conjugate vaccines on pneumococcal meningitis cases in France between 2001 and 2014: a time series analysis. BMC Med 2016;14(1):211.

16. Trotter CL, Lingani C, Fernandez K, et al. Impact of MenAfriVac in nine countries of the African meningitis belt, 2010-15: an analysis of surveillance data. Lancet Infect Dis 2017;17(8):867-72.

17. Whittaker R, Dias JG, Ramliden M, et al. The epidemiology of invasive meningococcal disease in EU/EEA countries, 2004-2014. Vaccine 2017;35(16):2034-41.

18. Campbell H, Edelstein M, Andrews N, et al. Emergency meningococcal ACWY vaccination program for teenagers to control group W meningococcal disease, England, 2015-2016. Emerg Infect Dis 2017;23(7):1184-7.

19. Bijlsma MW, Brouwer MC, Kasanmoentalib ES, et al. Community-acquired bacterial meningitis in adults in the Netherlands, 2006-14: a prospective cohort study. Lancet Infect Dis 2016;16(3):339-47.

20. Koopmans MM, Bijlsma MW, Brouwer MC, et al. Listeria monocytogenes meningitis in the Netherlands, 1985-2014: a nationwide surveillance study. J Infect 2017;75(1):12-9.

21. Kremer PH, Lees JA, Koopmans MM, et al. Benzalkonium tolerance genes and outcome in Listeria monocytogenes meningitis. Clin Microbiol Infect 2017;23(4): 265.e1-e7.

22. Brouwer MC, van de Beek D, Heckenberg SG, et al. Community-acquired Haemophilus influenzae meningitis in adults. Clin Microbiol Infect 2007;13(4):439-42.

23. Lucas MJ, Brouwer MC, van der Ende A, et al. Endocarditis in adults with bacterial meningitis. Circulation 2013;127(20):2056-62.

24. van Samkar A, Brouwer MC, Schultsz C, et al. Streptococcus suis meningitis: a systematic review and meta-analysis. PLoS Negl Trop Dis 2015;9(10):e0004191.
25. Adriani KS, Brouwer MC, van de Beek D. Risk factors for community-acquired bacterial meningitis in adults. Neth J Med 2015;73(2):53–60.
26. van Veen KE, Brouwer MC, van der Ende A, et al. Bacterial meningitis in alcoholic patients: a population-based prospective study. J Infect 2017;74(4):352–7.
27. van Veen KE, Brouwer MC, van der Ende A, et al. Bacterial meningitis in diabetes patients: a population-based prospective study. Sci Rep 2016;6:36996.
28. van Veen KEB, Brouwer MC, van der Ende A, et al. Bacterial meningitis in patients using immunosuppressive medication: a population-based prospective nationwide study. J Neuroimmune Pharmacol 2017;12(2):213–8.
29. van Veen KE, Brouwer MC, van der Ende A, et al. Bacterial meningitis in patients with HIV: a population-based prospective study. J Infect 2016;72(3):362–8.
30. Costerus JM, Brouwer MC, van der Ende A, et al. Community-acquired bacterial meningitis in adults with cancer or a history of cancer. Neurology 2016;86(9): 860–6.
31. Brouwer MC, de Gans J, Heckenberg SG, et al. Host genetic susceptibility to pneumococcal and meningococcal disease: a systematic review and meta-analysis. Lancet Infect Dis 2009;9(1):31–44.
32. Adriani KS, Brouwer MC, Geldhoff M, et al. Common polymorphisms in the complement system and susceptiblity to bacterial meningitis. J Infect 2013;66(3): 255–62.
33. Adriani KS, van de Beek D, Brouwer MC, et al. Community-acquired recurrent bacterial meningitis in adults. Clin Infect Dis 2007;45(5):e46–51.
34. van de Beek D, de Gans J, Tunkel AR, et al. Community-acquired bacterial meningitis in adults. N Engl J Med 2006;354(1):44–53.
35. Weisfelt M, van de Beek D, Spanjaard L, et al. Community-acquired bacterial meningitis in older people. J Am Geriatr Soc 2006;54(10):1500–7.
36. van de Beek D, de Gans J, Spanjaard L, et al. Clinical features and prognostic factors in adults with bacterial meningitis. N Engl J Med 2004;351(18):1849–59.
37. Weisfelt M, van de Beek D, Spanjaard L, et al. Clinical features, complications, and outcome in adults with pneumococcal meningitis: a prospective case series. Lancet Neurol 2006;5(2):123–9.
38. Weisfelt M, de Gans J, van der Poll T, et al. Pneumococcal meningitis in adults: new approaches to management and prevention. Lancet Neurol 2006;5(4): 332–42.
39. Heckenberg SG, Brouwer MC, van der Ende A, et al. Adjunctive dexamethasone in adults with meningococcal meningitis. Neurology 2012;79(15):1563–9.
40. Costerus JM, Brouwer MC, van de Beek D. Technological advances and changing indications for lumbar puncture in neurological disorders. Lancet Neurol 2018;17(3):268–78.
41. Fitch MT, van de Beek D. Emergency diagnosis and treatment of adult meningitis. Lancet Infect Dis 2007;7(3):191–200.
42. Khatib U, van de Beek D, Lees JA, et al. Adults with suspected central nervous system infection: a prospective study of diagnostic accuracy. J Infect 2017;74(1): 1–9.
43. Nigrovic LE, Kuppermann N, Macias CG, et al. Clinical prediction rule for identifying children with cerebrospinal fluid pleocytosis at very low risk of bacterial meningitis. JAMA 2007;297(1):52–60.

44. Costerus JM, Brouwer MC, Sprengers MES, et al. Cranial CT, Lumbar puncture, and clinical deterioration in bacterial meningitis: a nationwide cohort study. Clin Infect Dis 2018;1–7.

45. Hasbun R, Abrahams J, Jekel J, et al. Computed tomography of the head before lumbar puncture in adults with suspected meningitis. N Engl J Med 2001;345(24): 1727–33.

46. Leber AL, Everhart K, Balada-Llasat JM, et al. Multicenter evaluation of BioFire FilmArray meningitis/encephalitis panel for detection of bacteria, viruses, and yeast in cerebrospinal fluid specimens. J Clin Microbiol 2016;54(9):2251–61.

47. Schut ES, de Gans J, van de Beek D. Community-acquired bacterial meningitis in adults. Pract Neurol 2008;8(1):8–23.

48. Brouwer MC, Tunkel AR, McKhann GM 2nd, et al. Brain abscess. N Engl J Med 2014;371(5):447–56.

49. Jim KK, Brouwer MC, van der Ende A, et al. Subdural empyema in bacterial meningitis. Neurology 2012;79(21):2133–9.

50. Aronin SI, Peduzzi P, Quagliarello VJ. Community-acquired bacterial meningitis: risk stratification for adverse clinical outcome and effect of antibiotic timing. Ann Intern Med 1998;129(11):862–9.

51. Proulx N, Frechette D, Toye B, et al. Delays in the administration of antibiotics are associated with mortality from adult acute bacterial meningitis. QJM 2005;98(4): 291–8.

52. van de Beek D, Brouwer MC, Thwaites GE, et al. Advances in treatment of bacterial meningitis. Lancet 2012;380(9854):1693–702.

53. Bekker V, Bijlsma MW, van de Beek D, et al. Incidence of invasive group B streptococcal disease and pathogen genotype distribution in newborn babies in the Netherlands over 25 years: a nationwide surveillance study. Lancet Infect Dis 2014;14(11):1083–9.

54. Tunkel AR, Hartman BJ, Kaplan SL, et al. Practice guidelines for the management of bacterial meningitis. Clin Infect Dis 2004;39(9):1267–84.

55. Mook-Kanamori BB, Geldhoff M, van der Poll T, et al. Pathogenesis and pathophysiology of pneumococcal meningitis. Clin Microbiol Rev 2011;24(3):557–91.

56. van de Beek D, de Gans J, McIntyre P, et al. Corticosteroids in acute bacterial meningitis. Cochrane Database Syst Rev 2003;(3):CD004405.

57. van de Beek D, de Gans J. Dexamethasone in adults with community-acquired bacterial meningitis. Drugs 2006;66(4):415–27.

58. Molyneux EM, Walsh AL, Forsyth H, et al. Dexamethasone treatment in childhood bacterial meningitis in Malawi: a randomised controlled trial. Lancet 2002; 360(9328):211–8.

59. Peltola H, Roine I, Fernandez J, et al. Adjuvant glycerol and/or dexamethasone to improve the outcomes of childhood bacterial meningitis: a prospective, randomized, double-blind, placebo-controlled trial. Clin Infect Dis 2007;45(10):1277–86.

60. Brouwer MC, McIntyre P, Prasad K, et al. Corticosteroids for acute bacterial meningitis. Cochrane Database Syst Rev 2015;(9):CD004405.

61. de Gans J, van de Beek D, European Dexamethasone in Adulthood Bacterial Meningitis Study I. Dexamethasone in adults with bacterial meningitis. N Engl J Med 2002;347(20):1549–56.

62. van de Beek D, de Gans J. Dexamethasone and pneumococcal meningitis. Ann Intern Med 2004;141(4):327.

63. Fritz D, Brouwer MC, van de Beek D. Dexamethasone and long-term survival in bacterial meningitis. Neurology 2012;79(22):2177–9.

64. van de Beek D, de Gans J, McIntyre P, et al. Steroids in adults with acute bacterial meningitis: a systematic review. Lancet Infect Dis 2004;4(3):139–43.
65. Scarborough M, Gordon SB, Whitty CJ, et al. Corticosteroids for bacterial meningitis in adults in sub-Saharan Africa. N Engl J Med 2007;357(24):2441–50.
66. Nguyen TH, Tran TH, Thwaites G, et al. Dexamethasone in Vietnamese adolescents and adults with bacterial meningitis. N Engl J Med 2007;357(24):2431–40.
67. van de Beek D, Farrar JJ, de Gans J, et al. Adjunctive dexamethasone in bacterial meningitis: a meta-analysis of individual patient data. Lancet Neurol 2010; 9(3):254.
68. Brouwer MC, Heckenberg SG, de Gans J, et al. Nationwide implementation of adjunctive dexamethasone therapy for pneumococcal meningitis. Neurology 2010;75(17):1533–9.
69. Schut ES, Brouwer MC, de Gans J, et al. Delayed cerebral thrombosis after initial good recovery from pneumococcal meningitis. Neurology 2009;73(23):1988–95.
70. Lucas MJ, Brouwer MC, van de Beek D. Delayed cerebral thrombosis in bacterial meningitis: a prospective cohort study. Intensive Care Med 2013;39(5):866–71.
71. Engelen-Lee JY, Brouwer MC, Aronica E, et al. Pneumococcal meningitis: clinical-pathological correlations (MeninGene-Path). Acta Neuropathol Commun 2016;4:26.
72. Engelen-Lee JY, Brouwer MC, Aronica E, et al. Delayed cerebral thrombosis complicating pneumococcal meningitis: an autopsy study. Ann Intensive Care 2018;8(1):20.
73. Lucas MJ, Brouwer MC, van de Beek D. Neurological sequelae of bacterial meningitis. J Infect 2016;73(1):18–27.
74. Schut ES, Brouwer MC, Scarborough M, et al. Validation of a Dutch risk score predicting poor outcome in adults with bacterial meningitis in Vietnam and Malawi. PLoS One 2012;7(3):e34311.
75. Schut ES, Lucas MJ, Brouwer MC, et al. Cerebral infarction in adults with bacterial meningitis. Neurocrit Care 2012;16(3):421–7.
76. Jim KK, Brouwer MC, van der Ende A, et al. Cerebral abscesses in patients with bacterial meningitis. J Infect 2012;64(2):236–8.
77. Mook-Kanamori BB, Fritz D, Brouwer MC, et al. Intracerebral hemorrhages in adults with community associated bacterial meningitis in adults: should we reconsider anticoagulant therapy? PLoS One 2012;7(9):e45271.
78. Heckenberg SG, Brouwer MC, van der Ende A, et al. Hearing loss in adults surviving pneumococcal meningitis is associated with otitis and pneumococcal serotype. Clin Microbiol Infect 2012;18(9):849–55.
79. van de Beek D, Schmand B, de Gans J, et al. Cognitive impairment in adults with good recovery after bacterial meningitis. J Infect Dis 2002;186(7):1047–52.
80. Hoogman M, van de Beek D, Weisfelt M, et al. Cognitive outcome in adults after bacterial meningitis. J Neurol Neurosurg Psychiatry 2007;78(10):1092–6.
81. Weisfelt M, Hoogman M, van de Beek D, et al. Dexamethasone and long-term outcome in adults with bacterial meningitis. Ann Neurol 2006;60(4):456–68.
82. Alvis-Zakzuk N, Carrasquilla-Sotomayor M, Alvis-Guzman N, et al. Economic costs of bacterial meningitis: a systematic review. Value Health 2015;18(7):A807.

Neuroborreliosis

John J. Halperin, MD[a,b],*

KEYWORDS

- Lyme • Neuroborreliosis • *Borrelia burgdorferi* • *Borreliella*
- Mononeuropathy multiplex • Radiculoneuritis • Diagnosis • Treatment

KEY POINTS

- Nervous system Lyme disease, or Lyme neuroborreliosis (LNB), is qualitatively similar in Europe and the United States.
- Common manifestations include lymphocytic meningitis, cranial neuritis (particularly facial nerve palsy), painful radiculitis, and other forms of mononeuropathy multiplex.
- Cerebrospinal fluid (CSF) may be informative in central nervous system (CNS) infection, with a pleocytosis and often with intrathecal production of specific antibody (ITAb).
- ITAb measurement is a quite specific marker of CNS infection, past or present. CSF leukocyte count and potentially CXCL13 concentration are better markers of active infection.
- CNS LNB causes meningitis, a pseudotumor-like picture in children and rarely parenchymal inflammation of the brain or spinal cord.

INTRODUCTION

Perceptions of neuroborreliosis bring to mind Charles Lutwidge Dodgson's (AKA Lewis Carroll) "Through the Looking Glass," both because of alternative logic and because of the apparent wide application of one of Humpty Dumpty's many brilliant assertions that "When I use a word it means just what I choose it to mean—neither more nor less." Recent years have seen significant refinements in our understanding of Lyme disease in general and nervous system involvement in particular. Yet confusion remains due in large part to misinterpretation of a wide range of clinical phenomena as evidence of neurologic disease. A useful starting point is to define terms.

Disclosure: No commercial conflict. Occasional testimony in medical malpractice cases defending physicians in relation to Lyme disease diagnosis or treatment.
[a] Department of Neurosciences, Overlook Medical Center, 99 Beauvoir Avenue, Summit, NJ 07902, USA; [b] Sidney Kimmel Medical College, Thomas Jefferson University, 1025 Walnut Street, Philadelphia, PA 19107, USA
* Corresponding author. Department of Neurosciences, Overlook Medical Center, 99 Beauvoir Avenue, Summit, NJ 07902.
E-mail address: John.halperin@atlantichealth.org

Neurol Clin 36 (2018) 821–830
https://doi.org/10.1016/j.ncl.2018.06.006
0733-8619/18/© 2018 Elsevier Inc. All rights reserved.

neurologic.theclinics.com

HISTORIC BACKGROUND

The nervous system manifestations of infection with the tick-borne spirochetes, collectively referred to as *Borrelia burgdorferi sensu lato*, were first described in 1922 by Garin and Bujadoux. A sheep farmer and retired French Foreign Legionnaire developed acute multisegmental radicular pain coupled with dermatomal muscle weakness and atrophy and a cerebrospinal fluid (CSF) pleocytosis following a bite by a hard-shelled *Ixodes* tick. Based on a faintly positive reaginic test for syphilis, the investigators surmised this was caused by a tick-borne spirochete, treated the patient with arsenic, and symptoms rapidly improved.[1] Following the description of a large series of such patients by Bannwarth[2] (whose paper's title included mention of "rheumatism"), this became known as either Garin-Bujadoux-Bannwarth syndrome or more simply Bannwarth syndrome. Although European clinicians demonstrated that the disorder responded to penicillin in the 1950s, it was fully 6 decades after the initial report that the causative organism was identified—initially in the United States, where a similar clinical syndrome had been identified in the 1970s in relation to Lyme arthritis.[3] Further work led to the identification of *Borrelia burgdorferi sensu stricto*, virtually the only etiologic agent in the United States, and *Borrelia afzelii* and *Borrelia garinii*, the causative agents for most cases in Europe. The various story lines resulted in multiple names for these closely related nervous system disorders. Because the US infection was initially identified in relation to Lyme disease, the rheumatologic disorder occurring in children in Lyme, Connecticut, the preferred US term has been nervous system Lyme disease. European terminology evolved from Bannwarth syndrome, to neuroborreliosis, and now to Lyme neuroborreliosis (LNB). Although much has been made of the differences between European and North American LNB, there seems to be a convergence of opinion that the clinical phenomena are more similar than different[4]; hence the term LNB will be used here to describe both.

This simplification has several limitations. It is now known that there are additional pathogenic *Borrelia*, including *Borrelia miyamotoi* (which causes a relapsing fever-like illness[5]), *Borrelia mayonii* (identified in 6 patients in the upper Midwest with a Lyme disease–like illness but no nervous system involvement to date[6]), and *Borrelia bavariensis* in Europe. Some of these newer pathogens cause Lyme disease–like symptoms, whereas others are more akin to the relapsing fevers. This, combined with a greater understanding of the organisms' genomes, has resulted in creation of a new genus,[7] *Borreliella*, subsuming *B burgdorferi sensu stricto*, *B garinii*, *B afzelii*, and others, now distinguished from the relapsing feverlike organisms, which retain the name *Borrelia*. The group overall has now been divorced from the *Spirochaetaceae* and assigned to the new family *Borreliaceae*. What this does to the term "borreliosis" is a work in progress. The good news is that none of the newer *Borreliella* seems to cause nervous system involvement in immunocompetent humans; so for now the term "neuroborreliosis" will be retained as incorporating both North American nervous system Lyme disease and European LNB.

LYME DISEASE: CLINICAL

In Europe, the extracutaneous manifestations of this disorder were long viewed as primarily neurologic. In the United States, LNB was identified as an add-on to what was initially viewed as a pediatric rheumatologic disorder, then a multisystem infectious disease, and only subsequently one with fairly characteristic nervous system involvement. For that reason, understanding the broader clinical context is essential.

Lyme disease is a zoonosis—an infection that bridges multiple species. The causative pathogens detailed earlier—*B burgdorferi*, *B afzelii,* and *B garinii*—require a reservoir host, capable of sustaining a prolonged, relatively asymptomatic spirochete-mia. Human infection requires a vector capable of feeding on both reservoir hosts and humans and, in between, harboring the infection in a way that permits trans-species infection. The only vectors that meet this requirement are hard-shelled *Ixodes* ticks—primarily *Ixodes scapularis* in the United States, commonly known as the deer or bear tick, and *Ixodes ricinus,* the sheep tick, in much of Europe. Importantly the large mammal that lends its name to these ticks is irrelevant to the infection cycle. Ticks hatch from eggs uninfected and typically have 3 meals during their 2-year life cy-cle. If an uninfected larva feeds on a spirochetemic mouse (the main reservoir host in most of the world), some spirochetes will remain in the tick's gut after the feeding. Dur-ing the months following the feeding, the larva matures into a nymph, about the size of a period on this page, which will feed on a second host, potentially a human or any other convenient mammalian host. Just as with an uninfected larva, if the nymph were not previously infected but now feeds on a spirochetemic host, it can become infected. On the other hand, if it is already infected, ingested blood leads to prolifera-tion of spirochetes in the tick's gut, ultimately with dissemination within the tick, including to its salivary glands. During the several days of attachment required for feeding, the tick injects a variety of anticoagulants, antiinflammatories, and local anes-thetics so that it can remain undisturbed while finishing its meal. Once spirochetes have reached its salivary glands, they can be injected along with this cocktail, infecting this new host. At least with *B burgdorferi* this cycle requires at least 24 to 48 hours of attachment. Hence removal of a feeding tick before this, drastically reduces the risk of infection. Following this meal, the tick will again spend several months maturing into an adult, when it will partake of its final meal, which may be on a human, deer, sheep, or other species. Once again it can transmit infection to this host. However, because it will never feed again, whether or not the deer or sheep is infected is irrelevant; even if the tick now acquires the infection, there will be no subsequent opportunity for further transmission. Consequently, although these larger species are supportive of the ticks' lifecycle, they are irrelevant to disease transmission.

Extraneurologic Disease

Cutaneous

By far the most common manifestation of both European and North American Lyme dis-ease is the characteristic cutaneous lesion known as erythema migrans (EM). First described over a century ago, this typically arises at the site of the tick bite. Unlike the allergic reaction that, as with other arthropod bites, arises virtually immediately at the time of the bite and is typically quite pruritic, EM arises days to a few weeks after the inoc-ulation of spirochetes and is often asymptomatic. This slowly expanding erythroderma expands over the course of days to a few weeks and can reach many inches or even a foot or more in diameter. It can have central pallor, rings of pallor, or be uniformly erythematous; its outer margin represents the leading edge of spirochetes migrating centrifugally from the inoculation site. With strains prevalent in the United States, the rash can be multifocal in up to a quarter of patients, each remote site arising from a new focus of hematogenously disseminated spirochetes. In Europe, the proportion of pa-tients with multifocal EM is lower. The proportion with EM is challenging to estimate. Because the rash is often asymptomatic and may occur on the back or other areas that are difficult to see, it is likely many go unnoticed. In children, typically closely observed by their parents, EM is reported to occur in up to 90%. Similar-appearing rashes are otherwise quite unusual. Southern tick–associated rash illness occurs in cen-tral states and can look identical. However, this has no accompanying systemic symptoms and testing for a causative organism, including *B burgdorferi*, has been uniformly negative.

A second cutaneous abnormality, acrodermatitis chronica atrophicans, occurs in more long-standing infection. Although this occurs only with strains found in Europe, the phenomenology is informative from a neurologic perspective. Occurring months to years after acute infection, the skin of the involved limb first becomes purplish and red, then quite thin and "cigarette paper-like". Biopsies demonstrate large numbers of spirochetes. Antibiotic treatment eliminates the spirochetes but not necessarily the cutaneous and other changes.

Rheumatologic

The other prominent finding is Lyme arthritis, the phenomenon that led to the original identification of this illness in the United States. Originally described in children, this preferentially affects large joints (knee, hip, shoulder, and elbow), usually affecting one joint at a time. Symptoms begin spontaneously, resolve over days to weeks, and then can recur in a different joint weeks to months later. Although episodes diminish over time, antimicrobial therapy is effective. A small proportion of patients may continue to have recurrent arthritis after microbiologically effective treatment, thought to be an induced autoimmune phenomenon.[8]

Cardiac

Cardiac involvement, particularly otherwise unexplained heart block, was originally estimated to occur in about 5% of patients, a proportion that seems to have diminished over time. Although this is quite antibiotic responsive, patients with complete heart block may require a temporary pacemaker. Deaths from Lyme disease are extraordinarily rare; estimates are so low that it is difficult to know if this really does occur.[9] Certainly, cardiac involvement could put individuals at risk; this is assumed to be the cause of death in the small number of patients in whom Lyme disease was thought to be a contributory factor.[10]

Nervous System Involvement

Much of the controversy about Lyme disease stems from misunderstandings of what constitutes nervous system disease. Neurobehavioral changes are very common in medical illnesses—hyperglycemia, hyponatremia, and myriad other biochemical abnormalities alter behavior, as do intoxications (alcohol, opiates, benzodiazepines) and physiologic states such as fever or fatigue. Although these affect behavior and even neurologic function, in all but extreme circumstances these states do not entail focal nervous system damage or dysfunction, the defining characteristic of neurologic disease. In addition, bacterial (including spirochetal) nervous system infections are almost invariably accompanied by nervous system inflammation. If the central nervous system (CNS) is involved in a nervous system infection, there will usually be evidence of this in the CSF. If disease is limited to the peripheral nervous system (PNS), CSF will often be normal. Regardless, if part of the nervous system is affected by an infection, there should be objective evidence of nervous system damage—on neurologic examination, neuroimaging (CNS), or electrophysiologic testing (PNS). Absent abnormalities by any of these measures, nervous system infection is unlikely at best.

Early descriptions of nervous system involvement, both in Europe and the United States, emphasized 3 elements, occurring singly or in combination: lymphocytic meningitis, cranial neuritis, and radiculoneuritis. Clinical symptoms of the meningitis are highly variable, ranging from those indistinguishable from viral meningitis (with which there is considerable temporal overlap) to an asymptomatic pleocytosis identified while evaluating a cranial neuropathy or radiculopathy. The pleocytosis is typically lymphocyte-predominant, modest (50–250 lymphocytes/mm^3) with a comparably modest elevation in protein and normal CSF glucose. Subsequent work has shown early entry of B burgdorferi into the CNS,[11] a rapid increase in locally produced CXCL13 (a B cell attracting chemokine),[12] followed by B cell in-migration, and increasing intrathecal production of anti-Borreliella antibodies. Some works suggest that the early and quite marked elevation in CXCL13 could serve as a nonspecific confirmatory test for LNB[12–14]; because the level drops rapidly after successful treatment it might at least be a useful marker of treatment efficacy, although whether it is any better than a cell count remains to be seen.

Studies from Europe have highlighted the presence of oligoclonal bands and an overall increase in immunoglobulin G (IgG) synthesis within the CNS. This has been less consistently described in US patients. One unusual manifestation of the meningitis, particularly in children, is a pseudotumor cerebri–like syndrome,[15] with papilledema, visual obscurations, and even vision compromise. This should be considered in the appropriate context, with the raised intracranial pressure treated specifically, in addition to antimicrobial therapy of the infection.

Cranial neuropathy

Cranial neuropathy most commonly affects the seventh cranial nerve, causing Lyme-associated facial nerve palsy (LAFP). This can be bilateral in up to a quarter of instances. Idiopathic facial nerve palsy is so uncommon in young children that when facial nerve palsies occur, in an appropriate epidemiologic setting, LAFP should be seriously considered. Like EM, LAFP can occur very early in infection—on occasion before there is a measurable antibody response.[16] In the appropriate setting, obtaining acute and convalescent serologies should be considered. Notably, in highly endemic areas, in tick season, only about a fourth of facial nerve palsies are Lyme disease related.[16] The other three-fourths require corticosteroid treatment. The role of corticosteroid treatment in LAFP has never been studied and is controversial. Although a strong argument can be made for simultaneous treatment with antibiotics and steroids, some have expressed concern about the possible negative impact of steroids on the host immune response to this infection. On the other hand, in at least 1 model of neuroborreliosis, corticosteroids seem to lessen nervous system damage.[17]

Other cranial nerves can be involved, but less frequently. Those to the extraocular muscles are probably the next most frequent, then the trigeminal and acoustic-vestibular, although all of these are uncommon. If the optic nerve is ever involved this is rare.[18] Involvement of the lower cranial nerves (IX–XII) is anecdotal at best.

Radiculoneuropathy

Radiculoneuropathy is probably the most commonly missed diagnosis. Patients present with dermatomal pain indistinguishable from that in mechanical radiculopathies, often with objective weakness and even atrophy of affected muscles. It is not uncommon for several adjacent roots to be involved. MRI may show enhancing roots but may not. The key observation is that patients typically lack a structural abnormality likely to cause the radicular symptoms. CSF is often inflammatory but this is not universally the case. In addition to radiculopathies, patients may present with plexopathies, a mononeuropathy, mononeuropathy multiplex, or a confluent mononeuropathy multiplex. Detailed neurophysiologic studies suggest that all these conditions—from cranial neuropathy and radiculopathy to mononeuropathy multiplex—represent various presentations of a mononeuropathy multiplex.[19] Importantly, in the only animal model of neuroborreliosis, the experimentally infected rhesus macaque monkey, virtually all develop a mononeuropathy multiplex.[20]

One area that has caused considerable confusion was the early description of a confluent mononeuropathy multiplex in patients with Lyme arthritis of several years duration. Neither long-standing untreated Lyme arthritis nor this neuropathy is commonly seen anymore, leading some to question its existence. However, given that virtually the identical disorder has been described in patients with acrodermatitis,[21,22] the correspondingly chronic infection seen in Europe, and given the pathophysiologic similarity to what is seen in more acute neuroborreliosis, it is likely this entity, while now uncommon, is real.

Rare patients will develop parenchymal CNS inflammation. This most commonly is described in European patients with Bannwarth syndrome, in whom there may be spinal cord inflammation at the same segmental level as the involved roots. More rarely, there may be parenchymal brain inflammation with focal abnormalities on examination, on MRI, and potentially on PET scans.[23] Such parenchymal inflammation is almost always accompanied by inflammatory CSF, increased CSF IgG synthesis, and, in particular, intrathecal production of anti-*Borreliella* antibodies (see later discussion).

The final entity worth consideration is what has been termed *Lyme encephalopathy*. Like the more indolent late neuropathy, this was originally described in patients with long-standing Lyme arthritis.[24,25] Involving mild memory and cognitive impairment, this differs from the neuropathy in that abundant evidence now supports this being unrelated to nervous system infection. Rather, this seems to be a nonspecific correlate of chronic inflammation, comparable to what occurs in everything from the flu to bacterial pneumonia to chronic inflammatory bowel disease. Unfortunately, misunderstandings about this nonspecific phenomenon fed the notion that patients with chronic subjective cognitive and memory symptoms, but who are neurologically normal, could have this as evidence of Lyme disease in the absence of any other evidence to support this diagnosis. Because these symptoms are highly prevalent in the general population,[26] they have no positive predictive value for the diagnosis of Lyme disease. Consequently, a causal relationship in any given individual requires other compelling evidence of active infection.

This also led to the introduction of the concept of "post treatment Lyme disease syndrome" (PTLDS)—patients with similar symptoms either persisting or beginning after microbiologically curative therapy. Although there is reason to believe this is simply anchoring bias[27]; there is still legitimate debate as to whether or not this entity exists. That notwithstanding, 2 things are clear about patients with these symptoms. First, additional antimicrobial therapy offers no benefit[28] but does carry substantial risk.[29] Second, this state occurs rarely, if ever, in patients who have had unequivocal neuroborreliosis.[30–32] Although neurologic residua may persist as a result of focal damage, nonspecific symptoms are rare after treated neuroborreliosis.[33] Not only do such patients have no evidence of nervous system infection when these symptoms are present, they are very unlikely to have previously had nervous system infection. In fact, the best predictors of these symptoms seem to be the presence of multiple comorbidities[31] and a low level of resilience.[34] Similar chronic nonspecific symptoms are now being described in patients who have recovered from Q fever[35] or chikungunya virus.[36] Perhaps as we learn more about these postinfectious symptoms this will provide insights regarding PTLDS.

Laboratory testing Diagnosis of Lyme disease requires 3 elements: likely epidemiologic exposure, signs, and symptoms known to be associated with this infection, and confirmation of the diagnosis either by the presence of a physical finding with a high positive predictive value of the diagnosis (EM) or by laboratory confirmation. Other than EM, which occurs before the patient becomes seropositive over 50% of the time, no clinical manifestation has sufficient positive predictive value to warrant a diagnosis of Lyme disease and treatment. Outside the research setting, laboratory support of the diagnosis relies on demonstration of antibody that reacts with *B burgdorferi*. For more than 2 decades the recommended approach in the United States has been 2-tiered testing—an enzyme-linked immunosorbent assay (ELISA) that measures total *B burgdorferi*–binding antibody in serum, followed by a Western blot in those in whom the ELISA is either positive (value >3 standard deviations (SDs) greater than the mean) or borderline (2SDs). Western blots should not be performed if the ELISA is negative, because the interpretive criteria were not developed in that context and it is easy to overinterpret faint bands. Western blot criteria are based on statistical analyses of observations in large numbers of patients and controls; the presence of 2 of 3 defined IgM bands (21–24, 39, and 41 kDa) or 5 of 10 defined IgG bands (18, 21–24, 28, 30, 39, 41, 45, 58, 66, and 93 kDa) has a very high positive predictive value. Interpretation is not based on the uniqueness of specific immunoreactivities; it is not correct to state that the presence of 1 or 2 particular bands is diagnostic. Similarly, it is important to recognize that the IgM response is both highly cross-reactive and only relevant in very early disease. Once a patient has had infection for more than 3 to 6 weeks, there should be a prominent IgG response; in this setting the IgM response is both irrelevant and meaningless. If a patient with months of symptoms has only an IgM response, this is undoubtedly a cross-reactive false-positive.

Recent work has suggested ways to simplify testing. Assessing immunoreactivity to the C6 antigen of *Borreliella* seems to provide sensitivity and specificity comparable to the more widely used whole-cell sonicate ELISA assays[37] and may even be more sensitive in early (EM) Lyme disease.[38] Some are suggesting this could substitute for the Western blot in 2-tiered testing, providing a simpler assay with results available more rapidly. Importantly, C6 seems to be equally useful with both European and US strains, potentially eliminating some of the challenges in Europe, where the greater number of strains makes Western blot interpretation more challenging.[39]

When the CNS is involved an additional tool is useful. As in many other infections, the presence of a pathogen in the CNS leads to in-migration of reactive B cells, with production of antibody specific to that organism within the CNS. Measurement of this requires correction for the small amount of antibody that normally filters through the blood brain barrier. Three approaches are available to accomplish this; all require simultaneous measurement of specific antibody in CSF and serum. Performing this measurement with a capture assay intrinsically provides information about the proportion of total antibody in both fluids that is specific to the target organism; the ratio of the CSF:serum ELISAs provides an informative antibody index (AI). Alternative, the laboratory can measure CSF and serum IgG and then use 1 of 2 approaches. Both fluids can be diluted to the same final IgG concentration; measuring specific antibody in both will then again provide an AI that is elevated if antibody is being produced within the CNS compartment. Alternatively, the laboratory can measure specific antibody at standard dilutions and adjust mathematically for the known IgG and albumin concentrations, which is the preferred approach in European laboratories. Each method has its own advantages and disadvantages. The critical consideration is the determination of the proportion of antibody in the 2 fluids that is specific for the causative organism.

There are at least 2 limitations of this approach. First, absent another gold standard for diagnosis, there is no way to determine the true diagnostic sensitivity. Most current estimates place this at about 85% to 90%, but the logic may be at least partly circular.

Second, just as with peripheral blood serologies, the index may remain elevated for years after successful treatment, making it unreliable both as a measure of treatment success and for differentiating between current CNS LNB and past infection. Fortunately, CSF cell counts, and quite likely CXCL13 concentrations, are probably better markers of current active infection.

Treatment

The *Borreliella* responsible for Lyme disease and the related infections seen in Europe have never been shown to develop resistance to commonly used antimicrobial regimens. Although some have conjectured about the development of biofilms, cystlike forms, and other mechanisms of treatment evasion, there is no evidence that any of these mechanisms play any role in human disease. All evidence is that standard 2- to 4-week courses are effective in well more than 90% of treated patients.[40] Importantly, all studies that have compared the efficacy of appropriate oral versus parenteral therapy have show them to be equivalent, including European studies in Lyme meningitis, cranial neuropathy, and radiculoneuropathy.[40] There have not been systematic studies of the very rare phenomenon of parenchymal CNS involvement, nor have there been US studies of oral versus parenteral treatment of LNB. That notwithstanding, anecdotal evidence from the United States, coupled with microbiologic measures of required minimum inhibitory concentrations needed for US versus European strains, supports the same conclusions as European studies. Soon to be published Guidelines from the Infectious Diseases Society of America and the American Academy of Neurology are likely to recommend initial treatment of all but the most serious infections with oral doxycycline. Other effective regimens include amoxicillin or cefuroxime axetil. Doxycycline has generally been preferred in neuroborreliosis because of its excellent CNS penetration. However, it is worth noting that, because of concerns about dental staining in children aged 8 years or younger, doxycycline has been avoided in young children. However, untold thousands of children have been treated with oral amoxicillin or cefuroxime axetil for EM; none has been described as developing breakthrough neuroborreliosis following this treatment, strongly suggesting these agents are effective for this as well.

REFERENCES

1. Garin C, Bujadoux A. Paralysie par les tiques. J Med Lyon 1922;71:765–7.
2. Bannwarth A. Chronische lymphocytare meningitis, entzundliche polyneuritis und "rheumatismus". Arch Psychiatr Nervenkr 1941;113:284–376.
3. Reik L, Steere AC, Bartenhagen NH, et al. Neurologic abnormalities of Lyme disease. Medicine 1979;58(4):281–94.
4. Koedel U, Fingerle V, Pfister HW. Lyme neuroborreliosis-epidemiology, diagnosis and management. Nat Rev Neurol 2015;11(8):446–56.
5. Krause PJ, Barbour AG. Borrelia miyamotoi: the newest infection brought to us by deer ticks. Ann Intern Med 2015;163(2):141–2.
6. Pritt BS, Mead PS, Johnson DK, et al. Identification of a novel pathogenic Borrelia species causing Lyme borreliosis with unusually high spirochaetaemia: a descriptive study. Lancet Infect Dis 2016;16(5):556–64.
7. Barbour AG, Adeolu M, Gupta RS. Division of the genus Borrelia into two genera (corresponding to Lyme disease and relapsing fever groups) reflects their genetic and phenotypic distinctiveness and will lead to a better understanding of these two groups of microbes (Margos et al. (2016) There is inadequate evidence to support the division of the genus Borrelia. Int. J. Syst. Evol. Microbiol. doi: 10.1099/ijsem.0.001717). Int J Syst Evol Microbiol 2017;67(6):2058–67.

8. Steere AC, Strle F, Wormser GP, et al. Lyme borreliosis. Nat Rev Dis Primers 2016; 2:16090.
9. Kugeler KJ, Griffith KS, Gould LH, et al. A review of death certificates listing Lyme disease as a cause of death in the United States. Clin Infect Dis 2011;52(3): 364–7.
10. Centers for Disease Control and Prevention (CDC). Three sudden cardiac deaths associated with lyme carditis - United States, November 2012-July 2013. MMWR Morb Mortal Wkly Rep 2013;62(49):993–6.
11. Luft BJ, Steinman CR, Neimark HC, et al. Invasion of the central nervous system by Borrelia burgdorferi in acute disseminated infection. JAMA 1992;267(10): 1364–7.
12. Rupprecht TA, Lechner C, Tumani H, et al. CXCL13: a biomarker for acute Lyme neuroborreliosis: investigation of the predictive value in the clinical routine. Nervenarzt 2014;85(4):459–64 [in German].
13. Dersch R, Hottenrott T, Senel M, et al. The chemokine CXCL13 is elevated in the cerebrospinal fluid of patients with neurosyphilis. Fluids Barriers CNS 2015;12(1):1–5.
14. Barstad B, Tveitnes D, Noraas S, et al. Cerebrospinal fluid B-lymphocyte chemoattractant CXCL13 in the diagnosis of acute lyme neuroborreliosis in children. Pediatr Infect Dis J 2017;36(12):e286–92.
15. Ramgopal S, Obeid R, Zuccoli G, et al. Lyme disease-related intracranial hypertension in children: clinical and imaging findings. J Neurol 2016;263(3):500–7.
16. Halperin JJ, Golightly M. Lyme borreliosis in Bell's palsy. Long Island Neuroborreliosis Collaborative Study Group. Neurology 1992;42(7):1268–70.
17. Ramesh G, Martinez AN, Martin DS, et al. Effects of dexamethasone and meloxicam on Borrelia burgdorferi-induced inflammation in glial and neuronal cells of the central nervous system. J Neuroinflammation 2017;14(1):28.
18. Sibony P, Halperin J, Coyle P, et al. Reactive Lyme serology in patients with optic neuritis and papilledema. J Neuroophthalmol 2005;25(2):71–82.
19. Halperin JJ, Luft BJ, Volkman DJ, et al. Lyme neuroborreliosis - peripheral nervous system manifestations. Brain 1990;113:1207–21.
20. England JD, Bohm RP, Roberts ED, et al. Mononeuropathy multiplex in rhesus monkeys with chronic Lyme disease. Ann Neurol 1997;41(3):375–84.
21. Hopf HC. Peripheral neuropathy in acrodermatitis chronica atrophicans (Herxheimer). J Neurol Neurosurg Psychiatry 1975;38(5):452–8.
22. Kristoferitsch W, Sluga E, Graf M, et al. Neuropathy associated with acrodermatitis chronica atrophicans. Clinical and morphological features. Ann N Y Acad Sci 1988;539:35–45.
23. Kalina P, Decker A, Kornel E, et al. Lyme disease of the brainstem. Neuroradiology 2005;47(12):903–7.
24. Halperin JJ, Luft BJ, Anand AK, et al. Lyme neuroborreliosis: central nervous system manifestations. Neurology 1989;39(6):753–9.
25. Logigian EL, Kaplan RF, Steere AC. Chronic neurologic manifestations of Lyme disease. N Engl J Med 1990;323(21):1438–44.
26. Luo N, Johnson J, Shaw J, et al. Self-reported health status of the general adult U.S. population as assessed by the EQ-5D and Health Utilities Index. Med Care 2005;43(11):1078–86.
27. Halperin JJ. Neuroborreliosis. J Neurol 2016;264(6):1292–7.
28. Berende A, ter Hofstede HJ, Vos FJ, et al. Randomized trial of longer-term therapy for symptoms attributed to Lyme disease. N Engl J Med 2016;374(13): 1209–20.

29. Marzec NS, Nelson C, Waldron PR, et al. Serious bacterial infections acquired during treatment of patients given a diagnosis of chronic Lyme disease - United States. MMWR Morb Mortal Wkly Rep 2017;66(23):607–9.
30. Dersch R, Sommer H, Rauer S, et al. Prevalence and spectrum of residual symptoms in Lyme neuroborreliosis after pharmacological treatment: a systematic review. J Neurol 2016;263(1):17–24.
31. Wills AB, Spaulding AB, Adjemian J, et al. Long-term follow-up of patients with Lyme disease: longitudinal analysis of clinical and quality-of-life measures. Clin Infect Dis 2016;62(12):1546–51.
32. Roaldsnes E, Eikeland R, Berild D. Lyme neuroborreliosis in cases of non-specific neurological symptoms. Tidsskr Nor Laegeforen 2017;137(2):101–4.
33. Knudtzen FC, Andersen NS, Jensen TG, et al. Characteristics and clinical outcome of Lyme Neuroborreliosis in a high endemic area, 1995-2014: a retrospective cohort study in Denmark. Clin Infect Dis 2017;65(9):1489–95.
34. Hassett AL, Sigal LH. The psychology of 'post Lyme disease syndrome' and 'not Lyme'. In: Halperin JJ, editor. Lyme disease - an Evidence based approach. Wallingford (United Kingdom): CABI; 2011. p. 232–47.
35. Keijmel SP, Delsing CE, Bleijenberg G, et al. Effectiveness of long-term Doxycycline treatment and cognitive-behavioral therapy on fatigue severity in patients with Q Fever Fatigue Syndrome (Qure Study): a randomized controlled trial. Clin Infect Dis 2017;64(8):998–1005.
36. Elsinga J, Gerstenbluth I, van der Ploeg S, et al. Long-term Chikungunya Sequelae in Curacao: burden, determinants, and a novel classification tool. J Infect Dis 2017;216(5):573–81.
37. Lipsett SC, Branda JA, McAdam AJ, et al. Evaluation of the C6 Lyme enzyme immunoassay for the diagnosis of Lyme disease in children and adolescents. Clin Infect Dis 2016;63(7):922–8.
38. Branda JA, Strle K, Nigrovic LE, et al. Evaluation of modified 2-tiered Serodiagnostic testing algorithms for early Lyme disease. Clin Infect Dis 2017;64(8):1074–80.
39. Leeflang MMG, Ang CW, Berkhout J, et al. The diagnostic accuracy of serological tests for Lyme borreliosis in Europe: a systematic review and meta-analysis. BMC Infect Dis 2016;16(1):1–17.
40. Halperin JJ, Shapiro ED, Logigian EL, et al. Practice parameter: treatment of nervous system Lyme disease. Neurology 2007;69(1):91–102.

Diagnostic Approach to Chronic Meningitis

Kelly J. Baldwin, MD*, Jose David Avila, MD

KEYWORDS

- Chronic meningitis • Fungal meningitis • Cryptococcus • Tuberculosis • Syphilis
- Leptomeningeal carcinomatosis • Neuroborreliosis • Neurosarcoidosis

KEY POINTS

- Chronic meningitis is defined as cerebrospinal fluid pleocytosis that is persistent for at least 4 weeks without spontaneous resolution.
- The most common cause of chronic meningitis is infection followed by malignancy and autoimmune disease.
- Despite extensive evaluation, over a third of cases are deemed idiopathic.
- An algorithmic approach to chronic meningitis aids in the evaluation of this complex condition.
- The most important aspect in the evaluation of chronic meningitis is a thorough history, including immune status, exposures, geography and travel, and systemic symptoms.

INTRODUCTION

Central nervous system (CNS) infections remain one of the most challenging clinical scenarios for the neurologist, with more than a third of chronic meningitis cases and more than half of meningoencephalitis cases deemed idiopathic after extensive investigation.[1,2] Chronic meningitis is defined as inflammation in the cerebrospinal fluid (CSF) that persists for at least 1 month without spontaneous resolution. The most common CSF laboratory findings in chronic meningitis are leukocyte pleocytosis and elevated protein. Because clinicians rarely have CSF results from symptoms onset, most would agree that a clinical history of 1 months' duration with supporting CSF findings at any point during the disease course would suffice to meet the definition of chronic meningitis.[3] The cause of inflammation in the CSF is broad, encompassing infectious diseases, autoimmune disorders, and neoplastic conditions (**Fig. 1**). One retrospective review of previously healthy patients who were diagnosed with chronic meningitis found the most common cause was infectious disease followed by malignancy with more than a third of cases remaining idiopathic. It is

No disclosures.
Department of Neurology, Geisinger Commonwealth School of Medicine, Geisinger Medical Center, 100 North Academy Avenue, Danville, PA 17822, USA
* Corresponding author.
E-mail address: kjbaldwin@geisinger.edu

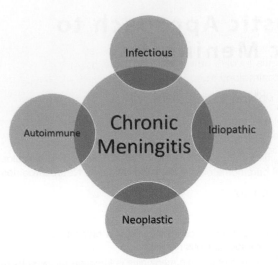

Fig. 1. Causes of chronic meningitis.

important to recognize that geographic differences may heavily affect these findings.[4] This review provides a detailed diagnostic approach to chronic meningitis, including history and physical examination pearls, diagnostic testing, and neuroimaging findings. Selected causes, including fungal meningitis, autoimmune meningitis, and neoplastic meningitis, are discussed in detail.

CLINICAL PRESENTATION

Inflammation in the CSF often affects multiple regions of the nervous system simultaneously, including brain, cranial nerves, nerve roots, and spinal cord. The most common presenting symptoms include headache, nausea, vomiting, cranial neuropathies, and polyradiculopathy. Occasionally, the inflammation is not limited to the CSF and may also cause cortical dysfunction or myelopathy.[5,6] Neurologic deficits gradually increase over the course of weeks before becoming severe, leading patients to seek medical attention. A comprehensive history is critical to determining a correct diagnosis and should include immunocompetence, social factors, drug use, geography and travel, hobbies, and animal and insect vector exposures. Discussion of systemic symptoms is important for clues about a neoplastic or rheumatologic diagnosis, including fever, weight loss, night sweats, shortness of breath, gastrointestinal issues, rashes, and joint involvement. Many infectious causes also have systemic symptoms; thus, a detailed review of symptoms is important for all patients presenting with chronic meningitis.

APPROACH TO INITIAL DIAGNOSIS AND MANAGEMENT

Once chronic meningitis is suspected based on the history and physical examination, the next step is to perform neuroimaging and CSF analysis. MRI brain scan with and without gadolinium is more sensitive than computerized tomography (CT) scan and is preferred in chronic meningitis. For patients with signs of myelopathy or polyradiculopathy, MRI spine scan with and without gadolinium should also be obtained. Lumbar puncture generally follows neuroimaging. Typical findings are elevated leukocytes and protein with normal or low glucose. Initial CSF testing should include measurement of opening pressure, cell count with differential, glucose, protein, bacterial culture, fungal culture, cryptococcal antigen, Gram stain, and cytology. Further testing should be tailored to potential exposures elicited during the clinic history.[6] Expert consultants are important to involve early on in a patient's presentation, because many causes of chronic meningitis involve other regions of the body. Important subspecialties to consider are ophthalmology, rheumatology, oncology, and neurosurgery. It is important to note that empiric antibiotics or antiviral medications are generally not indicated in cases of chronic meningitis because of the low likelihood of an acute bacterial process and the indolent nature of most infectious causes. The decision to initiate empiric therapy should be considered on a case-by-case basis and should consider factors such as spinal fluid formula abnormalities, immune status, recent exposure history, epidemiologic likely cause, and potential risks of treatment.

DIAGNOSTIC ALGORITHM

The initial history, physical examination, neuroimaging, and CSF analysis will establish the diagnosis of chronic meningitis. Identifying this clinical syndrome however is only the beginning of the more challenging quest for the cause to guide the initiation of an appropriate treatment regimen. With the rapid expansion of molecular diagnostics, antibody analysis, and next-generation sequencing, clinicians have additional tools available. By using a standardized algorithmic approach to each case, these tools can be used strategically and responsibly to yield accurate results and guide important treatment (**Fig. 2**).

- Step 1: Immunocompetence of the patient
  - The first step in the diagnostic algorithm is to identify the immunologic status of the patient. Immunocompromised patients from transplantation, immunosuppressive medications, or human immunodeficiency virus (HIV) are more likely to be suffering from infectious causes of chronic meningitis. Clinicians can narrow down each organism by cell deficiency (**Table 1**) to selectively guide CSF and serum testing. Immunocompetent patients may also have an infectious cause; however, autoimmune and neoplastic conditions must also be considered.

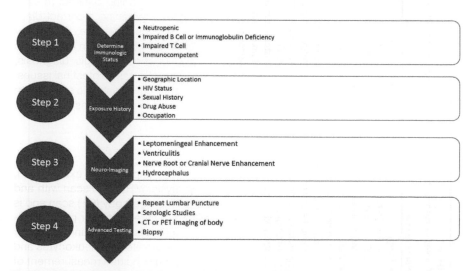

Fig. 2. Clinical algorithmic approach to chronic meningitis.

Table 1
Causes of chronic meningitis based on immunocompetence

Neutropenia	B-cell Deficiency	T-cell Deficiency	Immunocompetent
• Fungal	• Bacterial	• Bacterial	• Bacterial
○ A fumigatus	○ Otitis media and sinusitis	○ Listeria monocytogenes	○ B burgdorferi
○ C albicans	○ Leptospirosis	○ Nocardia asteroids	○ T pallidum
○ Mucoraceae	• Fungal	○ T pallidum	○ Mycobacterium
• Viral	○ C albicans	○ Mycobacterium	○ Bartonella
○ Cytomegalovirus	• Viral	• Fungal	• Fungal
○ Herpes simplex virus	○ Cytomegalovirus	○ Mucoraceae	○ C neoformans
○ Varicella zoster virus	○ Herpes simplex virus	○ C neoformans	○ C gattii
○ Human herpes virus 6 and 7	○ Varicella zoster virus	○ Histoplasma capsulatum	○ H capsulatum
○ Astrovirus	○ JC virus	○ Coccidioides immitis	○ C immitis
○ West Nile virus	○ Epstein-Barr virus	○ Blastomyces dermatitidis	○ B dermatitidis
	○ Human herpes virus 6 and 7	○ Aspergillus fumigatus	○ C albicans
	○ Astrovirus	• Viral	• Viral
		○ Cytomegalovirus	○ HIV
		○ Herpes simplex virus	○ Varicella zoster virus
		○ Varicella zoster virus	○ Herpes simplex virus 2 (Mollaret)
		○ JC virus	○ West Nile virus
		○ Epstein-Barr virus	• Neoplastic
		○ Human herpes virus 6 and 7	○ Lymphoma
		○ Astrovirus	○ Leptomeningeal carcinomatosis
		○ Neoplastic	○ Paraneoplastic
		○ Lymphoma	• Autoimmune
			○ Sarcoidosis
			○ NMO
			○ Sjogren
			○ Systemic lupus erythematous
			○ Behcet
			○ Primary angiitis of the CNS
			○ Periodic fever syndrome

- Step 2: Exposure history and associated symptoms
  - The key to identifying the cause for an immunocompetent patient is gathering a detailed exposure history and review of symptoms. Social history revealing farming or exposure to birds is an important risk factor for fungal infections, such as cryptococcus or histoplasmosis. An African American patient with pulmonary symptoms and endocrine abnormalities may lead the clinician toward a condition like sarcoidosis. A history of intravenous (IV) drug abuse suggests testing for HIV and syphilis and may place the patient at risk for *Candida albicans* meningitis (see example in later discussion).
- Step 3: Neuroimaging
  - MRI head scan in chronic meningitis can be normal or may demonstrate leptomeningeal and cranial nerve enhancement. There are several unique MRI patterns that may be helpful in narrowing the differential diagnosis if present (**Figs. 3** and **4**).
- Step 4: Advanced testing
  - Once steps 1 through 3 are completed, the clinician should have a narrowed differential diagnosis and list of advanced testing. Many patients will require at least 2 lumbar punctures to complete the diagnostic testing needed to fully evaluate for a diagnosis. For example, in a patient in whom leptomeningeal carcinomatous was suspected, 2 large-volume lumbar punctures may be needed for maximal sensitivity for cytology.[7] Other advanced serologic testing, body imaging, or biopsy may be required.

Applying the Algorithm

Case 1: A 62-year-old man presented with 1 month of bitemporal headache and 3 days of visual loss in the left eye. The patient was admitted to the hospital from

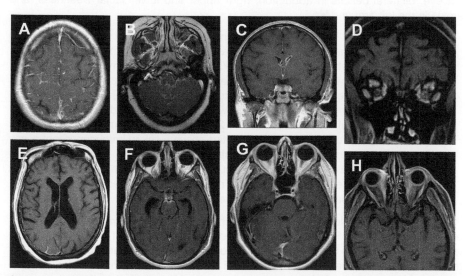

Fig. 3. Common brain MRI findings in chronic meningitis. Axial T1 postcontrast demonstrates different patterns of leptomeningeal enhancement, cortical (*A*), basilar (*B*), focal right occipital (*E*). Coronal T1 postcontrast demonstrates enhancement involving the lateral and third ventricles in a case of *C albicans* meningitis (*C*; see case 2). Coronal (*D*) and axial (*G, H*) T1 postcontrast demonstrate cranial nerve enhancement, bilateral optic nerve (*D, H*), asymmetric bilateral CN5, and left CN7 (*G*). Axial T1 postcontrast demonstrates peripontine enhancement and enlargement of the temporal horns of the lateral ventricles in a case of tuberculosis meningitis with hydrocephalus (*F*).

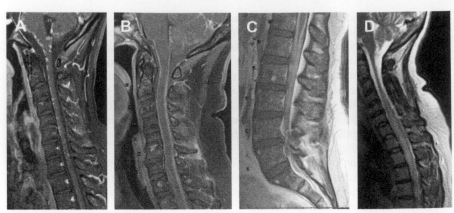

Fig. 4. Common spine MRI findings in chronic meningitis. Sagittal T1 postcontrast images demonstrate nodular leptomeningeal enhancement in a case of neurosarcoidosis (*A*) and diffuse, linear leptomeningeal enhancement in a case of neoplastic chronic meningitis (*B*, *C*; see case 5). Also note the enhancement of the cauda equina (*C*) and some vertebral bodies (*B*, *C*). Sagittal T2-weighted image demonstrates cord edema and longitudinally extensive transverse myelitis involving more than 3 spinal cord segments in a patient with NMOSD (*D*; see case 4).

the ophthalmology clinic, where he was found to have left disc edema. Neurology was consulted 2 days after admission due to development of diplopia and right facial weakness. General examination revealed a diaphoretic and tachycardic man in mild distress. Neurologic examination demonstrated an afferent pupillary defect in the left eye, bilateral deficits in abduction, right upper and lower facial weakness, and ataxia in the left arm and leg.

- Implementing the algorithm: An immunocompetent patient with negative HIV testing (step 1). The patient works as a landscaper in the northeast United States. He presents to the hospital in the summer. He has systemic symptoms of a macular rash on his trunk, fever, and tachycardia with symptomatic palpitations (step 2). Neuroimaging revealed cranial nerve and leptomeningeal enhancement (step 3). CSF revealed lymphocytic meningitis with 351 white blood cell count (WBC; 97% lymphocytes), elevated protein of 234 mg/dL, and normal glucose. Serum Lyme testing was completed with a positive enzyme-linked immunosorbent assay (ELISA) and confirmatory western blot (step 4).
  - Comments: By using an organized approach to this complex patient, clinicians rapidly diagnosed neuroborreliosis. Treatment was initiated with oral doxycycline, and the patient had complete recovery at 1 month.

Case 2: A 23-year-old man presented to the hospital with blurred vision in the left eye and headache for 1 month. Two days before, his vision went nearly black in the left eye, prompting him to see an ophthalmologist, and he was found to have endophthalmitis. The patient was sent to the hospital for further evaluation. Neurologic examination revealed mild nuchal rigidity, an afferent pupillary defect in the left eye with decreased visual acuity, and left arm ataxia.[8]

- Implementing the algorithm: An immunocompetent patient with negative HIV testing. However, he is a current IV drug user of brown heroin (step 1 and 2). Neuroimaging revealed extensive ventriculitis (**Fig. 3**C). Ophthalmologic examination revealed discrete fungal lesions in the vitreous with surrounding vitritis and optic nerve edema (step 3). CSF revealed a mixed pleocytosis with 7775 cu/mm WBC (53% polymorphonuclear leukocytes, 40% lymphocytes, 7% monocytes), 1150 cu/mm red blood cell count, glucose 9 mg/dL, protein 295 mg/dL (step 5).

o Comments: Social history was the key to this case, because the history of IV brown heroin use has been reported in a case series of more than 80 patients to be a risk factor for developing *C albicans* meningitis.[9] The supporting ophthalmologic findings of fungal uveitis were additional evidence that ultimately led the patient to be treated with intraocular amphotericin B and systemic voriconazole. After 2 months of treatment, the patient's neuroimaging and CSF improved. Although his other neurologic symptoms resolved, he did not regain vision of his left eye.

SELECTED INFECTIOUS CAUSES

Chronic meningitis can be caused by a variety of pathogens, including fungi, bacteria, viruses, and parasites. Available literature over the past few years alone has identified even more novel organisms causing chronic meningitis, such as *Nocardia* sp, *Mycobacterium abscessus*, *Sporothrix schenckii*, Cache valley virus, neuroleptospirosis, and astrovirus.[10–15] This section, however, focuses on the most common causes that the neurologist will encounter with patients presenting with infectious causes of chronic meningitis. Epidemiology, risk factors, clinical presentation, diagnosis, and treatment regimens for *Cryptococcus* spp, *Aspergillus* spp, and *Treponema pallidum* are discussed in detail. *Mycobacterium tuberculosis*, *Borrelia burgdorferi*, and HIV infections are common causes of chronic meningitis and are discussed elsewhere in this issue of *Neurologic Clinics*.

Cryptococcal Spp

Cryptococcal meningitis (CM) is the most common cause of chronic meningitis in the United States based on limited case series.[4] CM is caused by the encapsulated yeast organism *Cryptococcus neoformans*, which is primarily found in contaminated soil, avian excrement, and the bark of several tree species. Infection usually occurs by inhalation of the organism, followed by a respiratory illness and dissemination of the infection. CM is most common in people with impaired cell-mediated immunity, especially HIV infection, hematologic malignancies, transplantation, and patients on chronic corticosteroids or other immunosuppressive therapies. It is important to note that immunocompetent individuals can also become infected, particularly by the Cryptococcal species *Cryptococcus gattii*.[16,17]

Clinical presentation of CM is dependent on the host immune status. HIV patients with severe immunodeficiency may have little to no CNS symptoms, whereas the immunocompetent patient may have more typical symptoms of headache, fever, vomiting, and symptoms of elevated intracranial pressure. Lumbar puncture is often notable for a mononuclear pleocytosis as well as increased protein and low-glucose concentrations. Although India ink staining of centrifuged CSF is a cost-efficient and rapid test, the decreasing use of microscopic evaluation of CSF in high-income countries has led to a reliance on higher sensitivity antigen-based assays. The CSF cryptococcal capsular polysaccharide antigen (CRAg) assay is both sensitive and specific for CM and can provide a quantitative titer that is useful for prognostication but has limited value for measuring response to therapy. Fungal culture for the organism is less sensitive but is useful for both diagnosing infection and speciation.[18] Neuroimaging is important to acquire early in the disease course and may show hydrocephalus that requires additional emergent management. MRI findings are similar to other causes of chronic meningitis, including leptomeningeal enhancement, nodular enhancement, basilar brain perivascular space enlargement due to infiltration, or focal parenchymal lesions sometimes called cryptococcomas.

The most dangerous complication of CM is uncontrolled elevations in intracranial pressure. More than half of patients will develop intracranial hypertension. Intracranial pressure management is important and may require daily lumbar punctures, lumbar or external ventricular drain placement, or ventriculoperitoneal shunt placement for refractory cases. Refer to **Table 1** for antifungal treatment.[19,20]

Aspergillus Spp

Aspergillus is a ubiquitous organism found in soil, water, and decaying vegetation. Fungal spores are released into the atmosphere, and inhalation is the typical route of entry for infection. Inhalation of organisms rarely results in disease because the conidia are eliminated efficiently by host immune mechanisms. *Aspergillus* infection generally occurs in immunocompromised patients, particularly those with neutropenia whose barrier defenses are altered in the setting of transplantation or HIV infection. In this small percent of patients, infection can spread hematogenously to the CNS or can directly invade from nasal mucosa. *Aspergillus fumigatus* is the most common species to infect humans and has been reported in several cases to cause fungal chronic meningitis.[3,21]

Clinical presentations of CNS involvement are typically a gradually progressive chronic meningitis with more acute focal disturbances from vascular events. Aspergillus has a vascular predilection and thus may present as ischemic or hemorrhagic strokes. As with many invasive fungal CNS infections, diagnosis is often achieved through examination of the primary entry site of infection. Thus, in patients with suspected CNS aspergillosis, it is important to examine the lungs and sinuses for evidence of infection and potential sites for obtaining biopsy or culture material. Because of its slow growing nature and low organism burden, CSF yields poor culture results.[22–24] Neuroimaging can be helpful in the evaluation of CNS aspergillosis. MRI scan of the brain can demonstrate cerebral infarction, hemorrhagic lesions, solid-enhancing aspergillomas, or ring-enhancing abscesses. Dural enhancement is usually seen in lesions adjacent to infected paranasal sinuses and indicates direct extension of disease.[25] Several valuable serum laboratory markers can aid in the diagnosis of invasive aspergillus. ELISA testing for galactomannan and beta-glucan, fungal cell wall constituents, should be considered, although their sensitivities in spinal fluid analysis are undefined.[26,27]

Unfortunately, CNS aspergillosis, especially in an immunocompromised patient, is difficult to treat and has a high mortality. The antifungal agent voriconazole has reduced mortality in an infection previously associated with almost universal mortality. Clinical trials have demonstrated that voriconazole is more effective than amphotericin B as initial therapy for invasive aspergillosis.[28]

Treponema pallidum

Syphilis is caused by the thin, motile corkscrew bacterium *T pallidum*. This organism cannot be routinely cultured in the laboratory and is difficult to visualize using traditional light microscopy. Transmission is primarily via sexual contact with an infected individual or by vertical transmission from mother to fetus. Without treatment, the disease will inevitably progress through a series of clinical stages. *T pallidum* spreads hematogenously to the CNS early in the course of disease.

Clinical signs and symptoms of CNS involvement are evident throughout the course of disease and not limited by stage. Neurosyphilis can be either early or late disease.

The early stage typically manifests as asymptomatic or symptomatic meningitis and meningovascular disease. Late disease more often affects the brain parenchyma or spinal cord, leading to general paresis, psychiatric illness, memory deficits, tabes dorsalis, and gummatous masses. Although neurosyphilis has several manifestations, this article limits the discussion to syphilitic meningitis. Syphilitic meningitis typically presents as an early stage of neurosyphilis, usually within 2 years of acquiring infection. Although less common than other forms of neurosyphilis, meningitis occurs in up to 25% of patients. The most common presenting symptoms include headache, photophobia, nausea and vomiting, meningismus, and cranial nerve deficits. Although every cranial nerve can be affected, cranial nerves VII and VIII are most commonly affected.[3]

Serologic testing with venereal disease research laboratory (VDRL) and rapid plasma reagin (RPR) have been the gold standards for screening. The main limitations of nontreponemal tests are their reduced sensitivity in primary syphilis and late latent syphilis with up to 30% false negative rates, and false positive results due to cross-reactivity. Recently, enzyme immunoassays (EIA) and multiplex flow immunoassays (MFI) were introduced to assess serologic response to *T pallidum*. The assay is highly sensitive and specific and allows for an objective interpretation of results. Because of several factors, including the low prevalence of syphilis in the United States, the increased specificity of treponemal assays, and the objective interpretation of MFI and EIA technology, initial serologic testing by a treponemal-specific assay (eg, EIA or MFI) is now commonly performed in clinical laboratories. After a positive initial screening, fluorescent treponemal antibody absorption (FTA-ABS) test or *T pallidum* particle agglutination can be used to confirm infection.[29]

Lumbar puncture is recommended for patients with possible neurosyphilis. Abnormal CSF is present in 70% of early patients, typically demonstrating a lymphocytic or mononuclear pleocytosis and elevated protein. CSF VDRL testing is usually abnormal in syphilitic meningitis; however, in late disease the sensitivity may be only 30%. Therefore, a negative result does not rule out disease. CSF polymerase chain reaction (PCR) may be useful as an adjunctive test but is not widely available and has varying sensitivity.[30] Treatment of syphilitic and other infectious meningitis can be found in **Table 2**.[31–34]

AUTOIMMUNE CHRONIC MENINGITIS

Chronic meningitis may be the initial manifestation or occur during the course of autoimmune disorders. The latter represents a unique diagnostic challenge because these patients are usually on immunosuppressive drugs and are therefore immunocompromised (step 1 of the diagnostic algorithm). The initial investigations should be directed to exclude an opportunistic infection. This step is critical because if an infection is not recognized, meningeal involvement will likely be considered a manifestation of the underlying autoimmune condition and lead to escalation of immunosuppression, with a detrimental effect to the patient.

Early studies of chronic meningitis indicated that autoimmune conditions were less frequent than neoplasms.[4,35] However, there are a group of patients with idiopathic chronic meningitis that respond to corticosteroids, suggesting that autoimmune causes may be more prevalent that originally thought.[4,36,37] This review focuses on the most common forms of autoimmune chronic meningitis encountered by neurologists, namely neurosarcoidosis and neuromyelitis optica (NMO).

Case 3: A 46-year-old Caucasian man presented with 2 months of bilateral leg pain and weakness, difficulty urinating, and 2 weeks of left facial weakness, visual changes, and headache. Past medical history was significant for poorly controlled diabetes. Neurologic examination demonstrated left upper and lower facial weakness,

Table 2
Infectious chronic meningitis

Organism	Diagnostic Testing	Treatment
C neoformans/gattii	• ↑ Opening pressure on LP • CSF India ink stains • CSF fungal culture • CRAg LFA	Induction (14 d) Amphotericin B 0.7 mg/kg/d to 1 mg/kg/d IV plus flucytosine 100 mg/kg/d OR Liposomal AmB 3–4 mg/kg per day plus flucytosine 100 mg/kg/d[19,20]
A fumigatus	• Bronchoalveolar lavage with culture • Serum, tissue, or CSF culture • Serum galactomannan or β-glucan	Induction (2 doses): voriconazole 6 mg/kg IV twice on day 1 followed by 4 mg/kg IV twice daily Maintenance: voriconazole 200 mg every 12 h[28]
T pallidum	• Serum VDRL and RPR • Serum FTA-ABS • CSF-VDRL	First line (10–14 d) Aqueous penicillin G 3 million U to 4 million U IV every 4 h or as continuous infusion Alternative (10–14 d) Procaine penicillin 2.4 million U intramuscularly once daily plus probenecid 500 mg orally 4 times daily[31]
C albicans	• Serum, tissue, or CSF culture • Serum galactomannan or β-glucan	Induction: liposomal amphotericin B 5 mg/kg IV daily with or without flucytosine 25 mg/kg orally 4 times daily for several weeks Step down: fluconazole 400–800 mg (6–12 mg/kg) orally daily[32]
B burgdorferi	• Serum ELISA and confirmatory western blot • CSF: lymphocytic meningitis • CSF/Serum Antibody Index	Doxycycline 100 mg orally BID × 14 d or Ceftriaxone 2 g IV daily × 14 d[33]
M tuberculosis	• ↑ Opening pressure • Large-volume CSF microscopy with acid-fast stain • CSF cultures on Lowenstein-Jensen media, CSF PCR • Bronchoalveolar lavage with culture	Isoniazid, rifampin, pyrazinamide, and ethambutol in an initial 2-mo phase. After 2 mo of 4-drug treatment, for meningitis known or presumed to be caused by susceptible strains, PZA and EMB may be discontinued, and INH and RIF continued for an additional 7–10 mo, although the optimal duration of chemotherapy is not defined Adjunctive corticosteroid therapy with dexamethasone or prednisolone tapered over 6–8 wk[34]

Abbreviations: CRAg LFA, Cryptococcal Antigen Lateral Flow Assay; EMB, Ethambutol; INH, Isoniazid; PZA, Pyrazinamide.

decreased sensation in the left hemiface and trunk up to the level of the nipples, hyper-reflexia, and no objective weakness.

- Implementing the algorithm: The patient is a homosexual man and uses protection intermittently. HIV testing was negative (step 1). He works in a prison and reports low-grade fever and unintentional weight loss. He denies pulmonary symptoms (step 2). Initial brain MRI scan showed a few small, nonenhancing white matter hyperintensities. Repeat imaging 1 month later demonstrated multifocal bilateral cranial nerve enhancement, involving the optic, oculomotor, trigeminal, and facial nerves. Cervical spine MRI scan showed enhancement of the anterior cord from C1 to C4 (step 3) (**Fig. 4**A). He underwent an LP (Lumbar puncture) that demonstrated lymphocytic pleocytosis (387 WBC/mm^3 with 93% lymphocytes), elevated protein (357 mg/dL) and glucose (87 mg/dL, capillary glucose 172 mg/dL). Cytology was negative for malignant cells. Testing for multiple infections, including tuberculosis, was negative. CT scan of the chest, abdomen, and pelvis showed enlarged paraesophageal lymph nodes. Biopsy revealed noncaseating granulomas. Fungal and mycobacterial stains were negative (step 4).
  - Comments: The exposure history and systemic symptoms in this case were initially suspicious for an underlying immunocompromised state with a superimposed opportunistic infection, particularly tuberculosis. However, by following the diagnostic algorithm, these possibilities were excluded. The case illustrates the importance of advance testing (full-body imaging and tissue biopsy), which was fundamental to arrive to the final diagnosis of neurosarcoidosis. The patient was treated with IV methylprednisolone followed by prednisone. He had partial improvement. Methotrexate was added later as a steroid-sparing agent with marked clinical improvement.

NEUROSARCOIDOSIS

Sarcoidosis is a multisystem disorder characterized by granulomatous inflammation affecting multiple organs, particularly the lungs and lymph nodes. It has a prevalence of 4.7 to 64 per 100,000, and it is more common in African Americans.[38,39] Neurosarcoidosis refers to the central and/or peripheral nervous system involvement in systemic sarcoidosis, which is clinically apparent in 5% of patients.[40,41] In approximately half of those, neurologic manifestations constitute the initial presentation of the disease.[40]

The most common initial presentation of neurosarcoidosis is cranial neuropathy, occurring in more than half of cases. The facial and optic nerves are the most frequently affected. Multiple cranial nerve involvement is common.[39–41] Meningitis has been reported in 8% to 40% of cases, usually in the setting of cranial neuropathy. Other manifestations are myelopathy, different forms of neuropathy including small fiber neuropathy, and myopathy.[39,40,42] Hypothalamic and/or pituitary involvement may lead to endocrine disorders, and when present, they are an important clue to the diagnosis. Diabetes insipidus, hyperprolactinemia, and hypogonadism are the most common hormonal derangements.[39,41]

Brain MRI shows abnormalities in nearly 80% of patients.[40] Leptomeningeal thickening and enhancement occur in approximately 40% of patients and may be nodular or diffuse. There is preferential involvement of the basal meninges and cranial nerves. Other abnormalities, such as hydrocephalus and space-occupying lesions, are less frequent.[43] The imaging abnormalities may show complete or partial resolution with immunosuppressive treatment.[44,45]

CSF analysis typically demonstrates lymphocytic pleocytosis and elevated protein. Glucose may be low, and oligoclonal bands may be present. Serum and CSF angiotensin converting enzyme (ACE) have low sensitivity, being elevated in 29% to 65% and 24% to 55% of cases, respectively.[39–41] The gold standard for the diagnosis is the demonstration of noncaseating granulomas on tissue biopsy. Different imaging modalities may be used to look for a target for biopsy. Chest imaging is usually the initial test, and hilar lymphadenopathy is the most common finding. Brain or leptomeningeal biopsy is rarely necessary when no alternative site for biopsy is available. Ophthalmologic and hormonal evaluations should also be performed.[39,41] A set of diagnostic criteria has been proposed, which includes the clinical presentation and supportive ancillary testing.[46]

The first-line treatment of neurosarcoidosis is corticosteroids. Multiple other immunosuppressive drugs are used as second- or third-line agents. Cranial radiation is reserved for refractory cases (**Table 3**).[39–41]

Table 3
Autoimmune and neoplastic chronic meningitis

Disease	Diagnostic Testing	Treatment
Neurosarcoidosis	• Serum and CSF ACE • Chest radiograph or CT • [18]FDG-PET-CT • Tissue biopsy • Ophthalmologic evaluation • Hormonal testing	First-line: prednisone Second-line: • Methotrexate • Azathioprine • Hydroxychloroquine • Cyclosporine • Cyclophosphamide • Mycophenolate mofetil • Tumor necrosis alpha antagonists Refractory disease: cranial radiation
NMO	• Serum aquaporin 4 antibody IgG (NMO IgG) • CSF oligoclonal bands (typically absent) • CSF interleukin-6	Acute attack • Methylprednisolone 1 g IV per day for 3–5 d followed by oral steroid taper • Plasma exchange Disease-modifying therapy: • Rituximab • Mycophenolate mofetil • Azathioprine Emerging therapies: • Eculizumab • Tocilizumab
Neoplastic meningitis	• Opening pressure on LP • Large-volume LP • CSF cytology • CSF flow cytometry • Radioisotope CSF flow studies • Meningeal biopsy • Age-appropriate cancer screening • Blood smear • CT chest, abdomen, and pelvis • Skin survey • Testicular ultrasound • Tissue biopsy (lymph node, bone marrow, other)	Metastatic meningeal involvement: • Treatment of the underlying systemic malignancy if present Primary CNS neoplasms: • Intrathecal or intraventricular chemotherapy with or without systemic chemotherapy • Whole brain or spinal radiation • Ventriculoperitoneal shunt for hydrocephalus

Case 4: A 48-year-old woman presented with a 2-month history of right-sided visual loss and bilateral leg weakness. Neurologic examination demonstrated an unreactive pupil and decreased visual acuity on the right, bilateral leg weakness (3–4/5 in the Medical Research Council scale), hyperreflexia, and bilateral Babinski sign.

- Implementing the algorithm: She is immunocompetent and had negative HIV testing (step 1). She denies fever and other systemic symptoms as well as relevant occupational exposures (step 2). Brain MRI scan was normal. Spinal MRI scan showed extensive cord edema and T2 hyperintensity from C4 to the conus medullaris (step 3). CSF analysis revealed lymphocytic pleocytosis (187 WBC/mm³) and elevated protein (163 mg/dL). Workup for infectious causes of transverse myelitis was unremarkable. Serum aquaporin 4 antibodies were positive (step 4).
  - Comments: The characteristic clinical presentation and imaging pattern were highly suggestive of NMO in this case. The patient was treated empirically with IV methylprednisolone followed by a prednisone taper, plasma exchange, and rituximab. She had significant improvement of leg strength. Three years after the initial diagnosis, she developed left optic neuropathy.

NEUROMYELITIS OPTICA

NMO or the more collective term neuromyelitis optica spectrum disorders (NMOSD) are a group of rare autoimmune diseases of the CNS associated with serum immunoglobulin G (IgG) antibodies against the water channel aquaporin-4[4] (AQP4-IgG or NMO-IgG). Although typically considered a demyelinating disorder, up to 35% of patients have persistent pleocytosis, thus meeting the definition of chronic meningitis.[47,48]

The incidence of NMOSD in Caucasians is approximately 4.5 per 100,000. Women are more commonly affected, and the mean age of onset is 35 to 40 years.[49,50] The classic clinical presentation is bilateral optic neuritis and transverse myelitis. However, the clinical spectrum of NMOSD has recently expanded with the recognition of other distinctive manifestations. The area postrema syndrome, for example, consists of episodes of unexplained hiccups or nausea and vomiting. Other brainstem syndromes include oculomotor dysfunction, pruritus, and several cranial neuropathies.[47,51,52]

Imaging is extremely helpful because there are certain patterns that are highly suggestive of NMOSD. In acute optic neuritis, T2 hyperintensities and enhancement of the optic nerve are seen in 84% and 94% of cases, respectively. Lesions may be bilateral and spread to the optic chiasm. In transverse myelitis, the abnormalities characteristically extend over 3 or more spinal cord segments. They usually involve the gray matter, and there may be cord edema. Other patterns include lesions in the dorsal medulla (associated with the area postrema syndrome), periependymal brainstem regions, and diencephalic structures.[47,51]

CSF pleocytosis is present in approximately half of patients with NMOSD, and in 35% the cell count is >50 WBC/uL. Neutrophils and eosinophils may be present, and oligoclonal bands are typically absent. Because cellular pleocytosis persists until treatment, which can be weeks to months, a definition of chronic meningitis is established. Many times clinicians may be led to consider infectious causes in these cases of NMO due to the high CSF WBC pleocytosis and parenchymal findings on neuroimaging. Serum AQP4-IgG is highly specific for the disease (85%–100%). The sensitivity varies depending on the method used. Cell-based assays are preferred over indirect immunofluorescence and ELISA (sensitivity 76% vs 63%–64%). Testing for AQP4-IgG in the CSF has limited utility. A negative antibody does not exclude the condition because the 2015 diagnostic criteria for NMOSD defines seropositive and seronegative disease.[47,51,52] Treatment options for autoimmune disease are described in **Table 3**.

VASCULITIS

Chronic meningitis has been reported in most cases of systemic vasculitis.[6,53–55] A full description of each vasculitis is beyond the scope of this review, but the most common forms are mentioned briefly.

Aseptic meningitis is one of the neuropsychiatric syndromes observed in systemic lupus erythematosus, as defined by the American College of Rheumatology. It is generally rare, with an estimated frequency of less than 1%.[53,54] Behçet disease is characterized by the triad of recurrent oral and genital ulcers, and uveitis. It is rare in the Western Hemisphere and more prevalent in the Middle East. Neurologic involvement (Neuro-Behçet disease) occurs in 5% to 10% of patients, and meningoencephalitis is the most common manifestation.[3,55]

Primary angiitis of the CNS is a rare form of vasculitis isolated to the CNS vessels. The typical clinical presentation includes headache and focal deficits secondary to strokes. Cranial neuropathy is uncommon. CSF pleocytosis is present in 90% of cases, and cerebral angiography may show characteristic segmental narrowing and dilation of multiple vessels (beading pattern). Brain biopsy is the gold standard for diagnosis, but it is not always necessary in cases with typical angiographic findings.[56,57]

Case 5: A 52-year-old woman presented with 4 weeks of intermittent headache, dizziness, nausea, and disorientation. Initial examination demonstrated right and torsional beating nystagmus on Dix-Hallpike maneuver. Brain MRI scan was thought to be normal, and she was diagnosed with peripheral vertigo. She presented again 5 days later with convulsions. There was new left abducens and right facial paresis on repeated examination.

1. Implementing the algorithm: She is immunocompetent, and HIV testing was negative (step 1). She had no relevant exposures. Review of systems revealed back pain radiating to the left leg for which she was started on gabapentin. The drug was recently stopped because of lack of efficacy, and her current symptoms had been previously attributed to gabapentin withdrawal (step 2). Brain and spinal MRI scans demonstrated leptomeningeal enhancement affecting the pituitary infundibulum, brainstem, multiple cranial nerves, entire spinal cord, and cauda equina. There was also abnormal signal and diffuse enhancement of osseous structures (step 3; **Fig. 4**B, C). Further review of the initial MRI scan revealed subtle perimesencephalic enhancement. CSF was notable for lymphocytic pleocytosis (28 cells/mm³) and elevated protein (215 mg/dL). CT of the chest, abdomen, and pelvis demonstrated a hyperdense lesion in the right breast and multiple sclerotic changes in the axial and appendicular skeleton. CSF cytology was positive for malignant epithelial cells. Biopsy of the breast lesion revealed an invasive breast carcinoma (step 4).
   o Comments: This case illustrates some of the challenges in diagnosing chronic meningitis. The initial radicular pain was likely due to involvement of the cauda equina, but this was not fully investigated. Even though the CNS imaging findings were not specific for neoplastic chronic meningitis, the presence of breast and bone lesions made malignancy the most likely cause. This was later confirmed with advanced testing. The patient was treated with whole brain radiation. She was offered systemic chemotherapy but elected to withdraw support. She was discharged to home hospice and died a few months later.

NEOPLASTIC CHRONIC MENINGITIS

Malignancy is the second most commonly identified cause of chronic meningitis.[4,35] Neoplastic meningitis presents in 5% of patients with cancer and occurs with solid tumors, hematologic malignancies, and primary brain tumors. It is typically seen in patients with known neoplasms, but it may be the initial manifestation of cancer in 5% to 10% of cases.[58]

Leptomeningeal carcinomatosis or carcinomatous meningitis refers to meningeal involvement in solid tumors. Breast, small cell lung cancer, and melanoma are most commonly implicated. In the case of hematologic malignancies, lymphomatous meningitis has been reported in 5% to 15% of patients with high-grade, non-Hodgkin lymphoma. In primary brain tumors, 1% to 10% of patients develop neoplastic chronic meningitis.[58–61]

The clinical manifestations of chronic meningitis vary depending on the affected structures. Symptoms are multifocal in more than half of patients. Spinal symptoms (myelopathy and radiculopathy) are most common, followed by cerebral dysfunction and cranial neuropathies. The oculomotor nerves are the most frequently involved. Brain and/or spinal MRI scans are abnormal in approximately 60% of patients, demonstrating focal or diffuse leptomeningeal enhancement. Communicating hydrocephalus may be seen in up to 10% of cases.[62,63] CSF pleocytosis and elevated protein are detected in most patients, more often in those with solid tumors than hematologic malignancies. Initial CSF cytology demonstrates malignant cells in 67% to 89% of patients. Repeating an LP increases the yield by 25% to 30%.[58,62] A small proportion of patients have persistently normal CSF cytology despite multiple examinations. Meningeal biopsy may be necessary in these cases. When chronic meningitis is the initial manifestation of a systemic cancer, appropriate screening should be pursued to find the primary malignancy (see **Table 3**).

The treatment of neoplastic meningitis depends on the primary cancer and includes radiation, systemic and intrathecal or intraventricular chemotherapy, and ventriculoperitoneal shunting for hydrocephalus.[58] Neoplastic meningitis carries a poor prognosis. Median survival of untreated disease is 1 to 2 months for solid tumors and 4 to 5 months for lymphoma.[59,61]

RARE CAUSES OF CHRONIC MENINGITIS

Certain drugs are known to induce aseptic meningitis.[64] In most circumstances, this adverse effect is anticipated, and in some cases even prevented. However, if drug-induced aseptic meningitis goes unrecognized for weeks or months, it may present as chronic meningitis.[65]

Neonatal-onset multisystem inflammatory disease or chronic infantile neurologic, cutaneous, and articular syndrome is the most severe form of the cryopyrin-associated periodic syndromes. It is an autosomal dominant disorder caused by mutations in the NLRP3 gene, and it is characterized by neonatal onset of fever, urticarial rash, and chronic aseptic meningitis.[66] Periodic fever syndromes and chronic meningitis have also been reported in adult patients and have responded well to treatment with anakinra.[67]

Fabry disease is a rare, X-linked lysosomal storage disorder caused by mutations in the gene encoding alpha-galactosidase A. The most common neurologic manifestation is acroparesthesia due to small fiber neuropathy. Steroid-responsive chronic meningitis has been reported in a few cases.[68,69]

IgG4-related disease is a recently recognized immune-mediated disorder that may affect the central and peripheral nervous system. Meningeal involvement manifests as a hypertrophic pachymeningitis on MRI scan. CSF analysis demonstrates mild lymphocytic pleocytosis. Corticosteroids have limited utility, and rituximab is recommended for severe cases.[70]

IDIOPATHIC CHRONIC MENINGITIS

Up to 30% of patients with chronic meningitis will have no discernible cause after exhaustive testing. Literature is sparse on this population of patients, with only one retrospective review that reports good clinical outcomes in 85% of patients. Corticosteroid therapy was effective in 52% of patients, but there are no data if this would affect outcomes.[37] With advances in knowledge and testing, such as next-generation sequencing, the number of idiopathic cases is likely to decrease. Clinicians should exhaust all efforts to identify treatable causes of chronic meningitis before labeling a patient as idiopathic.

DISCUSSION

Chronic meningitis is a common diagnostic challenge for neurologists. The differential diagnosis for CSF pleocytosis that is persistent for more than 1 month is large and encompasses infectious, neoplastic, idiopathic, and other rare causes. By using a standardized algorithmic approach, as outlined in this article, many patients can be accurately diagnosed and treated appropriately. In the minority of cases whereby a cause cannot be ascertained despite complete evaluation, empiric treatment with steroids is reasonable.

ACKNOWLEDGMENTS

The authors thank Na Tosha Gatson, MD, PhD and Taimur Malik, MD for providing 2 of the cases presented in this article.

REFERENCES

1. Colombe B, Derradji M, Bosseray A, et al. Chronic meningitis: aetiologies, diagnosis and treatment. Rev Med Interne 2003;24:24–33.
2. Glaser CA, Gilliam S, Schnurr D, et al. In search of encephalitis etiologies: diagnostic challenges in the California Encephalitis Project, 1998-2000. Clin Infect Dis 2003;36:731–42.
3. Zunt JRM, Baldwin KJ. Chronic and subacute meningitis. Contin lifelong learn. Neuro 2012;18:1290–318.
4. Anderson NE, Willoughby EW. Chronic meningitis without predisposing illness – a review of 83 cases. Q J Med 1987;63:283–95.
5. Ginsberg L, Kidd D. Chronic and recurrent meningitis. Pract Neurol 2008;8: 348–61.
6. Baldwin KJ, Zunt JR. Evaluation and treatment of chronic meningitis. Neurohospitalist 2014;4:185–95.
7. Glass JP, Melamed M, Chernik NL, et al. Malignant cells in the cerebrospinal fluid (CSF): the meaning of a positive CSF cytology. Neurology 1979;29(20):1369–75.
8. Elfiky N, Baldwin K. Brown heroin-associated candida albicans ventriculitis and endophthalmitis treated with voriconazole. Case Rep Neurol 2016;8(2):151–5.
9. Bisbe J, Miro JM, Latorre X, et al. Disseminated candidiasis in addicts who use brown heroin: report of 83 cases and review. Clin Infect Dis 1992;15:910–23.
10. Yamamoto F, Yamashita S, Kawano H, et al. Meningitis and ventriculitis due to *Nocardia araoensis* infection. Intern Med 2017;56(7):853–9.
11. Baidya A, Tripathi M, Pandey P, et al. Mycobacterium abscessus as a cause of chronic meningitis: a rare clinical entity. Am J Med Sci 2016; 351(4):437–9.

12. Hessler C, Kauffman CA, Chow FC. The upside of bias: a case of chronic meningitis due to sporothrix schenckii in an immunocompetent host. Neurohospitalist 2017;7(1):30–4.
13. Wilson MR, Suan D, Duggins A, et al. A novel cause of chronic viral meningoencephalitis: Cache Valley virus. Ann Neurol 2017;82:105–14.
14. Wilson MR, Naccache SN, Samayoa E, et al. Actionable diagnosis of neuroleptospirosis by next-generation sequencing. N Engl J Med 2014;370:2408–17.
15. Naccache SN, Peggs KS, Mattes FM, et al. Diagnosis of neuroinvasive astrovirus infection in an immunocompromised adult with encephalitis by unbiased next-generation sequencing. Clin Infect Dis 2015;60:919–23.
16. Chayakulkeeree M, Perfect JR. Cryptococcosis. Infect Dis Clin North Am 2006; 20(3):507–44.
17. Chen S, Sorrell T, Nimmo G, et al. Epidemiology and host- and variety-dependent characteristics of infection due to Cryptococcus neoformans in Australia and New Zealand. Australasian Cryptococcal Study Group. Clin Infect Dis 2003; 31(2):499–508.
18. Day J. Cryptococcal meningitis. Pract Neurol 2004;4:274–85.
19. Graybill JR, Sobel J, Saag M, et al. Diagnosis and management of increased intracranial pressure in patients with AIDS and cryptococcal meningitis. The NIAID mycoses study group and AIDS cooperative treatment groups. Clin Infect Dis 2000;30(1):47–54.
20. Day JN, Chau TTH, Wolbers M, et al. Combination antifungal therapy for cryptococcal meningitis. N Engl J Med 2013;368(14):1291–302.
21. Pichler MR, Parisi JE, Klaas JP. A woman in her 60s with chronic meningitis. JAMA Neurol 2017;74(3):348–52.
22. Latge JP. Aspergillus fumigatus and aspergillosis. Clin Microbiol Rev 1999;12(2): 310–50.
23. Denning DW. Invasive aspergillosis. Clin Infect Dis 1998;26(4):781–803.
24. Kleinschmidt-DeMasters BK. Central nervous system aspergillosis: a 20-year retrospective series. Hum Pathol 2002;33(1):116–24.
25. Jain KK, Mittal SK, Kuman S, et al. Imaging feature of central nervous system fungal infections. Neurol India 2007;55(3):214–50.
26. Herbrecht R, Letscher-Bru V, Oprea C, et al. Aspergillus galactomannan detection in the diagnosis of invasive aspergillosis in cancer patients. J Clin Oncol 2002;20(7):1898–906.
27. Odabasi Z, Mattiuzzi G, Estey E, et al. Beta-D-glucan as a diagnostic adjunct for invasive fungal infections: validation, cutoff development, and performance in patients with acute myelogenous leukemiaand myelodysplastic syndrome. Clin Infect Dis 2004;39(2):199–205.
28. Herbrecht R, Denning DW, Patterson TF, et al. Voriconazole versus amphotericin B for primary therapy of invasive aspergillosis. N Engl J Med 2002;347(6):408–15.
29. U.S. Preventive Services Task Force. Screening for syphilis infection: recommendation statement. Ann Fam Med 2004;2:362–5.
30. Marra CM, Tantalo LC, Maxwell CL, et al. Alternative cerebrospinal fluid tests to diagnose neurosyphilis in HIV-infected individuals. Neurology 2004;63(1):85–8.
31. Workowski KA, Bolan GA, Centers for Disease Control and Prevention. Sexually transmitted diseases treatment guidelines. MMWR Recomm Rep 2015;64(RR-03): 1–137.
32. Pappas PG, Kauffman CA, Andes DR, et al. Clinical practice guideline for the management of candidiasis: 2016 update by the infectious diseases Society of America. Clin Infect Dis 2016;62(4):e1–50.

33. Wormser GP, Dattwyler RJ, Shapiro ED, et al. The clinical assessment, treatment, and prevention of lyme disease, human granulocytic anaplasmosis, and babesiosis: clinical practice guidelines by the infectious diseases Society of America. Clin Infect Dis 2006;43:1089–134.
34. Nahid P, Dorman SE, Alipanah N, et al. Official American Thoracic Society/Centers for Disease Control and Prevention/Infectious Diseases Society of America clinical practice guidelines: treatment of drug-susceptible tuberculosis. Clin Infect Dis 2016;63:e147–95.
35. Ellner JJ, Bennett JE. Chronic meningitis. Medicine (Baltimore) 1976;55:341–69.
36. Charleston AJ, Anderson NE, Willoughby EW. Idiopathic steroid responsive chronic lymphocytic meningitis–clinical features and long-term outcome in 17 patients. Aust N Z J Med 1998;28:784–9.
37. Smith JE, Aksamit AJ Jr. Outcome of chronic idiopathic meningitis. Mayo Clin Proc 1994;69(6):548–56.
38. Valeyre D, Prasse A, Nunes H, et al. Sarcoidosis. Lancet 2014;383:1155–67.
39. Lacomis D. Neurosarcoidosis. Curr Neuropharmacol 2011;9:429–36.
40. Fritz D, van de Beek D, Brouwer MC. Clinical features, treatment and outcome in neurosarcoidosis: systematic review and meta-analysis. BMC Neurol 2016; 16:220.
41. Carlson ML, White JR Jr, Espahbodi M, et al. Cranial base manifestations of neurosarcoidosis: a review of 305 patients. Otol Neurotol 2015;36:156–66.
42. Tavee JO, Karwa K, Ahmed Z, et al. Sarcoidosis-associated small fiber neuropathy in a large cohort: clinical aspects and response to IVIG and anti-TNF alpha treatment. Respir Med 2017;126:135–8.
43. Smith JK, Matheus MG, Castillo M. Imaging manifestations of neurosarcoidosis. AJR Am J Roentgenol 2004;182:289–95.
44. Lexa FJ, Grossman RI. MR of sarcoidosis in the head and spine: spectrum of manifestations and radiographic response to steroid therapy. AJNR Am J Neuroradiol 1994;15:973–82.
45. Avila JD, Bucelli RC. Nodular leptomeningeal enhancement in neurosarcoidosis: before and after treatment. Neurohospitalist 2017;7:NP1–2.
46. Zajicek JP, Scolding NJ, Foster O, et al. Central nervous system sarcoidosis–diagnosis and management. QJM 1999;92:103–17.
47. Patterson SL, Goglin SE. Neuromyelitis Optica. Rheum Dis Clin North Am 2017; 43:579–91.
48. Jarius S, Paul F, Franciotta D, et al. Cerebrospinal fluid findings in aquaporin-4 antibody positive neuromyelitis optica: results from 211 lumbar punctures. J Neurol Sci 2011;306:82–90.
49. Asgari N, Lillevang ST, Skejoe HP, et al. A population-based study of neuromyelitis optica in Caucasians. Neurology 2011;76:1589–95.
50. Mealy MA, Wingerchuk DM, Greenberg BM, et al. Epidemiology of neuromyelitis optica in the United States: a multicenter analysis. Arch Neurol 2012;69:1176–80.
51. Wingerchuk DM, Banwell B, Bennett JL, et al. International consensus diagnostic criteria for neuromyelitis optica spectrum disorders. Neurology 2015;85:177–89.
52. Kremer L, Mealy M, Jacob A, et al. Brainstem manifestations in neuromyelitis optica: a multicenter study of 258 patients. Mult Scler 2014;20:843–7.
53. The American College of Rheumatology nomenclature and case definitions for neuropsychiatric lupus syndromes. Arthritis Rheum 1999;42:599–608.
54. Kim JM, Kim KJ, Yoon HS, et al. Meningitis in Korean patients with systemic lupus erythematosus: analysis of demographics, clinical features and outcomes;

experience from affiliated hospitals of the Catholic University of Korea. Lupus 2011;20:531–6.

55. Kalra S, Silman A, Akman-Demir G, et al. Diagnosis and management of Neuro-Behçet's disease: international consensus recommendations. J Neurol 2014;261: 1662–76.

56. Hajj-Ali RA, Singhal AB, Benseler S, et al. Primary angiitis of the CNS. Lancet Neurol 2011;10:561–72.

57. Salvarani C, Brown RD Jr, Calamia KT, et al. Primary central nervous system vasculitis: analysis of 101 patients. Ann Neurol 2007;62:442–51.

58. Gleissner B, Chamberlain MC. Neoplastic meningitis. Lancet Neurol 2006;5: 443–52.

59. Le Rhun E, Taillibert S, Chamberlain MC. Neoplastic meningitis due to lung, breast, and melanoma metastases. Cancer Control 2017;24:22–32.

60. Chowdhary S, Damlo S, Chamberlain MC. Cerebrospinal fluid dissemination and neoplastic meningitis in primary brain tumors. Cancer Control 2017;24:S1–16.

61. Taylor JW, Flanagan EP, O'Neill BP, et al. Primary leptomeningeal lymphoma: International primary CNS lymphoma collaborative group report. Neurology 2013; 81:1690–6.

62. van Oostenbrugge RJ, Twijnstra A. Presenting features and value of diagnostic procedures in leptomeningeal metastases. Neurology 1999;53:382–5.

63. Chamberlain MC. Comprehensive neuraxis imaging in leptomeningeal metastasis: a retrospective case series. CNS Oncol 2013;2:121–8.

64. Holle D, Obermann M. Headache in drug-induced aseptic meningitis. Curr Pain Headache Rep 2015;19:29.

65. Ashton D, Kim P, Griffiths N, et al. Cognitive decline with chronic meningitis secondary to a COX-2 inhibitor. Age Ageing 2004;33:408–9.

66. Finetti M, Omenetti A, Federici S, et al. Chronic infantile neurological cutaneous and articular (CINCA) syndrome: a review. Orphanet J Rare Dis 2016;11:167.

67. Novroski AR, Baldwin KJ. Chronic autoimmune meningoencephalitis and periodic fever syndrome treated with anakinra. Case Rep Neurol 2017;9(1):91–7.

68. Uyama E, Ueno N, Uchino M, et al. Headache associated with aseptic meningeal reaction as clinical onset of Fabry's disease. Headache 1995;35:498–501.

69. Lidove O, Chauveheid MP, Benoist L, et al. Chronic meningitis and thalamic involvement in a woman: Fabry disease expanding phenotype. J Neurol Neurosurg Psychiatry 2007;78:1007.

70. AbdelRazek M, Stone JH. Neurologic features of immunoglobulin G4-related disease. Rheum Dis Clin North Am 2017;43:621–31.

Neurocysticercosis

Hector H. Garcia, MD, PhD[a,b,]*

KEYWORDS

- Cysticercosis • Neurocysticercosis • *Taenia solium* • Epilepsy
- Nervous system infections • Albendazole • Praziquantel

KEY POINTS

- Neurocysticercosis (NCC) is a major contributor to the burden of seizure disorders and epilepsy in most of the world.
- NCC encompasses a variety of clinical presentations, greatly depending on the characteristics of infection (number, location, size, and involutive stage of lesions) as well as on the inflammatory response of the host.
- Diagnosis and therapy should be tailored to the specific type of NCC.
- Medical therapy for NCC should first cover appropriate symptom control and then use of antiparasitic agents should be considered. Antiparasitic treatment is of benefit in most cases of viable and degenerating NCC.
- Active interventions in endemic regions have resulted in temporal elimination of transmission, setting the foundations for widespread elimination and eventual eradication of the disease.

INTRODUCTION

In most poor societies, with exception of Muslim countries, villagers raise pigs as a cheap and easy source of meat. Coexistence of pigs and humans in poor sanitary conditions provides the perfect setting for the establishment of the cycle of *Taenia solium*, the pork tapeworm (discussed later). The larvae of *T solium* can invade the human nervous system causing neurocysticercosis (NCC), which is a frequent condition affecting 10% to 20% of villagers in endemic regions.[1,2] Although most NCC infections seem asymptomatic, a minority of symptomatic patients still result in a sizable burden of disease, contributing to approximately 30% of all seizure disorders in *T solium*–endemic regions.[1,3,4] Travel and migration make NCC an occasional diagnosis in nonendemic countries, with more than 1000 cases per year in the United States only.[5,6]

BIOLOGY OF THE PARASITE

In the usual life cycle, humans carry the intestinal adult tapeworm that results from ingestion of improperly cooked pork with cysts. The tapeworm is highly infectious.

a Cysticercosis Unit, Instituto Nacional de Ciencias Neurologicas, Jr Ancash 1271, Lima 1, Peru;
b Center for Global Health, Universidad Peruana Cayetano Heredia, SMP, Lima 31, Peru
* Center for Global Health, Universidad Peruana Cayetano Heredia, SMP, Lima 31, Peru.
E-mail address: hgarcia@jhsph.edu

Neurol Clin 36 (2018) 851–864
https://doi.org/10.1016/j.ncl.2018.07.003

A single segment or proglottid may contain 30,000 infectious eggs and the tapeworm can expel with the carrier stools several proglottids in a day. In places lacking appropriate sanitation, pigs access and ingest these contaminated stools, become infected with tapeworm eggs, and develop cystic larvae in their flesh and other tissues (porcine cysticercosis) (**Fig. 1**).[7] Unfortunately, humans are exposed to tapeworm eggs by microscopic fecal contamination and can develop cysticercosis too. Human cysticercosis infection is usually dependent on close contact with a tapeworm carrier[8–10] and does not involve ingestion of infected pork with cysts (so a tapeworm carrier can originate NCC cases even in a noncysticercosis–endemic region).[11] Most studies have found few *T solium* eggs in flies, water, or short stem vegetables, so infection through these sources seems unlikely.[12] Human infection is not exclusive of the nervous system.

HUMAN CENTRAL NERVOUS SYSTEM INFECTION AND TYPES OF NEUROCYSTICERCOSIS

After ingestion, tapeworm eggs hatch in the digestive system and liberate the infective oncospheres that cross the intestinal mucosa and distribute to all tissues by the blood stream. Although there is minimal or no information of the natural course of human infection, it seems that most cysts are destroyed by the immune response of the host and die soon after infection, likely in weeks or months.[13] CNS cysts are a minority of all cysts distributed in the body and probably those that survive are because of blood-brain barrier protection from the host immunity.

The location of the parasite in the CNS and its expansion toward the inside of the brain parenchyma or toward the subarachnoid and ventricular spaces is a major determinant of its process of evolution and the subsequent clinical manifestations.

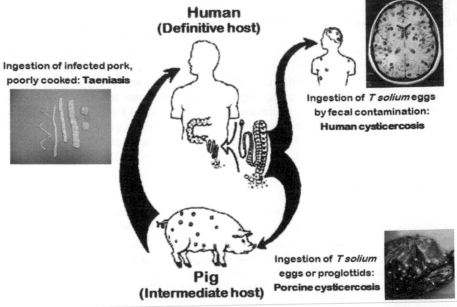

Human (Definitive host)

Ingestion of infected pork, poorly cooked: Taeniasis

Ingestion of *T solium* eggs by fecal contamination: Human cysticercosis

Ingestion of *T solium* eggs or proglottids: Porcine cysticercosis

Pig (Intermediate host)

Fig. 1. Life cycle of the pork tapeworm *T solium*. (*Adapted from* Garcia HH, Martinez SM. *Taenia solium* taeniasis/cysticercosis. Lima (Peru): Ed. Universo; 1999. p. 346; with permission.)

Intraparenchymal Cysts

Cysticerci in the brain parenchyma establish initially as viable cysts usually measuring 0.5 cm to 1.5 cm in diameter, with a clear liquid content. Cysts may survive in this quiescent stage for many years thanks to active immune evasion mechanisms. Eventually, the host's immune system detects the parasite and launches a cellular response with local inflammation that disrupts the cyst membranes and affects its homeostasis, leading to a progressively increasing density of cyst contents, to then collapse the cyst into a granulomatous lesion that is later cleared completely or replaced by a calcified scar[14] (**Fig. 2**). In more classical literature, the cystic form used to be named *Cysticercus cellulosae*.

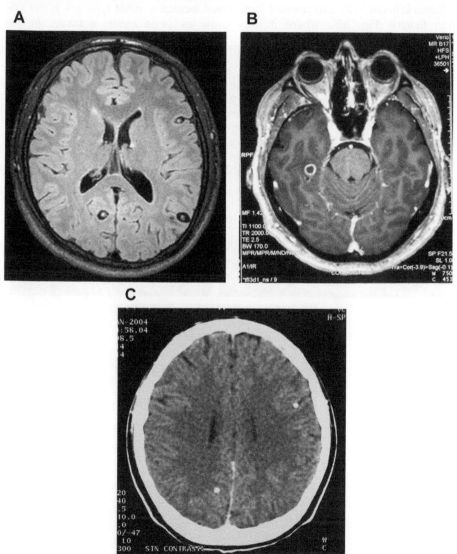

Fig. 2. Parenchymal neurocysticercosis. (*A*) Viable cysts (MRI, fluid-attenuated inversion recovery sequence); (*B*) degenerating cyst (cysticercal granuloma, postcontrast T1 MRI sequence); and (*C*) calcified lesions (noncontrasted CT).

Extraparenchymal Cysts

The information on the natural evolution of cysts inside the ventricular cavities (ventricular NCC) is limited by their clinical expression. Ventricular cysts frequently block the circulation of cerebrospinal fluid (CSF) causing obstructive hydrocephalus, and some of them, in particular those attached to a ventricular wall and not blocking the CSF flow, follow an involutive course, similar to the one described previously for intraparenchymal cysts, and eventually resolve (**Fig. 3**A). Cysts in the subarachnoid space, on the contrary, tend to grow and expand their membranes forming vesicular clusters that involve the neighboring spaces.[14,15] These lesions were called *racemose cysticercosis* in the classic literature, in reference to their similarity with a bunch of grapes (racemus).

Subarachnoid NCC can present in different locations, most typically in the sylvian fissure (**Fig. 3**B), where it may grow as large cystic masses, in the

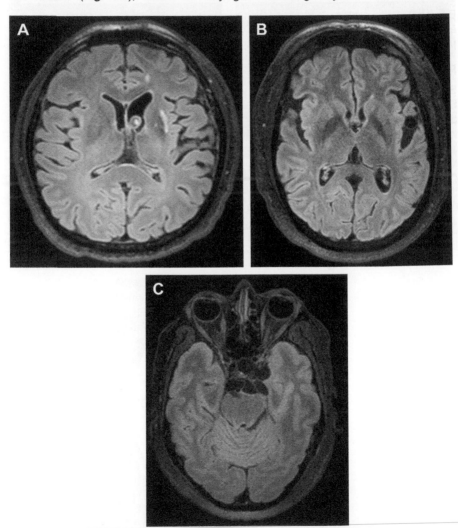

Fig. 3. Extraparenchymal neurocysticercosis. (*A*) ventricular cysts; (*B*) cystic mass in the sylvian fissure; (*C*) basal subarachnoid NCC. All images are MRI in fluid-attenuated inversion recovery sequence.

interhemispheric spaces, or in the basal cisterns. The latter (basal subarachnoid NCC [**Fig. 3**C]) is associated with extensive parasitic infiltration and a marked inflammatory response evident in neuroimaging and CSF examinations. Although not formally demonstrated, most experts consider that subarachnoid NCC is progressive and associated with significant mortality, reported to be more than 20% even in well-equipped centers.[15–17]

Because cysticerci reach the brain via the blood stream, most of them grow from the gray-white matter interphase. Small cysts partially embedded in the parenchyma but growing toward the subarachnoid spaces behave as intraparenchymal rather than as subarachnoid cysts.

SYMPTOMS

Because of its potential to locate in diverse areas of the CNS, NCC has been associated with a wide variety of neurologic symptoms. The most frequent clinical manifestations are seizures, intracranial hypertension, focal deficits, and cognitive alterations.

Seizures and Epilepsy

Seizures are the most characteristic symptom of parenchymal brain cysticercosis. Seizures may appear in any stage of the parasite, from viable noninflamed cysts, degenerating cysts, or calcified lesions. Seizure activity is more frequent in patients with degenerating cysts and rare in patients with only viable, noninflamed cysts. The semiology of seizures frequently correlates with the anatomic location of one of the brain parasites.[18] When and whether an epileptogenic circuit is formed around a cysticerci is unclear, but patients frequently present repeated episodes of the same type of seizure, in many cases even years after the parasitic larvae has died and become calcified.

Headache and Intracranial Hypertension

Headache in NCC also may occur as a postictal manifestation after a seizure episode or as an isolated symptom, although its most conspicuous presentation is as part of an intracranial hypertension syndrome. Extraparenchymal NCC frequently presents with intracranial hypertension that can evolve from diverse mechanisms. One of the most frequent causes is obstructive hydrocephalus resulting from external compression of the CSF pathways by cystic masses, from internal blockage by intraventricular cysts, or from residual arachnoiditis in chronic cases.[19] Intracranial hypertension also may result from large cyst masses in the sylvian fissures or interhemispheric spaces,[20] or more rarely from an acute, diffuse encephalitis-like reaction to massive cyst infections. The later, termed *cysticercotic encephalitis*, is a rare condition that occurs more frequently in young female patients and may be life-threatening.[21]

Mass Effect and Focal Deficits

Large cysts or cyst clusters in the subarachnoid spaces may cause mass effects leading to intracranial hypertension or focal deficits.[20] Mass effect also can result from perilesional edema in calcified NCC. In these cases, MRI examination after a seizure episode unveils large areas of edema surrounding 1 or more calcified parasites.[22] Perilesional edema may manifest with focal deficits associated with headache without seizures.[23] Increased neurologic symptoms during antiparasitic therapy likely result from a similar mechanism resulting in perilesional inflammation and edema around a degenerating cyst. Focal deficits may occur after repeated partial seizures, from Todd paralysis, and may take a few days to resolve.

Cognitive Alterations and Psychiatric Symptoms

Ancient NCC case descriptions have frequently noted mood alterations in the NCC patients,[24] and series of NCC cases with psychiatric alterations can be found in the literature.[25] More recently, the association between NCC and cognitive alterations has been more systematically assessed in series from Brazil and other endemic regions.[26] Depression also seems a common event in NCC.[27] The real prevalence of cognitive alterations and psychiatric symptoms by type of NCC, however, is yet unknown.

DIAGNOSIS

A diagnosis of NCC is based on neuroimaging examinations and supported by specific serologic assays.

Neuroimaging

Imaging techniques (CT and MRI) are crucial because they provide information on the presence, number, location, size, and stage of the parasite as well as on the immune response of the host visible as perilesional or diffuse inflammation and blood-brain barrier dysfunction shown by focal contrast enhancement. In addition, it may demonstrate other associated conditions, such as hydrocephalus or stroke.[28,29] Ideally, a patient with suspected NCC should have both CT and MRI performed because MRI provides better imaging of small lesions and those close to the skull and in the posterior fossa and gives more information on parenchymal inflammation or periventricular effusion in hydrocephalus. CT is much better to detect calcifications,[30] however, and it is not uncommon to miss calcified cysts if MRI alone is used. In endemic countries, however, economic factors limit the access to neuroimaging and many times CT is the only available tool.

On imaging, viable intraparenchymal cysts are seen as well-defined, rounded cystic structures with liquid contents which signal similar to CSF, with minimal or no surrounding inflammation. Once the parasite is detected by the immune system of the host, inflammation is initially noticeable as pericystic edema and contrast enhancement, followed by the collapse of the cyst into a small annular or nodular lesion that resolves and then eventually reappears in most cases as a small nodular calcified lesion[28,29] (see **Fig. 2**). Intraventricular cysts are poorly defined on CT but appear on MRI also as well-defined viable or degenerating cysts. Cysts in the subarachnoid space are less defined in shape and tend to accommodate to the available spaces where they distort the normal anatomy. These lesions may grow and occupy large spaces, particularly in the sylvian fissures and in the basal cisterns (see **Fig. 3**). Balanced steady state gradient-echo sequences (Fast Imaging Employing Steady-state Acquisition [FIESTA], Balanced Fast Field Echo [BFFE], True Fast Imaging with Steady state Precession [TrueFISP], FIESTA-C, and Constructive Interference Steady State [CISS], depending on the magnetic resonance company) do a better job in defining the parasitic lesions in the subarachnoid space.[31] Perilesional inflammation is uncommon in subarachnoid NCC except in cases where a region of residual arachnoiditis replace the cysts.

Immunodiagnosis

Serology for NCC aims to detect specific antibodies to the parasite or circulating parasite antigens. Up to the early 1980s, the performance of antibody detection in NCC was disappointing. The introduction of ELISA assays improved assay sensitivity and specificity[32] but the use of crude antigens resulted in significant rates of cross-reactions with other parasite infections (such as hydatid disease and hymenolepiasis) that are frequent in cysticercosis-endemic regions, significantly affecting their specificity when used in these populations.[33–36] The enzyme-linked immunoelectrotransfer blot (EITB)–Western blot assay using lentil-lectin purified antigens (LLGP), developed at the Centers for Disease Control and Prevention and introduced in 1989,[37] provided a much better performing tool with no known cross-reactions with other infections of humans, and a very high (approximately 98%) sensitivity in individuals with 2 or more brain cysts, although it may be lower for cases with a single brain lesion.[38]

Antibody detection, however, has limitations. Between 10% and 20% of all individuals in endemic populations may present specific antibody reactions not only in those with viable NCC infections but also due to infections outside the CNS, from passive transfer from their mothers, from exposure without infection, or from infections that resolved spontaneously. Detecting specific circulating parasite antigens confirms the presence of viable parasites and overcomes these limitations. Two ELISA assays based on monoclonal antibodies (originally produced against the closely related beef tapeworm *T saginata*) have been reported to work for this purpose.[39,40] As expected, the sensitivity of antigen detection is lower than that for antibody detection, and negative results in individuals with few brain cysts are frequent.[38]

Appropriately used, LLGP-EITB antibody detection and monoclonal antibody–based ELISA antigen detection may be extremely useful to support a diagnosis of NCC or to rule out nonconclusive imaging diagnoses. In particular, individuals with viable cyst infections should be positive on LLGP-EITB,[41] and individuals with calcified lesions only should be antigen negative.[42] A remaining caveat of serology occurs with a seronegative individual with a single brain cyst or single degenerating nodule. In this case, there is no alternative form to confirm the diagnosis of NCC, unless a *T solium* carrier can be found in the household.

A chart of diagnostic criteria for NCC was initially prepared in 1996 and revisited in 2001[43,44] and more recently in 2017 (Del Brutto's diagnostic criteria [**Box 1**]),[45] nicely assembling different diagnostic information in categories and degrees of certainty. The criteria approach is based on neuroimaging studies as the essential tool for NCC diagnosis, with other information providing indirect evidence in favor of the diagnosis. Validation by an external group demonstrated a sensitivity of 93.6% and a specificity of 81.1% for the 2001 version. Although some groups have proposed specific adaptations for particular scenarios,[46–48] systematic use of the practical definitions in this set of criteria should help to uniformize the diagnosis of NCC in diverse settings.

PROGNOSIS

In general, parenchymal NCC seems to carry a benign prognosis if adequate symptomatic therapy is provided. Destruction of cysts by means of antiparasitic agents is recommended to reduce the likelihood of future seizure relapses and to decrease the risk of disease progression.[49] Extraparenchymal NCC, on the other hand, is not benign. Intraventricular cysts may lead to obstructive hydrocephalus and even to sudden death, and subarachnoid NCC may also progress to kill the patient. Past estimates of lethality of subarachnoid NCC ranged between 20% and 50% of cases.[50] Although these rates are likely much lower now, this type of NCC still carries significant risks even in the best available management conditions.

MANAGEMENT
Symptomatic Treatment

NCC is a chronic infection and patients present symptoms months or years after infection.[24] It follows that destroying the parasite is not an emergency and thus

Box 1
Diagnostic criteria for neurocysticercosis

Absolute criteria

- Histologic demonstration of the parasite from biopsy of a brain or spinal cord lesion
- Visualization of subretinal cysticercus
- Conclusive demonstration of a scolex within a cystic lesion on neuroimaging studies

Neuroimaging criteria

Major neuroimaging criteria
- Cystic lesions without a discernible scolex
- Enhancing lesions
- Multilobulated cystic lesions in the subarachnoid space
- Typical parenchymal brain calcifications

Confirmative neuroimaging criteria
- Resolution of cystic lesions after cysticidal drug therapy
- Spontaneous resolution of single small enhancing lesions
- Migration of ventricular cysts documented on sequential neuroimaging studies

Minor neuroimaging criteria
- Obstructive hydrocephalus (symmetric or asymmetric) or abnormal enhancement of basal leptomeninges

Clinical/exposure criteria

Major clinical/exposure
- Detection of specific anticysticercal antibodies or cysticercal antigens by well-standardized immunodiagnostic tests
- Cysticercosis outside the central nervous system
- Evidence of a household contact with T solium infection

Minor clinical/exposure
- Clinical manifestations suggestive of neurocysticercosis
- Individuals coming from or living in an area where cysticercosis is endemic

A definitive diagnosis is defined by (1) 1 absolute criterion; (2) 2 major neuroimaging criteria plus any clinical/exposure criteria; (3) 1 major and 2 confirmative neuroimaging criteria plus any clinical/exposure criteria; or (4) 1 major neuroimaging criteria plus 2 clinical/exposure criteria (including at least 1 major clinical/exposure criterion), together with the exclusion of other pathologies producing similar neuroimaging findings. A probable diagnosis is defined by (1) 1 major neuroimaging criteria plus any 2 clinical/exposure criteria or (2) 1 minor neuroimaging criteria plus at least one major clinical/exposure criteria.
From Del Brutto OH, Nash TE, White AC Jr, et al. Revised diagnostic criteria for neurocysticercosis. J Neurol Sci 2017;372:204; with permission.

the initial approach to a patient with NCC should be appropriate symptom control. Analgesics and antiepileptic drugs should be used as indicated in general practice.[51] Control of intracranial hypertension may require steroids, acetazolamide, mannitol, or surgery (either neuroendoscopic approaches with fenestration of the anterior wall of the third ventricle or shunt placement; rarely, excision of a large lesion or lesion conglomerate).[52]

Antiparasitic Treatment

One of the most controversial points in the cysticercosis literature is the use of antiparasitic agents to kill brain cysts. Before 1979, there was no specific therapy for NCC. The introduction of praziquantel (PZQ), initially described by Robles and Chavarria Chavarria,[53] provided the first cysticidal agent. Its efficacy was demonstrated by brain imaging, and clinical benefits were evident in most patients. Unfortunately, as PZQ was more widely used, some patients experienced serious exacerbations of their neurologic symptoms, including several deaths. This phenomenon was rapidly recognized as an inflammatory response to the death of the parasites and concomitant use of steroids was added with satisfactory results.[54] Some groups, however, argued that the risk of treatment-associated symptoms was unnecessary because the parasite had already begun to resolve. Now a large body of evidence confirms that parasitic cysts do not spontaneously resolve in the short term, that antiparasitic agents are effective in destroying the cysts, and that cyst destruction is associated with fewer seizure relapses in the follow-up.[49,55,56] Currently most regimens use albendazole (ABZ) alone or combined with PZQ, with concomitant steroid therapy (**Table 1**).[17] The initial inflammatory response that follows the onset of antiparasitic treatment, however, may be severe in patients with many cysts or those with large lesions or lesions located in delicate areas of the encephalon.

The efficacy of a first course of antiparasitic treatment (usually ABZ) in parenchymal NCC is approximately 60% to 80% in terms of cyst destruction and 30% to 40% in terms of complete resolution of all lesions. Although there are no large series or controlled studies, the efficacy of the initial course of antiparasitic drugs to clear subarachnoid NCC seems even lower. Again, there are no controlled studies comparing the efficacy of a second course of ABZ versus switching to PZQ or using combined ABZ plus PZQ in patients who fail an initial treatment. In the absence of safety data for higher doses of ABZ, a longer course of ABZ or combined ABZ plus PZQ seem the most logical alternative.

Anti-inflammatory Treatment

Inflammation in NCC occurs as part of the natural evolution of the parasites and is also triggered by antiparasitic treatment. Steroids have been used in many different schemes varying the agent, dose, and length of treatment. Dexamethasone is frequently used in doses ranging between 0.1 mg/kg/d and 0.2 mg/kg/d, although higher doses may be required.[57,58] Abrupt steroid withdrawal may be associated with a rebound in inflammation so gradual tapering is recommended.[59] Methotrexate has been successfully used as a steroid-sparing agent although there are no precise indications and the number of cases is still limited.[60]

Surgery

Surgical intervention may be needed in cases of obstructive hydrocephalus caused by intraventricular cysts or cysts in the basal cisterns or in large cysts or cysts clusters. Hydrocephalus is usually resolved by means of ventriculo-peritoneal shunt or by neuroendoscopic excision of intraventricular lesions with fenestration of the anterior wall of the third ventricle. Medical treatment of large cysts or cyst clusters may cause

Table 1 Treatment of neurocysticercosis			
Parenchymal cysts	Viable cysts	Single	ABZ, 15 mg/k/d × 1 week with steroids
		Multiple	ABZ, 15 mg/k/d plus PZQ 50 mg/k/d × 10 days with steroids
	Degenerating	Single or multiple	ABZ, 15 mg/k/d × 1 week with steroids
Extra Parenchymal NCC	Intraventricular		Neuroendoscopic excision
	Subarachnoid		ABZ, 15 mg/k/d × 1 month with high-dose steroids

perilesional inflammation with edema and worsen the mass effects, with the risk of herniation and death. Excision of large cysts or cysts clusters is thus a reasonable complementary approach or an alternative to medical treatment in these cases.[52]

DISEASE COMPLICATIONS

The natural evolution of the disease may place patients at risk of death, mostly in cases with subarachnoid NCC, where hydrocephalus and intracranial hypertension may gradually or acutely deteriorate. Risks associated with seizures, however, are always present in individuals with parenchymal NCC and should not be neglected. Both these conditions may present or worsen during the initial days of anti-parasitic treatment as a result of the inflammatory response of the host against the parasite (or by the time of withdrawing steroids) but are usually well managed with steroids, mannitol, or surgery, if needed.

CONTROL AND POTENTIAL ELIMINATION

T solium has been signaled as potentially eradicable for more than 30 years,[61] but systematic evidence of the feasibility of actively interrupting its transmission was only recently obtained in a large field program in Northern Peru. This elimination program using multiple rounds of human deworming with niclosamide, antiparasitic treatment of pigs with oxfendazole, and pig vaccination with the TSOL18 vaccine was able to interrupt active transmission in 104 of 107 villages.[62] Follow-up of previously intervened villages suggested that the effect of elimination persisted for at least 1 year without further intervention. Albeit preliminary, this evidence opens the way for large-scale elimination programs and hopefully the eventual eradication of the disease.

CONTROVERSIES

Some investigators question if there is any benefit of using antiparasitic agents to destroy intraparenchymal cysticerci, based on the concept that these lesions eventually resolve by natural involution. To date, there is a substantial body of evidence demonstrating that viable cysts do not resolve in the short term, that patients with viable NCC may continue having viable cysts and seizures for many years, and that patients in whom the lesions are destroyed by antiparasitic treatment have fewer seizures in the long term.[24,49,55,56,63,64] Seizure freedom, however, is not the rule and seizures do relapse in a significant proportion of individuals even after all cysts have resolved. Residual lesion calcification seems to be a major risk factor for future seizure relapses.[65]

In recent years, the study of individuals with refractory epilepsy and NCC being evaluated in surgical centers[66] and a large imaging study of asymptomatic villagers in a rural Ecuadorian village[67] have shown an association between calcified NCC and mesial temporal sclerosis. Whether there is a causal relation and what the mechanisms are behind it are still unknown. This finding may be of importance for the understanding of secondary epileptogenesis in the human brain.[68]

REFERENCES

1. Montano SM, Villaran MV, Ylquimiche L, et al. Neurocysticercosis: association between seizures, serology, and brain CT in rural Peru. Neurology 2005;65(2): 229–34.
2. Cruz ME, Schantz PM, Cruz I, et al. Epilepsy and neurocysticercosis in an Andean community. Int J Epidemiol 1999;28(4):799–803.

3. Ndimubanzi PC, Carabin H, Budke CM, et al. A systematic review of the frequency of neurocyticercosis with a focus on people with epilepsy. PLoS Negl Trop Dis 2010;4(11):e870.

4. Newton CR, Garcia HH. Epilepsy in poor regions of the world. Lancet 2012; 380(9848):1193–201.

5. Coyle CM, Mahanty S, Zunt JR, et al. Neurocysticercosis: neglected but not forgotten. PLoS Negl Trop Dis 2012;6(5):e1500.

6. O'Neal SE, Flecker RH. Hospitalization frequency and charges for neurocysticercosis, United States, 2003–2012. Emerg Infect Dis 2015;21(6):969–76.

7. Flisser A. Taeniasis and cysticercosis due to Taenia solium. Prog Clin Parasitol 1994;4:77–116.

8. Sarti-Gutierrez EJ, Schantz PM, Lara-Aguilera R, et al. Taenia solium taeniasis and cysticercosis in a Mexican village. Trop Med Parasitol 1988;39(3):194–8.

9. Lescano AG, Garcia HH, Gilman RH, et al. Taenia solium cysticercosis hotspots surrounding tapeworm carriers: Clustering on human seroprevalence but not on seizures. PLoS Negl Trop Dis 2009;3(1):e371.

10. Oneal SE, Moyano LM, Ayvar V, et al. Geographic correlation between tapeworm carriers and heavily infected cysticercotic pigs. Am J Trop Med Hyg 2012;87(5): 326–7.

11. Schantz PM, Moore AC, Munoz JL, et al. Neurocysticercosis in an Orthodox Jewish community in New York City. N Engl J Med 1992;327(10):692–5.

12. Martinez MJ, de Aluja AS, Gemmell M. Failure to incriminate domestic flies (Diptera: Muscidae) as mechanical vectors of Taenia eggs (Cyclophyllidea: Taeniidae) in rural Mexico. J Med Entomol 2000;37(4):489–91.

13. Gonzales I, Rivera JT, Garcia HH. Pathogenesis of Taenia solium taeniasis and cysticercosis. Parasite Immunol 2016;38(3):136–46.

14. Escobar A. The pathology of neurocysticercosis. In: Palacios E, Rodriguez-Carbajal J, Taveras JM, editors. Cysticercosis of the central nervous system. Springfield (MA): Charles C. Thomas; 1983. p. 27–54.

15. Fleury A, Carrillo-Mezo R, Flisser A, et al. Subarachnoid basal neurocysticercosis: A focus on the most severe form of the disease. Expert Rev Anti Infect Ther 2011; 9(1):123–33.

16. Bandres JC, White AC Jr, Samo T, et al. Extraparenchymal neurocysticercosis: report of five cases and review of management. Clin Infect Dis 1992;15(5): 799–811.

17. White AC Jr, Coyle CM, Rajshekhar V, et al. Diagnosis and Treatment of Neurocysticercosis: 2017 Clinical Practice Guidelines by the Infectious Diseases Society of America (IDSA) and the American Society of Tropical Medicine and Hygiene (ASTMH). Clin Infect Dis 2018;66(8):1159–63.

18. Nash TE, Bustos JA, Garcia HH. Disease centered around calcified taenia solium granuloma. Trends Parasitol 2017;33(1):65–73.

19. Lobato RD, Lamas E, Portillo JM. Hydrocephalus in cerebral cysticercosis. Pathogenic and therapeutic considerations. J Neurosurg 1981;55(5):786–93.

20. Proaño JV, Madrazo I, Avelar F, et al. Medical treatment for neurocysticercosis characterized by giant subarachnoid cysts. N Engl J Med 2001;345(12):879–85.

21. Del Brutto OH, Campos X. Massive neurocysticercosis: encephalitic versus non-encephalitic. Am J Trop Med Hyg 2012;87(3):381.

22. Nash TE, Pretell EJ, Lescano AG, et al. Perilesional brain oedema and seizure activity in patients with calcified neurocysticercosis: a prospective cohort and nested case-control study. Lancet Neurol 2008;7(12):1099–105.

23. Nash TE, Patronas NJ. Edema associated with calcified lesions in neurocysticercosis. Neurology 1999;53(4):777–81.
24. Dixon HB, Lipscomb FM. Cysticercosis: an analysis and follow-up of 450 cases. In: Her Majesty's Stationery Office. London: Medical Research Council; 1961.
25. Forlenza OV, Vieira Filho AHG, Nobrega JPS, et al. Psychiatric manifestations of neurocysticercosis: A study of 38 patients from a neurology clinic in Brazil. J Neurol Neurosurg Psychiatry 1997;62(6):612–6.
26. Bianchin MM, Dal Pizzol A, Scotta Cabral L, et al. Cognitive impairment and dementia in neurocysticercosis: a cross-sectional controlled study. Neurology 2010; 75(11):1028.
27. de Almeida SM, Gurjão SA. Frequency of depression among patients with neurocysticercosis. Arq Neuropsiquiatr 2010;68(1):76–80.
28. Dumas JL, Visy JM, Belin C, et al. Parenchymal neurocysticercosis: follow-up and staging by MRI. Neuroradiology 1997;39(1):12–8.
29. García HH, Del Brutto OH. Imaging findings in neurocysticercosis. Acta Trop 2003;87(1):71–8.
30. Nash TE, Del Brutto OH, Butman JA, et al. Calcific neurocysticercosis and epileptogenesis. Neurology 2004;62(11):1934–8.
31. Carrillo Mezo R, Lara Garcia J, Arroyo M, et al. Relevance of 3D magnetic resonance imaging sequences in diagnosing basal subarachnoid neurocysticercosis. Acta Trop 2015;152:60–5.
32. Arambulo PV 3rd, Walls KW, Bullock S, et al. Serodiagnosis of human cysticercosis by microplate enzyme-linked immunospecific assay (ELISA). Acta Trop 1978;35(1):63–7.
33. Coker-Vann M, Brown P, Gajdusek DC. Serodiagnosis of human cysticercosis using a chromatofocused antigenic preparation of Taenia solium cysticerci in an enzyme-linked immunosorbent assay (ELISA). Trans R Soc Trop Med Hyg 1984;78(4):492–6.
34. Pammenter MD, Rossouw EJ. Serological techniques for the diagnosis of cysticercosis. S Afr Med J 1984;65(22):875–8.
35. Tellez Giron E, Ramos MC, Dufour L, et al. Use of the ELISA method in the diagnosis of cysticercosis. Bol Oficina Sanit Panam 1984;97(1):8–13 [in Spanish]. Aplicacion del metodo ELISA para el diagnostico de la cisticercosis.
36. Mohammad IN, Heiner DC, Miller BL, et al. Enzyme-linked immunosorbent assay for the diagnosis of cerebral cysticercosis. J Clin Microbiol 1984; 20(4):775–9.
37. Tsang VC, Brand JA, Boyer AE. An enzyme-linked immunoelectrotransfer blot assay and glycoprotein antigens for diagnosing human cysticercosis (Taenia solium). J Infect Dis 1989;159(1):50–9.
38. Rodriguez S, Wilkins P, Dorny P. Immunological and molecular diagnosis of cysticercosis. Pathog Glob Health 2012;106(5):286–98.
39. Harrison LJS, Joshua GWP, Wright SH, et al. Specific detection of circulating surface/secreted glycoproteins of viable cysticerci in Taenia saginata cysticercosis. Parasite Immunol 1989;11(4):351–70.
40. Brandt JRA, Geerts S, De Deken R, et al. A monoclonal antibody-based ELISA for the detection of circulating excretory-secretory antigens in Taenia saginata cysticercosis. Int J Parasitol 1992;22(4):471–7.
41. Arroyo G, Rodriguez S, Lescano AG, et al. Antibody banding patterns of the Enzyme-linked Immunoelectrotransfer Blot (EITB) and brain imaging findings in patients with neurocysticercosis. Clin Infect Dis 2018;66(2):282–8.

42. Zea-Vera A, Cordova EG, Rodriguez S, et al. Parasite antigen in serum predicts the presence of viable brain parasites in patients with apparently calcified cysticercosis only. Clin Infect Dis 2013;57(7):e154–9.
43. Del Brutto OH, Rajshekhar V, White AC Jr, et al. Proposed diagnostic criteria for neurocysticercosis. Neurology 2001;57(2):177–83.
44. Del Brutto OH, Wadia NH, Dumas M, et al. Proposal of diagnostic criteria for human cysticercosis and neurocysticercosis. J Neurol Sci 1996;142(1–2):1–6.
45. Del Brutto OH, Nash TE, White AC Jr, et al. Revised diagnostic criteria for neurocysticercosis. J Neurol Sci 2017;372:202–10.
46. Garg RK. Diagnostic criteria for neurocysticercosis: some modifications are needed for Indian patients. Neurol India 2004;52(2):171–7.
47. Carpio A, Fleury A, Romo ML, et al. New diagnostic criteria for neurocysticercosis: Reliability and validity. Ann Neurol 2016;80(3):434–42.
48. Gabriel S, Blocher J, Dorny P, et al. Added value of antigen ELISA in the diagnosis of neurocysticercosis in resource poor settings. PLoS Negl Trop Dis 2012;6(10):e1851.
49. Garcia HH, Pretell EJ, Gilman RH, et al. A trial of antiparasitic treatment to reduce the rate of seizures due to cerebral cysticercosis. N Engl J Med 2004;350(3):249–58.
50. DeGiorgio CM, Houston I, Oviedo S, et al. Deaths associated with cysticercosis. Report of three cases and review of the literature. Neurosurg Focus 2002;12(6):e2.
51. Bustos JA, Garcia HH, Del Brutto OH. Antiepileptic drug therapy and recommendations for withdrawal in patients with seizures and epilepsy due to neurocysticercosis. Expert Rev Neurother 2016;16(9):1079–85.
52. Rajshekhar V. Surgical management of neurocysticercosis. Int J Surg 2010;8(2):100–4.
53. Robles C, Chavarria Chavarria M. Report of a clinical case of cerebral cysticercosis treated medically with a new drug: praziquantel. Salud Publica Mex 1979;21(5):603–18 [in Spanish]. Presentacion de un caso clinico de cisticercosis cerebral tratado medicamente con un nuevo farmaco: praziquantel.
54. Spina-Franca A, Nobrega JPS, Livramento JA, et al. Administration of praziquantel in neurocysticercosis. Tropenmed Parasitol 1982;33(1):1–4.
55. Romo ML, Carpio A, Wyka K, et al. Effect of albendazole on seizures in patients with symptomatic neurocysticercosis. Am J Trop Med Hyg 2014;91(5):363–4.
56. Garcia HH, Gonzales I, Lescano AG, et al. Efficacy of combined antiparasitic therapy with praziquantel and albendazole for neurocysticercosis: a double-blind, randomised controlled trial. Lancet Infect Dis 2014;14(8):687–95.
57. Nash TE, Mahanty S, Garcia HH. Corticosteroid use in neurocysticercosis. Expert Rev Neurother 2011;11(8):1175–83.
58. Garcia HH, Gonzales I, Lescano AG, et al. Enhanced steroid dosing reduces seizures during antiparasitic treatment for cysticercosis and early after. Epilepsia 2014;55(9):1452–9.
59. Poeschl P, Janzen A, Schuierer G, et al. Calcified neurocysticercosis lesions trigger symptomatic inflammation during antiparasitic therapy. AJNR Am J Neuroradiol 2006;27(3):653–5.
60. Mitre E, Talaat KR, Sperling MR, et al. Methotrexate as a corticosteroid-sparing agent in complicated neurocysticercosis. Clin Infect Dis 2007;44(4):549–53.
61. Schantz PM, Cruz M, Sarti E, et al. Potential eradicability of taeniasis and cysticercosis. Bull Pan Am Health Organ 1993;27(4):397–403.
62. Garcia HH, Gonzalez AE, Tsang VCW, et al. Elimination of Taenia solium transmission in northern Peru. N Engl J Med 2016;374(24):2335–44.

63. Vazquez V, Sotelo J. The course of seizures after treatment for cerebral cysticercosis. N Engl J Med 1992;327(10):696–701.
64. Del Brutto OH, Santibanez R, Noboa CA, et al. Epilepsy due to neurocysticercosis: analysis of 203 patients. Neurology 1992;42(2):389–92.
65. Del Brutto OH. Prognostic factors for seizure recurrence after withdrawal of antiepileptic drugs in patients with neurocysticercosis. Neurology 1994;44(9):1706–9.
66. Bianchin MM, Velasco TR, Wichert-Ana L, et al. Neuroimaging observations linking neurocysticercosis and mesial temporal lobe epilepsy with hippocampal sclerosis. Epilepsy Res 2015;116:34–9.
67. Del Brutto OH, Salgado P, Lama J, et al. Calcified neurocysticercosis associates with hippocampal atrophy: a population-based study. Am J Trop Med Hyg 2015;92(1):64–8.
68. Del Brutto OH, Engel J Jr, Eliashiv DS, et al. Hippocampal sclerosis: the missing link of cysticercosis epileptogenesis? Epilepsia 2014;55(12):2077–8.

Prion Diseases

Boon Lead Tee, MD, MS[a,b], Erika Mariana Longoria Ibarrola, MD[a,c],
Michael D. Geschwind, MD, PhD[d],*

KEYWORDS

- Creutzfeldt-Jakob disease • CJD • Jakob-Creutzfeldt disease
- Rapidly progressive dementia • Protein misfolding disorders
- Transmissible spongiform encephalopathies

KEY POINTS

- Prion diseases are caused by templated misfolding of normal cellular proteins, leading to neurodegeneration.
- Novel diagnostic techniques, such as real-time quaking-induced conversion assay applied to cerebrospinal fluid (and possibly other bodily tissues), have significantly improved specificity of premortem diagnosis of sporadic Jakob-Creutzfeldt disease.
- Protein aggregates found in most neurodegenerative diseases exhibit prion-like seeding with cell-to-cell transmission of misfolded proteins.
- Although prion diseases are uniformly fatal and incurable, promising therapies now being applied to other neurodegenerative diseases, such as antisense oligonucleotides, may hold hope for prion diseases.

INTRODUCTION

Prion diseases (PrDs) are a group of neurodegenerative conditions resulting from the conversion of the normal brain prion protein, the cellular form of prion-related protein (PrP^C), into misfolded disease-causing forms called prions, commonly referred to as PrP^{Sc} (Sc stands for scrapie, the PrD of sheep and goats).

In 1920, the German neurologist Hans Gerhard Creutzfeldt described a 23-year-old woman with fluctuating neuropsychological symptoms since adolescence and more

Disclosure Statement: See last page of article
[a] Global Brain Health Institute, University of California, San Francisco, 675 Nelson Rising Lane, Suite 190, San Francisco, CA 94518, USA; [b] Department of Neurology, Buddhist Tzu Chi General Hospital, No. 707, Section 3, Zhong Yang Road, Hualien City, Hualien County 97002, Taiwan; [c] Dementia Department, National Institute of Neurology and Neurosurgery Manuel Velasco Suarez, Av. Insurgentes Sur 3877, Col. La Fama, Del. Tlalpan, Ciudad de México. C.P. 14269, Mexico; [d] Memory and Aging Center, Department of Neurology, University of California, San Francisco, 675 Nelson Rising Lane, Suite 190, San Francisco, CA 94158, USA
* Corresponding author. Memory and Aging Center, University of California, San Francisco, 675 Nelson Rising Lane, Suite 190, San Francisco, CA 94158.
E-mail address: Michael.geschwind@ucsf.edu

recent onset of spastic paraparesis, dystonia, and cerebellar ataxia and status epilepticus.[1] Between 1921 and 1923, Alfons Maria Jakob described 5 other cases he thought were similar to Creutzfeldt's case.[2] For many decades the disease was known as Jakob's syndrome, Jakob-Creutzfeldt disease (JCD), or Creutzfeldt-Jakob disease, but in the late 1960s, a prominent researcher in the field, Clarence J. Gibbs, began favoring the term Creutzfeldt-Jakob because the initials were closer to his own, which helped this term to become the one more commonly used.[3] Through later pathologic analysis of the 5 original cases, however, it was determined that Creutzfeldt's case was not PrD,[4] whereas at least 2 of Jakob's 5 cases were PrD.[5] In view of this finding and the fact that, clinically, Creutzfeldt's case was not typical of JCD, it would be more appropriate to use the term Jakob's disease or Jakob-Creutzfeldt disease (JCD), instead of Creutzfeldt-Jakob disease (CJD).[6] Therefore, in this article, we use the term Jakob-Creutzfeldt disease or JCD.

Based on the modes in which human PrDs occur, PrDs can be classified into 3 different categories: sporadic (spontaneous), genetic (familial, inherited), and acquired (infectious, transmitted). Eighty-five to 90% of cases are sporadic JCD (sJCD), 10% to 15% are genetic (familial JCD, Gerstmann-Sträussler-Scheinker syndrome, and fatal familial insomnia), and less than 1% are acquired cases (kuru, variant JCD [vJCD], and iatrogenic JCD [iJCD]).[3,6–10] sJCD is thought to occur through spontaneous misfolding of the prion protein (PrP^C) into a disease-causing form called the prion (also called PrP^{Sc}. This process is believed to occur either spontaneously or possibly through a spontaneous somatic mutation of the prion protein gene, *PRNP*, which results in PrP^C being more susceptible to misfolding into PrP^{Sc}. Genetic PrD occurs due to a mutation in *PRNP* (usually inherited, rarely de novo).[11,12] Acquired PrD results from the unintentional transmission of prions to a person through medical procedures (iJCD), consumption of prion-contaminated beef (vJCD) or cannibalism (kuru).

This article provides a general introduction to PrDs, with a particular focus on the sporadic and acquired PrDs. It discusses common and uncommon clinical presentations, updated diagnostic criteria, infection control issues, and novel diagnostic methods.

EPIDEMIOLOGY OF HUMAN PRION DISEASES

The annual incidence of human PrD is estimated to be around 1.0 to 1.5 per million population worldwide, varying somewhat between countries. The incidence has increased in most countries over the past 2 decades, likely owing to improved diagnostic methods and the expanding aging population, resulting in a greater number of people reaching the age range in which PrD commonly occurs.[13–15] Most types of PrDs occur in late adulthood, usually in people in their 50s to 70s. Although there can be great variation in age of onset, on average sJCD has a median age of onset in the mid-60s;[16,17] genetic PrDs have a median age of onset in the mid-50s[18–20]; and acquired JCD has an average onset, but is generally earlier than that for sJCD. Because PrDs tend to occur in late middle-age – an age most persons in the developing world will live through – a person's lifetime risk of dying from PrD is much higher than the incidence, around 1 in 5000 to tens of thousands.[21]

SPORADIC JAKOB-CREUTZFELDT DISEASE

Although the peak age of onset for sJCD is in the 60s,[16,17,22,23] there is high variability, ranging from 12 to 96 years of age.[9,24] The most common or early manifestations include cognitive decline, ataxia, and myoclonus, particularly startle-provoked myoclonus.[17,22,23,25] Cognitive impairment may manifest in the form of memory loss, aphasia, dysexecutive symptoms, disorientation, visuospatial impairment, decreased alertness, and/or apraxia. Almost all reported cases of neuropathologic sJCD had cognitive decline throughout their disease course.[22] In a study at our center of about 100 sJCD cases, 40% first manifested clinically with cognitive symptoms, about 20% first manifested with cerebellar, constitutional, or behavioral symptoms, and about 10% or fewer first manifested with motor, visual, or sensory symptoms.[26] Although myoclonus occurs in more than 78% of the sJCD cases during their disease course, fewer than 10% have motor symptoms, including myoclonus, as first symptoms.[22,23,25,26] Other common clinical manifestations include cerebellar symptoms (gait disturbance, limb ataxia), constitutional symptoms (dizziness/vertigo, fatigue/lethargy, headache, sleep or eating changes, urinary incontinence, weight loss), behavioral changes (agitation, depression, aggression, apathy, personality changes), other motor symptoms (pyramidal, extrapyramidal, myoclonus, and tremor), abnormal sensory symptoms, and visual disturbance.[22,23,25,26] Focal cortical involvement can manifests as cortical blindness (Heidenhain variant), rapid primary progressive aphasia, or cortico basal syndrome with or without alien limb phenomenon. More than half of patients with sJCD have cerebellar symptoms during their disease course, with more than 20% having it as their first or initial symptom.[23,26] Owing to its wide variation in clinical presentation, sJCD is sometimes referred to as "the great mimicker."[9,24,27] Almost all PrD cases exhibit akinetic mutism at the last stage of the disease.[9] The mean survival in sJCD cases is around 6 months, with a median of 5 months. Most patients die within the first year from onset, although a minority live past 1 year and some even a few years.[16,17,28]

The most common subclassification of sJCD is based on 2 factors: the genetic polymorphism at codon 129 in the host patient's prion protein gene PRNP, and the electrophoretic mobility of PrP^{Sc} extracted from affected brain after being cleaved by proteases and run on a Western blot. Codon 129 can either be a methionine (M) or valine (V). Cleavage of type 1 prions occurs at more distal cleavage sites than type 2, generating a 21-kDA unglycosylated fragment and a 19-kDa unglycosylated fragment, respectively.[17,29] With the 3 possible codon 129 polymorphism combinations and 2 types of prions, there are 6 molecular subtypes of sJCD: MM1, MV1, VV1, MM2, MV2, and VV2. Because MM1 and MV1 are very similar clinically and pathologically, they are often grouped as a single subtype. MM2 is often divided into a cortical and a thalamic subtype. Each subtype has different clinical and pathologic presentations with varying sensitivity to diagnostic tests discussed elsewhere in this article.[16,17,30] About 6% of sJCD cases have both type 1 and type 2 prions and present along a spectrum between both prion types, the phenotype of which depends on their relative ratio.[7,16]

sJCD can be challenging to diagnose, particularly in early stages. Researchers have identified certain ancillary tests that can support an sJCD diagnosis. The first biomarker used was periodic sharp-wave complexes of electroencephalogram (EEG), but this finding only has a sensitivity of about 60%. The specificity is higher, but this finding is often only present in advanced stages of the disease.[16,31]

Since the late 1990s, cerebrospinal fluid (CSF) proteins that reflect rapid neuronal damage have been reported as diagnostic biomarkers for JCD. CSF 14-3-3 protein was among the first protein biomakrers to be reported, and the literature has shown varying degrees of diagnostic performance.[16,32–35] In 2012, the American Academy of Neurology conducted a systematic review that pooled a total of 1,849 patients suspected to have sJCD; the CSF 14-3-3 protein was reported to have 92% sensitivity and 80% specificity.[36] That study concluded that an elevated CSF 14-3-3 is highly suggestive of sJCD only if clinical features were compatible, but has low negative predicting value and does not exclude sJCD in atypical cases. The sensitivity and specificity of CSF 14-3-3 varies greatly among cohorts, but overall has come down over time with sensitivity around 82% and specificity around 63%.[30,37–40] Importantly, CSF 14-3-3 is elevated in many conditions with rapid neuronal injury, such as stroke, multiple sclerosis, brain tumors, or neurodegenerative diseases such as Alzheimer's disease or frontotemporal dementia,[34,41–45] some of which overlap clinically with sJCD;[30,34,46–48] thus, a positive CSF 14-3-3 must be interpreted with caution and in clinical context. Other nonspecific CSF biomarkers such as neuron-specific enolase (NSE), total-tau (t-tau), and S100ß generally have higher diagnostic accuracy than CSF 14-3-3.[30,38,40,49–53] CSF t-tau typically demonstrates a sensitivity and specificity of about 90%.[38,49] The sensitivity and specificity for NSE ranges from 53% to 80% and 92% to 98%, respectively.[33,51,54] For S100ß the sensitivity ranges from approximately 65% to 94%, but with much more variable specificity, ranging from 40% to 85%.[35,54–56] Several studies have suggested that ratio of phosphorylated tau and t-tau has the best diagnostic accuracy of surrogate CSF biomarkers in sJCD, in particular in differentiating sJCD from Alzheimer's disease.[40,57–59]

These proteins are not actually testing for PrP^{Sc}, however, and thus are surrogate markers, because they are biomarkers for rapid neuronal injury.[9,40,60] A relatively new test, the real-time quaking-induced conversion assay (RT-QuIC), enables prion protein detection through a method of amplification by mixing the sample with a substrate containing PrP^{C} (either recombinantly derived or from healthy rodent brain). With continuous shaking, the PrP^{Sc} in samples come in contact with PrP^{C}, converting it into PrP^{Sc} which aggregate into amyloid fibrils. The PrP^{Sc} amyloid fibrils can be detected using thioflavin T, which binds amyloid and emits fluorescent signal.[61,62] This technique can be applied to several tissues, including brain, CSF, olfactory mucosa, and skin (discussed elsewhere in this article). The sensitivity of RT-QuIC in sJCD CSF varies greatly in the literature and between molecular subtypes of sJCD (discussed elsewhere in this article),[40,63] but generally ranges around 80% with a specificity of about 98%.[30,40,56,61,62,64–66] Thus, a negative test does not exclude disease, but a positive test in the right clinical context has great diagnostic value.

The first findings reported on brain MRI in sJCD were increased signal in deep nuclei, primarily striatum, on T2-weighted images.[67,68] Later, it was found that the most sensitive findings are diffusion restriction signal in the cerebral cortex or deep gray matter nuclei, usually being most evident in the diffusion-weighted imaging (DWI) or apparent diffusion coefficient (ADC) sequences.[69–73] The cortical abnormal hyperintensity is also commonly known as "cortical ribboning" (**Fig. 1**). Brain diffusion MRI has high diagnostic usefulness utility in sJCD, with a sensitivity ranging from 92% to 96% and a specificity of about 93% to 94%.[73–75] In comparison with the CSF biomarkers such as CSF 14-3-3 protein, t-tau, and NSE, we found visual assessment of DWI and ADC sequences had by far the highest diagnostic accuracy, at around 97% when read by those with knowledge of sJCD MRI findings.[51] Unfortunately, DWI MRIs in sJCD are often misread by radiologists.[76,77] MRI findings also vary with different molecular subtypes. Basal ganglia hyperintensities are more commonly seen in the MV2, VV2, and MM1 subtypes whereas abnormal diffuse cortical ribboning signal is more common in the VV1, MM2, and MV1 subtypes, and thalamic hyperintensity is often seen in the VV2 and MV2 subtypes.[78] DWI usually is much more sensitive than the fluid-attenuated inversion recovery (FLAIR) sequence in detecting the hyperintensity abnormalities in sJCD.[73–75,79] We have found that MRI diagnosis is improved by high-quality acquisition, use of specific MRI sequences (axially and coronal

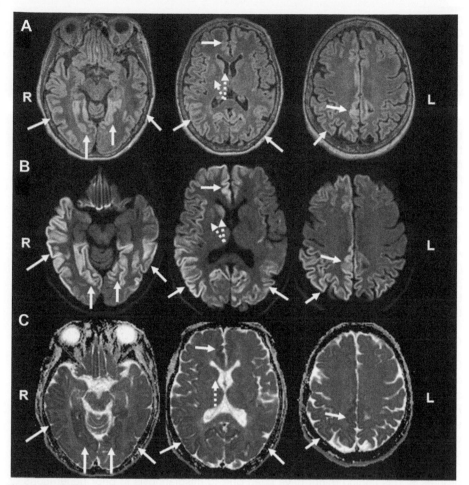

Fig. 1. Typical sporadic Jakob–Creutzfeldt disease (sJCD) brain MRI. (*A*) Axial fluid-attenuated inversion recovery (FLAIR) and (*B*) diffusion-weighted imaging (DWI) cortical ribboning and striatal hyperintensities. (*C*) Corresponding apparent diffusion coefficient (ADC) map hypointensities. Dashed arrows indicate striatal abnormalities. Solid arrows indicate some of the regions with cortical ribboning abnormalities. Note the mild asymmetry of MRI findings and that the ADC hypointensities generally correspond to DWI hyperintensities, which confirms restricted diffusion, consistent with prion disease.[75,80,81] This MRI shows both cortical and deep nuclei involvement, although sJCD cases also can have either finding alone. Orientation is radiological (right side of figure is left side of brain); R, right side of brain; L, left side of brain.

acquired b2000 DWI and ADC map) to reduce any air–brain artifact, evaluation of specific cortical and subcortical areas more commonly involved in JCD, having MRIs read by someone familiar with MRI findings in PrD, and noting the presence of sJCD-relevant symptoms in when ordering the MRI.[9,75,80,81]

To date, a definite diagnosis for sJCD relies on a neuropathologic diagnosis with identification of PrP[Sc] via immunohistochemistry or Western blot.[9,82] Classic neuropathologic findings of PrDs consist of vacuolation (formerly referred to as spongiform changes) in the upper layers of cortex, neuronal loss without inflammation in the cortical layers III and IV, and PrP[Sc] deposition.[82] Several clinical diagnostic criteria for probable sJCD have been proposed (**Table 1**), with the University of California–San Francisco (UCSF)[83] and European MRI-CJD Consortium criteria[84] perhaps being the most commonly used. Both were derived from 1998 World Health Organization (WHO) diagnostic criteria that were established to retrospectively identify through medical records nonpathologically confirmed sJCD cases for surveillance purposes. Thus, the WHO criteria are reasonably good for retrospective diagnosis, but not very sensitive for living patients, particularly those in early stages of the disease.[85] The UCSF criteria in 2007 modified symptoms/signs, emphasized the importance of diffusion-weighted brain MRI findings and eliminated the use of the CSF 14-3-3 protein owing to concern with its low specificity.[83] In 2009, the European Consortium criteria modified the 1998 WHO criteria by including DWI or FLAIR brain MRI findings as an ancillary test; we feel, however, that these MRI criteria are inadequate because for two primary reasons: FLAIR MRI is not sensitive nor specific enough for JCD diagnosis, and the criteria do not include frontal lobe involvement as the study had many false positives due to hyperintensities on FLAIR and DWI in this region. To overcome these issues, UCSF MRI criteria use DWI and ADC maps as well as T2/FLAIR imaging; these criteria continue to be modified (**Table 2**).[74,75,80] The 2017 revised European CJD Consortium criteria allow for a probable sJCD diagnosis in any progressive neurologic syndrome with a positive RT-QuIC from any tissue.[86] This strategy, however, could lead to some false positives, because even RT-QuIC is not 100% specific.

GENETIC PRION DISEASES

Genetic PrDs, causing about 10% to 15% of human PrDs, are due to autosomal-dominant mutations in *PRNP*. Most are due to mutations are missense although some are insertions or stop-codons, and there is at least 1 deletion. More than 40 PRNP mutations have been associated with PrD; most are 100% penetrant, but some have very low penetrance (<1%) and might just be risk factors.[87,88] Several detailed reviews discuss the spectrum of genetic PrDs.[19,20,87] Importantly, a large study found that almost one-half of the cases found to be genetic through European CJD Surveillance programs had no family history of PrD or other neurologic syndromes.[20] This finding might have been due to misdiagnosis in prior generations or reduced penetrance of some mutations. Although at least some genetic PrDs are known to be transmissible by direct inoculation into animals,[89,90] human-to-human transmission of genetic PrD has not been reported. It is not known if genetic PrD can be transmitted by blood. Although persons with a *PRNP* mutation have it from birth, it is not known when prions begin to form, and we do not know if and when there are sufficient prions in the blood to be transmissible even in symptomatic patients. As a conservative precautionary measure, persons with a blood relative with PrD are not allowed to donate blood in many countries, including the United States.[91]

ACQUIRED JAKOB-CREUTZFELDT DISEASE

Acquired PrDs can be categorized into vJCD, iJCD, and Kuru; this section focuses on vJCD and iJCD, because Kuru is essentially extinct.[92] An important finding, however, regarding kuru, the PrD of the Fore ethnic group in Papua New Guinea, was the identification of a *PRNP* polymorphism at codon 127 among survivors of the kuru epidemic that seems to lead to resistance to PrD in animal models.[93] Understanding or mimicking the effect of this polymorphism in preventing PrP^C from misfolding into PrP^{Sc} could be relevant for the development of treatments for human PrD. Of note, although PrDs are considered infectious, they are not contagious.[94]

Table 1
Several commonly used diagnostic criteria for probable sICD

	1998 WHO Revised Criteria[85]	2007 UCSF Criteria[74,83]	2009 European Consortium[84]	2017 European Consortium[86]
Clinical features	Progressive dementia with 2 of the following: • Myoclonus • Visual or cerebellar disturbance • Pyramidal/extrapyramidal signs • Akinetic mutism	Rapidly progressive dementia with 2 of the following: • Myoclonus • Visual disturbance • Cerebellar signs • Pyramidal/extrapyramidal signs • Akinetic mutism • Focal cortical signal (eg, neglect, aphasia, acalculia, apraxia)	Progressive dementia with 2 of the following: • Myoclonus • Visual or cerebellar disturbance • Pyramidal or extrapyramidal signs • Akinetic mutism	Rapidly progressive cognitive impairment with 2 of the following: • Myoclonus • Visual or cerebellar disturbance • Pyramidal or extrapyramidal signs • Akinetic mutism
Diagnostic test	• Typical EEG[a] Or • Elevated CSF protein 14-3-3 (with total disease duration <2 y)	• Typical EEG[a] Or • Typical MRI[b]	• Typical EEG[a] Or • Elevated CSF protein 14-3-3 (with total disease duration <2 y) Or • Typical MRI[c]	• Typical EEG[a] Or • Typical MRI[b] Or • Elevated CSF protein 14-3-3 Or • Positive RT-QuIC in CSF or other tissues in setting of any progressive neurologic condition[d]
Other	• Routine investigations should not suggest an alternative diagnosis	• Routine investigations should not suggest an alternative diagnosis	• Routine investigations should not suggest an alternative diagnosis	• Routine investigations should not suggest an alternative diagnosis

Abbreviations: CSF, cerebrospinal fluid; EEG, electroencephalography; RT-QuIC, real-time quaking-induced conversion assay; sJCD, sporadic Jakob-Creutzfeldt disease; UCSF, University of California–San Francisco; WHO, World Health Organization.

[a] Typical EEG: periodic sharp waves complexes.

[b] Typical MRI for UCSF MRI criteria initially required diffusion-weighted imaging brighter than fluid-attenuated inversion recovery hyperintensity in the cingulate, striatum, and/or more than 1 neocortical gyrus, ideally with sparing of the precentral gyrus and apparent diffusion coefficient map supporting restricted diffusion. (See Table 1 in Vitali P, et al. 2011 Neurology). UCSF MRI criteria were updated in 2017 (see Table 2).[80]

[c] Typical MRI for European criteria: high signal abnormalities in caudate nuclear and putamen or at least 2 cortical regions (temporal-parietal-occipital, but not frontal, cingulate, insular, or hippocampal) either on diffusion-weighted imaging or fluid-attenuated inversion recovery MRI.

[d] Probable sJCD diagnosis by a positive RT-QuIC does not require the combination of specific symptoms noted above, just any progressive neurologic condition.

Table 2
UCSF 2017 sJCD MRI criteria

Diagnosis	Criteria[75]

MRI definitely JCD	DWI > FLAIR[a] cortical ribboning[b] hyperintensity in:
	1. Classic pathognomonic: cingulate,[c] striatum, and >1 neocortical gyrus (often precuneus, angular, superior parietal, superior, or middle frontal gyrus)
	  a. Supportive for subcortical[d] involvement
	    i. Striatum with decreasing anterior-posterior gradient
	    ii. Corresponding ADC hypointensity
	  b. Supportive for cortical involvement
	    i. Asymmetric involvement of midline neocortex or cingulate[4]
	    ii. Sparing of precentral gyrus[e]
	    iii. Corresponding ADC cortical ribboning hypointensity
	2. Cortex only (>3 gyri); see supportive for cortex (above)

MRI probably JCD	1. Unilateral striatum or cortex (≤3 gyri); see supportive for subcortical and cortex (above) 2. Bilateral striatum (see supportive for subcortical) or posteromesial thalamus; see supportive for subcortical (above) 3. DWI > FLAIR hyperintensities only in limbic areas, with corresponding ADC hypointensity[f]
MRI probably not JCD	1. Only FLAIR/DWI abnormalities only in limbic areas, where hyperintensity can be normal (eg, insula, anterior cingulate, hippocampi), and ADC map does not show corresponding restricted diffusion (hypointensity) 2. DWI hyperintensities owing to artifact (signal distortion); see other MRI issues (below) 3. FLAIR > DWI hyperintensities[g]; see other MRI issues (below)
MRI definitely not JCD	1. Normal 2. Abnormalities not consistent with JCD
Other MRI issues	In prolonged courses of sJCD (approximately >1 y) brain MRI might show significant atrophy with loss of DWI hyperintensity, particularly in areas previously with restricted diffusion To help distinguish abnormality from artifact, obtain b2000 diffusion sequences in multiple directions (eg, axial and coronal)

Abbreviations: ADC, apparent diffusion coefficient; DWI, diffusion-weighted imaging; FLAIR, fluid-attenuated inversion recovery; sJCD, sporadic Jakob-Creutzfeldt disease; UCSF, University of California–San Francisco.

[a] Recommended minimum standard diffusion sequence parameters to best identify cortical ribboning: axial and coronal DWI/ADC b = 1000 s/cm^2 or b = 2000 s/cm^2, depending on scanner field strength and capabilities to achieve satisfactory image quality. At 3 Tesla, b = 2000 may be preferred owing to the higher contrast to background for abnormal gray matter diffusion.

[b] Involvement of cortical gray matter with sparing of underlying or adjacent white matter.

[c] Mid and posterior cingulate preferred over anterior owing to anterior air–brain artifact, especially on axial acquisition (anterior acceptable if coronal acquisition). Can be symmetric, but if so prefer ADC hypointensity correlate.

[d] Subcortical = deep nuclei, in decreasing order of frequency: caudate, putamen, thalamus (posteriomesial or diffuse), and globus pallidus (rare). ADC often shows corresponding and earlier involvement than DWI.

[e] If precentral gyrus is preferentially involved consider nonprion diagnoses (eg, seizures, Wernicke's).

[f] DWI > FLAIR with reduced ADC in limbic or other cortical regions also can occur in herpes simplex virus encephalitis[80] and seizures.[226,227] Depending on clinical picture, these should be ruled out.

[g] Consider T2-shine through.[228]

From Staffaroni AM, Elahi FM, McDermott D, et al. Neuroimaging in dementia. Semin Neurol 2017;37(5):510–37. p. 522; with permission.

Variant Jakob-Creutzfeldt Disease

In 1995, vJCD was first identified in a 16-year-old who developed sensory symptoms in 1994, followed within several months by cognitive decline and cerebellar symptoms, and an 18-year-old with cognitive and behavioral/psychiatric symptoms developing over a few months, followed by cerebellar symptoms and myoclonus. Both patients had atypical prion neuropathology and did not have *PRNP* mutations.[95,96] In 1996, 8 more cases were published (in addition to the first two).[97] Based on the first 100 cases, the initial typical symptoms are psychiatric, with features such as dysphoria, anxiety, withdrawal, anhedonia, irritability, and insomnia. Ataxia also is common. These symptoms are often followed or accompanied by sensory disturbances and cognitive decline and motor symptoms such as chorea, dystonia, or myoclonus.[98] In only about 15% of the cases did the neurologic symptoms precede the psychiatric features.[98] Compared with sJCD, vJCD tends to occur at a younger age (median 26.5 years; range 12–74 years) and have longer survival (approximately 14 months).[99]

As of 2017, there have been 231 deaths from vJCD reported worldwide: 178 in the United Kingdom, 27 in France, 5 in Spain, 4 in Ireland, 4 in the United States, 3 in Italy, 3 in the Netherlands, 2 in Canada, 2 in Portugal, and 1 each in Japan, Taiwan, and Saudi Arabia (**Fig. 2**).[100] Most patients were exposed to prions and acquired their illness in the UK or less commonly in France. Some patients developed symptomatic disease in a country different from where they were exposed. The 6 North American cases, for example, are thought to all have been exposed outside North America, four in the UK and 2 in Saudi Arabia.[101,102] The vast majority of vJCD cases occurred through inadvertent consumption of meat or offal contaminated with prions from bovine spongiform encephalopathy (BSE), colloquially known as mad cow disease.[103]

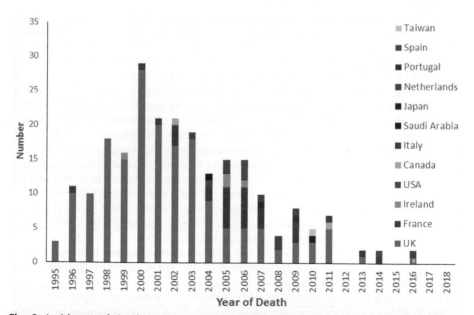

Fig. 2. Incidence of death owing to variant Jakob–Creutzfeldt disease (vJCD) worldwide from 1995 to 2018. The vJCD cases (n = 231) are color coded by the countries that diagnosed and reported cases. Not all cases contracted disease in the same country in which they were diagnosed and/or died (see text). [a] MV at codon129 of the *PRNP* gene (*Courtesy of* National CJD Surveillance Unit, Edinburgh, UK; with permission.)

Evidence suggests that BSE occurred because of the practice of feeding sheep parts that likely were unknowingly contaminated with scrapie, the PrD of sheep and goats, being fed to cattle, which are normally herbivores.[104,105] Epidemiologic and laboratory evidence suggests that most cases of vJCD occurred from exposure to BSE.[94,106,107] The incidence of vJCD peaked in 2000 (see **Fig. 2**), about 8 years after the peak of the BSE epidemic in 1992,[105] and has declined dramatically since then, with no new cases reported in 2017 through at least May 2018. The decreased incidences of BSE and vCJD are believed to be due to the strong implementation of import control policies, ban-feed regulations and offal, and cattle nervous system disposal measures.[105,108]

Several tests are helpful for the premortem diagnosis of vJCD. A hallmark feature on brain MRI imaging is the pulvinar sign, in which the pulvinar (posterior thalamus) is brighter on T2-weighted sequences than the anterior putamen; this sign is seen in about 78% of cases (**Fig. 3**).[109] These findings are also present on diffusion sequences, but initial MRI studies did not include diffusion MRI, so it is possible that sensitivity is higher with DWI sequences. The pulvinar sign is relatively specific, but rarely is seen in sJCD,[110] metabolic disorders,[111–113] autoimmune encephalitis,[114–116] and acute demyelinating disease.[117] Another common, yet less specific MRI finding is the double hockey stick sign, in which bilateral medial-dorsal and posterior thalami are bright on T2- or diffusion-weighted sequences (**Fig. 4**).[109,118] The double hockey stick sign also has been reported on T2- and/or diffusion-weighted MRI in a variety of conditions, including sJCD,[119,120] metabolic disorders such as Wernicke's encephalopathy,[111,112] paraneoplastic limbic encephalitis,[115,116] and thalamic infarcts. As vJCD progresses, the pulvinar sign and other MRI findings may disappear in late stages of disease.[118,121] Most vJCD cases have abnormal slow wave activity on EEGs,[122] but typical periodic sharp waves complexes found in sJCD are rare in vJCD, and only seen in the end stage of disease.[121,123]

One study of 45 pathology-proven vJCD cases found that CSF 14-3-3 was even less sensitive, around 50%, than in sJCD; other CSF biomarkers, however, had higher sensitivity than 14-3-3: NSE, 52%; t-tau, 80%; and S-100b, 81%.[124] The specificities of these biomarkers with 34 controls who were initially diagnosed and erroneously referred as JCD to the UK CJD Research & Surveillance Center (but later shown to have other diagnoses) ranged between 73% and 94%.[124] In clinical practice, none of these surrogate biomarkers are specific for PrD, including vJCD, so they should be only interpreted in the proper clinical context.[124,125] To our knowledge, as of early 2018 no vJCD cases have tested positive by CSF RT-QuIC, although the test only became available in the UK after most vJCD cases had died, so many cases might not have been tested.[126]

Variant JCD has distinct neuropathologic and Western blot features that differentiate it from other prion disorders.[127,128] On brain immunohistochemistry, the pattern of prions in vJCD is relatively distinct, forming a florid plaque, which is an amyloid plaque of prions surrounded by vacuoles (spongiform change) that give a flower or floridlike appearance.[97,128] Because vJCD is primarily acquired orally, PrP^Sc from the gut accumulates in the lymphoreticular system, including the spleen, lymph nodes, tonsils, and appendix. Thus, vJCD prions can be detected in these tissues by immunohistochemistry and Western blot.[129,130] Tonsil biopsy has been used diagnostically for probable diagnosis.

Based on ruling out other conditions, clinical course, symptoms and signs, EEG, neuroimaging and/or tonsil biopsy results, vJCD is categorized as meeting possible or probable diagnostic criteria; however, definite criteria require neuropathologic evidence of vJCD (**Table 3**).[86] Per 1 study of 106 definite vJCD cases and 45 controls (referred to the UK CJD Surveillance unit as vCJD, but pathology proven to not be vCJD) the probable/possible criteria have 89% sensitivity and close to 100% specificity.[131]

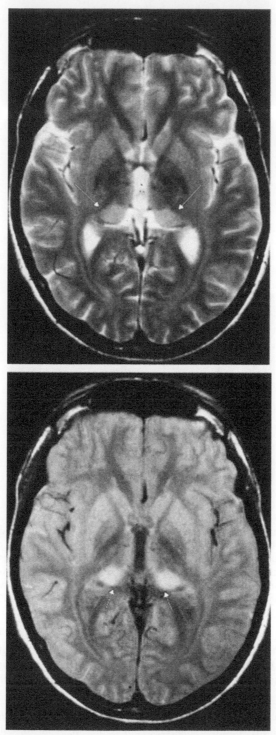

Fig. 3. The pulvinar sign in a histologically confirmed case of variant Jakob–Creutzfeldt disease (vJCD). (*Top*) T2-weighted axial MRI section of brain showing high signal changes in the

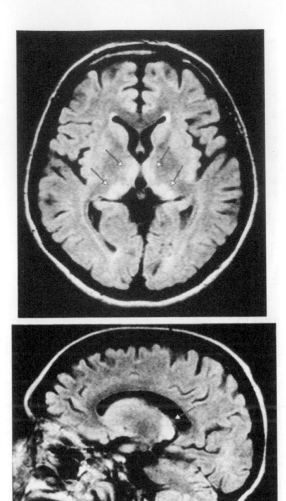

Fig. 4. Fluid-attenuated inversion recovery (FLAIR) MRI sections of a histologically confirmed case of variant Jakob–Creutzfeldt disease (vCJD). (*Top*) Axial image showing characteristic high signal in both the pulvinar and the dorsomedial nuclei of the thalamus giving the "hockey stick" sign (two arrows each side). (*Bottom*) Sagittal image showing well-defined anterior border to the thalamic changes (arrow). (*From* Zeidler M, Sellar RJ, Collie DA, et al. The pulvinar sign on magnetic resonance imaging in variant Creutzfeldt-Jakob disease. Lancet 2000;355(9213):1415; with permission.)

To date, all but 2 vJCD clinical cases have been codon 129 MM[132]; 2 cases were codon 129 MV, one probable, and the other definite vJCD.[132,133] This finding suggests that persons with the codon 129 MV polymorphism (possibly VV as well) are less likely (if ever in the case of those whom are codon 129 VV) to develop clinical vJCD, but

---

pulvinar of the thalamus (*arrows*). (*Bottom*) These changes were consistently more conspicuous on proton density-weighted images. (*From* Zeidler M, Sellar RJ, Collie DA, et al. The pulvinar sign on magnetic resonance imaging in variant Creutzfeldt-Jakob disease. Lancet 2000;355(9213):1415; with permission.)

Table 3		
Variant JCD diagnostic clinical criteria		
I	A	Progressive neuropsychiatric disorder
	B	Duration of illness >6 mo
	C	Routine investigations do not suggest an alternative diagnosis
	D	No history of potential iatrogenic exposure
	E	No evidence of a familial form of transmissible spongiform encephalopathy
II	A	Early psychiatric symptoms[a]
	B	Persistent painful sensory symptoms[b]
	C	Ataxia
	D	Myoclonus or chorea or dystonia
	E	Dementia
III	A	EEG does not show the typical appearance of sporadic JCD[c] in the early stages of illness
	B	Bilateral pulvinar high signal on MRI scan
IV	A	Positive tonsil biopsy[d]
Definite	IA + neuropathologic confirmation of vJCD[e]	
Probable	I and 4/5 II and IIIA and IIIB	
	OR I and IVA	
Possible	I and 4/5 II and IIIA	

Abbreviations: EEG, electroencephalogram; sJCD, sporadic Jakob–Creutzfeldt disease; vJCD, variant Jakob–Creutzfeldt disease.

[a] Depression, anxiety, apathy, withdrawal, delusions.

[b] Frank pain and/or dysesthesia.

[c] The typical appearance of the EEG in sporadic JCD consists of generalized triphasic periodic complexes at approximately 1 per second. These may occasionally be seen in the late stages of vCJD.

[d] Tonsil biopsy is not recommended routinely, nor in cases with EEG appearances typical of sporadic CJD, but may be useful in suspect cases in which the clinical features are compatible with vCJD and MRI does not show bilateral pulvinar high signal.

[e] Spongiform change and extensive prion-related protein deposition with florid plaques throughout the cerebrum and cerebellum.

Courtesy of National CJD Research and Surveillance Center, UK 2018 (https://www.cjd.ed.ac.uk); with permission.

could be carriers of the disease with a significant transmission risk. Alternatively, codon 129 MV (and possibly VV) individuals might just have longer incubation periods than persons who are MM at codon 129.[94]

Because PrP^{Sc} in vJCD is present in the lymphoreticular system, this probably results in more prions in the blood, making the blood more infectious than with other human PrDs. Three clinical vCJD cases and 2 additional cases of asymptomatic infection in the UK were likely acquired through blood product transfusion.[134] Data on the cases suspected to be transfusion-related are shown in **Table 4**. The 3 transfusion-associated vJCD cases developed symptoms 6.5 to 8.3 years after receiving nonleukodepleted blood transfusion from vJCD donors.[135–137] The donors were 17 to 40 months before onset of symptoms when they donated blood, which was already infective.[134–138] The 2 asymptomatic recipients of vJCD-contaminated blood died of nonneurologic causes, but had vJCD prions in their lymphoreticular system at autopsy.[139,140] It is unclear if these 2 asymptomatic cases ever would have developed vJCD had they lived longer.[134] Notably, all 3 symptomatic cases were MM homozygotes, and both asymptomatic cases were MV heterozygotes.[134] Studies from the UK and the United States suggest there is no evidence of transmission from blood donors who later developed sJCD, although 1 study from Italy suggested blood transfusion might be a risk for subsequent sJCD.[141–143]

Table 4
Variant JCD infection cases likely transmitted through blood or blood product transfusion

	Donor		Recipient				
No.	Age of Onset (y)	Interval Between Transfusion and Symptom Onset (mo)	Age of Onset (y)	Codon 129	Interval Between Transfusion and Symptom Onset	Transfusion Product	References
vJCD symptomatic (neurologic) cases							
1	24[b]	40	62[b]	MM	6.5 y	Nonleuko-depleted pRBCs	134,136,137
2	N/A	20	23[b]	MM	7.5 y	Nonleuko-depleted pRBCs	134,135
3	N/A	17[a]	N/A	MM	8.5 y	Nonleuko-depleted pRBC	134,137
Asymptomatic carriers of vCJD prions outside of CNS via blood transfusion							
4	N/A	18	Elderly	MV	5 y[d]	Nonleuko-depleted pRBCs	134,139
5	N/A	N/A	73[c]	MV	12–14 y[d]	Hemophilia, factor VIII	134,140

Abbreviations: CNS, central nervous system; N/A, not available; pRBCs, packed red blood cells; vCJD, variant Creutzfeld–Jakob disease.
[a] Same donor as in case 2.
[b] Age at time of donation.
[c] Age when deceased.
[d] Interval between transfusion and deceased.

In vJCD, PrP^{Sc} can be detected in lymphoreticular tissues, blood, and urine specimens. This allows tonsil biopsy to be included in diagnostic criteria for probable vJCD.[130,144,145] In a cohort of 8 neuropathologically confirmed vJCD, all tonsil biopsy samples were positive for PrP^{Sc} immunohistochemistry staining.[144] PrP^{Sc} was also reported to be present in the appendix tissue of UK birth cohort.[146,147] With the protein misfolding cyclic amplification (PMCA) technique of amplifying prions (the method on which RT-QuIC is partially based), PrP^{Sc} could be detected in the urine of 13 of 14 vJCD cases providing a sensitivity of 92.9% (95% confidence interval, 66.1–99.8).[148] A different assay has been developed, using a solid-state binding matrix to capture and concentrate PrP^{Sc}, to detect vJCD prions in blood. This test has a sensitivity of about 70% and a specificity of close to 100% (albiet not tested in very large numbers of controls), with only sJCD showing a few false positives. Ultimately, such a test might be applied for both vJCD diagnosis and blood supply screening.[149,150] To date, neither of these urine or blood tests are available clinically.

Frighteningly, a sizable minority of the UK population seem to be carriers of vJCD prions in their lymphoreticular system. Based on sampling from a bank of anonymized tonsil and appendix tissue, vJCD PrP^{Sc} was identified by immunohistochemistry in appendix tissue from 1 in 4000 of UK individuals.[151] A follow-up study found 1 in 2000 individuals to have vCJD PrP^{Sc} in their appendices.[147] It is not known if these carriers might eventually develop the disease or be capable of transmitting it.[152,153] This finding is why persons whom have spent certain minimum periods of time in

BSE-affected countries, particularly during the peak period of the BSE epidemic, are prohibited from donating blood in the United States and why the United Kingdom primarily uses blood products from the United States.

Iatrogenic Jakob-Creutzfeldt Disease

In contrast to most cases of vJCD, iJCD is a human-to-human transmission PrD. The first case was reported in 1974 in a corneal transplant recipient from an infected cadaver.[154] As of July 2017, more than 492 iJCD cases have been reported worldwide.[155] Transmission of iJCD can occur through the administration of cadaveric human pituitary hormones (growth hormone and gonadotrophic hormone), dura mater graft transplants, corneal transplants, liver transplants (unclear if this was the etiology of JCD), and the use of contaminated neurosurgical instruments or EEG stereotactic depth electrodes (**Table 5**).

There are an estimated 238 human growth hormone (hGH)-associated iJCD cases worldwide, with majority of them found at France, the UK, and the United States.[18,155] Among all, 119 of the cases originated from a French cohort of 1170 patients that received treatment for short stature between December 1983 and July 1985.[18] No cases have been reported since 2008 in France (up to 2012).[18] In the UK, there were 75 reported cases with no evident cohort pattern.[155] In the United States, there were 31 reported growth hormone-related iJCD cases. All but one of them can be traced back to the US National Hormone and Pituitary Program.[18,156] No reported cases received growth hormone after 1977, the year when a highly selective column chromatography step was included in the purification protocol.[18,155] The mean incubation period for growth hormone related iJCD is 17 years (range, 5–24 years).[18] Individuals with growth hormone related iJCD mainly present with cerebellar symptoms, and if dementia occurred, it was in the late stages. As with sJCD, there is a higher proportion of the MM homozygous genotype among the iJCD population, suggesting that these individuals have a higher susceptibility for iJCD.[18] In Australia, between 1964 and 1985, the human pituitary hormone program supplied hGH for 664 children with short stature and pituitary gonadotrophin for 1447 adults with infertility. As many as 800 cadaver pituitary glands were pooled to provide a single batch. Unfortunately, 4 women who received gonadotrophins died from iJCD,[18,157] as well as 1 possible case from growth hormone (not in official counts).[158] Many persons were potentially exposed to cadaver-derived prion-contaminated pituitary hormones in worldwide and it remains uncertain if they will ever develop iJCD or could be carriers.

Another common transmission medium of iJCD is has been dura mater. The first case was described in 1987[159] and there are at least 238 reported cases worldwide.[155] Most dura mater–transmitted iJCD (dJCD) cases received dura mater grafts named Lyodura, which is manufactured by the German company B. Braun Melsungen AG. Lyodura had been distributed worldwide and used most widely used in Japan, which led to roughly 60% of the reported cases occurring in Japan.[155] The mean incubation period for dJCD ranges between 1.3 and 30.0 years (mean 12 years).[18] Generally, the clinical course of dJCD cases are similar to that of sJCD, although in Japan they found dJCD cases could be classified into 2 distinct clinicopathological types: two-thirds had typical features of sJCD and without PrPSc plaques in the brain, and one-third were considered atypical cases with a slower progression, without periodic sharp wave complexes on EEG, and with plaque formation in the brain.[160,161] The atypical form might arise because those persons are infected by prions from individuals with sJCD with VV2 or MV2 PrPSc, whereas the typical form of dJCD is transmitted from individuals with sJCD with MM1 or MV1 PrPSc.[162]

To date, there have been 4 cases of neurosurgical instrument transmitted iCJD cases documented in the literature—3 in the UK and 1 in France.[18,108] All underwent

Table 5
Iatrogenic JCD cases through July 2017

Transmission Source	No. of Cases	Countries Reporting	Average Incubation Period in Years (Range)	Prominent Clinical Signs	References
Growth hormone	238	Majority in France, UK, and US	17 (5–42)	Cerebellar	18,100,155
Gonadotrophins	4	Australia	13.5 (12.0–16.0)	Cerebellar	157,229,230
Dura mater grafts	238	Japan, France, Germany, Spain, UK, Australia, Canada, Italy, and US in descending order	12.0 (1.3–30.0)	Cerebellar, visual, dementia	155,159
Corneal transplant	2	US, Germany	15.75 (1.50–30.00)	Dementia, cerebellar	163–165
Neurosurgical instruments	4	UK and France	1.6 (1.4–2.2)	Visual, dementia, cerebellar	108,231
EEG brain depth electrodes	2	Switzerland	1.5 (1.3–1.7)	Dementia, cerebellar	155,166
Nonleukodepleted packed red blood cells	3[a]	UK	7.53 (6.5–8.3)	Psychiatric, sensory, dementia, cerebellar	135,136,139

Abbreviation: JCD, Jakob–Creutzfeldt disease.

[a] This does not include the 2 asymptomatic persons in **Table 4** with vJCD prions outside the CNS. [134,139,140]

Data from Brown P, Brandel JP, Sato T, et al. Iatrogenic Creutzfeldt-Jakob disease, final assessment. Emerg Infect Dis. 2012;18(6):901–7 and Bonda DJ, Manjila S, Mehndiratta P, et al. Human prion diseases: surgical lessons learned from iatrogenic prion transmission. Neurosurg Focus. 2016;41(1):E10.

cranial surgery and developed symptoms between 1.4 and 2.2 years after surgery.[18,155] Between 1998 and 2012, there were 19 cases of suspected JCD exposure from contaminated surgical instruments (2 ophthalmological and 17 neurosurgical) reported to the US Centers for Disease Control and Prevention. In all cases, the patients had not been identified as JCD at the time of the operation, so no prion-precautions were used and the surgical instruments were placed in the normal sterilization cycle and then reused on subsequent patients; the risk to the patients exposed to this potentially contaminated equipment is not fully-known.[155]

Other modes of transmission for iJCD include corneal transplantation,[163–165] EEG depth electrodes,[155,166] blood transfusion,[135,136,139] and possibly (albeit unlikely) liver transplantion The only JCD case that was associated with liver transplantation developed JCD symptoms 2 years after transplant surgery, but the donor was never pathologically confirmed and the recipient had also received albumin transfusion from a donor with rapid progressive dementia.[167] All reported blood transfusion-related iJCD have been from vJCD donors, and there is no known case of sJCD or genetic PrD transmitted through blood products.

CHRONIC WASTING DISEASE

Chronic wasting disease (CWD) is a PrD first identified in 1967 in infected mule deer on a breeding farm in Colorado. As of 2018, CWD has been detected in at least 23 US states, 2 provinces in Canada, as well as in South Korea, Finland, and Norway (**Fig. 5**). CWD is found in the cervids family, specifically in; mule; red, sika, Muntjac, and white-tailed deer; Rocky Mountain elk; and, less frequently, moose. Clinical signs include emaciation, head tremors, excessive drinking and urination, reduced feeding, behavioral changes such as depression and isolation from herd, and, during the terminal stages, hyperexcitability.[168–171] Unlike many other PrDs, in CWD PrP^{Sc} is found not only in central nervous system (CNS), but also in the peripheral nervous system and research has shown it can be transmitted through secretion products such as saliva, urine, and feces.[172–174] There is concern of zoologic transmission from cervids to humans, although no case has been reported to date. Some animal studies reported that CWD brain homogenate can be transmitted to squirrel monkeys via intracranial inoculation and oral exposure. One study found that CWD brain homogenate was not transmitted to *Cynomolgus macaques*, which is evolutionary closer to human than the squirrel monkey by intracerebral or oral route.[175] An ongoing, not yet published, study from the Canadian Food Inspection Institute, however, reported at the 2017 International Prion meeting (Prion2017) in Edinburgh that they were able to transmit CWD to macaques only by feeding them CWD meat/muscle from white-tailed deer. This latter finding raises concern for the possibility of transmission of CWD to humans. One reason the US Centers for Disease Control and Prevention funds the US National Prion Disease Pathology Surveillance Center (NPDPSC; www.cjdsurveillance.com) to conduct free autopsies on all suspected PrD cases in the United States is to determine if CWD might be being transmitted to people, as well as to make sure there is not an outbreak of vJCD or other novel human PrDs in the United States.

NEW FINDINGS IN THE FIELD DIAGNOSTICS

To date, neuropathologic diagnosis remains the gold standard for human PrDs. Novel diagnostic tests and biomarkers, however, are helping with earlier and more accurate diagnosis of JCD. Recent data suggests that pre-mortem, minimally-invasive testing of certain tissues might have greater diagnostic accuracy than CSF. A 2003 study showed that PrP^{Sc} was present postmortem by olfactory mucosa biopsy in 8 of 9 cadavers with sJCD,[176] and in 2004 nasal mucosa biopsy

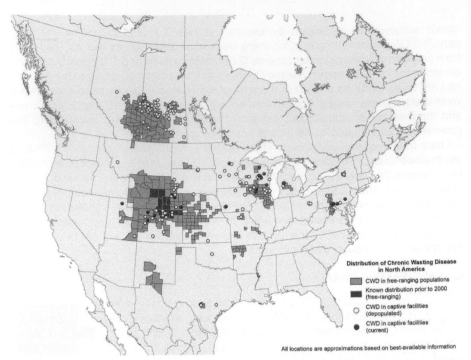

Fig. 5. Distribution of chronic wasting disease (CWD) in North America of April 1, 2018. (*Courtesy of* Bryan Richards, US Geological Service (USGS) National Wildlife Health Center. Public domain. Available at: https://www.usgs.gov/media/images/distribution-chronic-wasting-disease-north-america-april-2018. Accessed July 21, 2018.)

found prions premortem in a late stage rapidly progressive sJCD case.[177] In a study published in 2017 with 30 definite sJCD, 31 probable sJCD and 17 control (who had been initially misdiagnosed as JCD) pre-mortem cases, RT-QuIC on olfactory mucosa swabs or brushings had a sensitivity of 90% to 95% for detecting prions, about 5% to 10% higher sensitivity than on CSF in the same cases.[65] Thus, RT-QuIC on olfactory mucosa swab samples might be a minimally invasive method for prion diagnosis; to our knowledge, as of mid-2018 it is only being used clinically on olfactory mucosal swabs in Italy.

Several epidemiologic studies have correlated sJCD incidence with non-CNS surgery.[178–181] In vJCD, prion protein is detected in multiple organs including skin, uterus, ovary, pancreas, liver, and kidney.[182] A study published in 2017 detected PrP^{Sc} in postmortem skin tissue using Western blot in 1 of 5 sJCD and 1 of 2 vJCD cases. RT-QuIC seeeemed to show much higher sensitivity, detecting prion seeding activity in at least 1 (of several) skin samples from each of 21 sJCD cadavers and 2 vJCD cadavers and was negative in all from skin biopsies non-JCD living cases.[183] When the skin samples of 2 sJCD cadavers were directly inoculated into transgenic mice, all 12 mice exhibited symptoms by 564 days.[183] This finding does not mean, however, that skin is infectious by surgery or certainly by casual contact, only that prions can be present in some skin samples post-mortem.

INFECTION CONTROL PROTOCOL FOR PRION DISEASES

In PrDs, the titers of misfolded PrP^{Sc} are generally parallel with the infectivity of the tissues.[184,185] Based on past reported cases and level of detected PrP^{Sc}, in 2005

WHO classified tissues into high, low, or no infectivity. High infectivity tissues included CNS tissues that attain a high titer of infectivity in the later stages of all PrDs and certain tissues that are anatomically associated with the CNS. Lower infectivity tissues included peripheral tissues that have tested positive for infectivity and/or PrP^{Sc} in at least 1 form of PrD. Tissues with no detectable infectivity included tissues that have been examined for infectivity and/or PrP^{Sc} with negative results. High infectivity tissues mainly include CNS tissues such as the brain, spinal cord, retina, optic nerve, spinal ganglia, trigeminal ganglia, pituitary, and dura mater.[186] Tissues in the peripheral nervous system, lymphoreticular system, skin, lung, liver, kidney, adrenal, pancreas, skeletal muscle, blood vessels, cornea, nasal mucosa, and part of the alimentary tract and reproductive tissues are considered low infectivity. These WHO criteria do not make sense to these authors because blood and CSF are classified as low infectivity, even for vJCD,[186] despite vJCD blood being known to be infectious.[134] Most bodily fluids, including saliva, feces, and urine, from CWD and scrapie are known vectors for transmission between animals, but these fluids have not shown to be infective in humans.

Because of the large number of patients with PrD we evaluate at our center, we use special precautions for handling CSF (and will also for olfactory mucosa) and we have very strict neurosurgical operating room procedures for suspected PrD cases.[187] Admittedly, some of these conservative precautions were due to medicolegal more than true infection risk reasons. Nevertheless, when dealing with bodily fluids from someone with PrD, particularly in the later stages of the disease, universal precautions (ie, gloves and gowns) are recommended.[187] It is important to note that infectivity does not equate the risk of infection, because factors including the route of transmission and amount of exposure should be taken into consideration.[186]

Prions are proteins and not nucleic acid; thus, traditional sterilizing methods that work for viruses and bacteria by destroying nucleic acid are not applicable for decontamination of prions. Because prions are resistant to conventional disinfection measurements, specific methods are adopted for the sterilization of prion-contaminated medical instruments. The WHO has published their recommended most effective sterilization methods. Most important, moist sterilization at higher temperatures and for longer time periods than stardard infection control are required for prions.[188] When possible, feasible, and safe, it is recommended to use disposable surgical tools, particularly when dealing with high-risk tissues. The use of disposable equipment, however, must weigh the risk of transmission of PrD against the risk of causing harm by using inadequate equipment. All disposable waste, instruments, and high (and in some circumstances low) infectivity tissues should be incinerated. Surfaces and heat-sensitive nondisposable instruments that were in contact with infective tissues should be sterilized by soaking in 2N NaOH or undiluted sodium hypochlorite for 1 hour and then rinsed with water.[188] The UK and Australia both have excellent guidelines for managing PrD in health care settings.[189,190]

The risk of JCD transmission through blood transfusion (or even nonneurosurgical procedures) for non-vJCD forms of PrD remains unknown. The long incubation period and rarity of JCD hinders investigation on delineating the risks.[191] Only a few vJCD cases have occurred through blood product transfusion transmission and none has ever been reported in sJCD.[134–140] The American Red Cross and the National Creutzfeldt-Jakob Disease Research and Surveillance Unit in the UK studied 817 and 211 sJCD blood recipients, 1 and 15 familial JCD (fJCD) blood recipients, respectively, and none has developed JCD symptoms.[141,191,192] Owing to the certain fatality of the disease, further surveillance of transfusion transmission is warranted.

IMPORTANCE OF AUTOPSY

Brain autopsy in cases of suspected PrD is important for many reasons, including accurate disease surveillance and identifying possible new forms of PrD (such as vJCD or transmission of CWD), confirming the clinical diagnosis, and assessing the risk of transmission in possible exposure cases. As noted, many cases of suspected PrD turned out to have nonprion disorders at autopsy, a large minority of which turn out to be treatable.[193–195] In many countries, brain autopsies in cases of suspected PrD are free through national prion surveillance programs.

PRION-LIKE MECHANISMS OF NEURODEGENERATIVE DISEASES

Much research now shows that nonprion neurodegenerative disorders (NDDs) also have nervous system proteins that can act in a prion-like manner with misfolded proteins spreading from cell to cell. NDDs and PrDs also have common characteristics. Both genetic forms of PrDs and nonprion NDDs manifest symptoms in adulthood. This implies that the quantity of the pathologic proteins have to exceed a certain threshold for the pathologic process to be unabated.[196,197] PrD occurs when PrP^{Sc} acts as a template and transforms adjacent PrP^C into PrP^{Sc} eventually becoming an exponential process.[198] Similar seeding properties can be found in the pathogenic proteins of nonprion NDDs, such as Aβ-amyloid, tau, synuclein, huntingtin, and TDP-43, proteins that play major roles in the pathophysiology of Alzheimer's disease, Parkinson's disease, Huntington's disease, and frontotemporal lobar degeneration.[199–203]

When transgenic mice expressing human amyloid precursor protein are inoculated intracerebrally or intraperitoneally with Aβ-amyloid–rich brain extracts from patients with Alzheimer's disease, these mice displayed premature formation of amyloid plaque and cerebral amyloid angiopathy in the brain.[204–207] In mice, Aβ deposition appears to start locally at the inoculation site and progressively spread toward adjacent axonally-connected brain regions, resembling the self-propagating nature of PrP^{Sc}.[208,209] In humans, 1 US study showed that 52% of 21 iJCD (hGH or dura mater) cases had amyloid β deposition in the brain (most commonly in the form of cerebral amyloid angiopathy),[210] which is higher than the 17% of 266 sJCD cases we found with Alzheimer's disease-like neuropathologic changes in our sJCD cohort.[211] Furthermore, in the UK, investigators found more amyloid-β and cerebral amyloid angiopathy than they expected in 8 hGH iJCD cases.[212,213] These data suggest amyloid-β is prionlike and may be transmissible when injected peripherally.

Analogous phenomena of spreading of misfolded proteins can also be observed with tau and α-synuclein.[214–216] Additionally, PrDs and nonprion NDDs pathogenic proteins tend to aggregate into toxic oligomeric and polymeric forms, and adopt β sheet structure and stack into amyloid fibrils, a process commonly referred to as amyloidosis.[196,217] Proteins in such amyloid state are thermodynamically highly stable and resistant to proteolysis, and often affect cells function and survival. As with prions, these other proteins can self-propagate and facilitate spreading between cells and species.[196,197] To date, there are more than 30 amyloidogenic proteins.[218,219] Notably, α-synuclein depositions were found in the transplanted fetal dopaminergic neurons of individuals with Parkinson's disease 11 to 16 years after transplantation, suggestive of cell–cell propagation of pathologic α-synuclein into grafted neurons that induce prion-like seeding process.[220–222] α-Synuclein derived from patients with multiple system atrophy has also shown to be transmissible in animal models and cause a neurodegenerative disease.[223,224] It is still inconclusive whether NDDs proteins are infectious in the same way that prions are. Human-to-human transmission of PrDs remains as a relatively small fraction of all PrD cases.[18,92] Factors such as protein durability, the method of transmission, and host susceptibility may all affect the infectivity of nonprion NDDs proteins. To date, despite NDDs proteins exhibiting prion-like features, there is no direct evidence supporting NDDs protein as infectious agents with human to human transmission.[203,225] Whether or not these other proteins by acting in a prion-like manner are actually infectious, studying the common disease mechanisms of protein misfolding and aggregation might lead to common treatments for all of these proteinopathies.

SUMMARY

The discovery of the prion opened a new chapter in the field of infectious diseases. Recent discoveries on the prion-like manner of other NDD proteins underline the fact that both PrDs and non-prion NDDs may share common pathophysiological mechanisms. Thus, understanding the pathophysiology of one may help to decipher the pathophysiology of other diseases. Advancements in diagnostic tests for PrD, such as diffusion MRI and RT-QuIC, have greatly increased our ability to make a premortem diagnosis. Techniques such as RT-QuIC or protein misfolding cyclic amplification for amplifying misfolded proteins may be adaptable for nonprion NDDs as well. Lastly, treatments targeting common characteristics between PrDs and nonprion NDDs may be effective for both groups of disorders.

DISCLOSURE STATEMENT

M.D. Geschwind is or has been a consultant for Grand Rounds Inc., Advanced Medical Inc., Best Doctors Inc., Gerson Lehrman Group Inc., Guidepoint Global, MEDACorp, LCN Consulting, Optio Biopharma Solutions, Biohaven Pharmaceuticals Inc., Quest Diagnostics Inc., and has done various medicolegal consulting. M.D. Geschwind received speaking honoraria from various medical centers, the American Academy of Neurology, and Oakstone Publishing, Inc. M.D. Geschwind currently receives research support from the NIH/NIA (grant R01 AG AG031189), Alliance Biosecure and the Michael J. Homer Family Fund. He has received research support from CurePSP, the Tau Consortium, Quest Diagnostics, and the NIH. He serves on the board of directors for San Francisco Bay Area Physicians for Social Responsibility and on the editorial board of *Dementia & Neuropsychologia*. The other authors report no conflicts of interest.

REFERENCES

1. Creutzfeldt HG. On a particular focal disease of the central nervous system (preliminary communication), 1920. Alzheimer Dis Assoc Disord 1989;3(1–2): 3–25.
2. Jakob A. Concerning a disorder of the central nervous system clinically resembling multiple sclerosis with remarkable anatomic findings (spastic pseudosclerosis). Report of a fourth case. Med Klin 1921;17:372–6.
3. Gibbs CJ Jr. Spongiform encephalopathies - slow, latent, and temperate virus infections - in retrospect. In: Prusiner SB, Collinge J, Powell J, et al, editors. Prion diseases of humans and animals. London: Ellis Horwood; 1992. p. 53–62.
4. Richardson EP Jr. Introduction to myoclonic dementia. In: Rottenber DA, Hochberg FH, editors. Neurological classics in modern translation. New York: Haffner Press; 1977. p. 95–6.
5. Masters CL, Gadjusek DC. The spectrum of Creutzfeldt-Jakob disease and the virus-induced subacute spongiform encephalopathies. In: Smith WT,

Cavanagh JB, editors. Recent advances in neuropathology. Number 2. Edinburgh (Scotland): Churchill Livingstone; 1982. p. 139–63.

6. Katscher F. It's Jakob's disease, not Creutzfeldt's. Nature 1998;393(6680):11.
7. Puoti G, Bizzi A, Forloni G, et al. Sporadic human prion diseases: molecular insights and diagnosis. Lancet Neurol 2012;11(7):618–28.
8. Masters CL, Harris JO, Gajdusek DC, et al. Creutzfeldt-Jakob disease: patterns of worldwide occurrence and the significance of familial and sporadic clustering. Ann Neurol 1979;5(2):177–88.
9. Geschwind MD. Prion diseases. Continuum (Minneap Minn) 2015;21(6 Neuroinfectious Disease):1612–38.
10. Takada LT, Kim MO, Metcalf S, et al. Prion disease. Handb Clin Neurol 2018;148:441–64.
11. Dagvadorj A, Petersen RB, Lee HS, et al. Spontaneous mutations in the prion protein gene causing transmissible spongiform encephalopathy. Ann Neurol 2002;52(3):355–9.
12. Takada LT, Kim M-O, Metcalf S, et al. Prion disease. In: Geschwind D, Paulson H, Klein K, editors. Neurogenetics, Part II of the handbook of clinical neurology, vol. 148. San Diego (CA): Elsevier; 2018. p. 441–66.
13. Ladogana A, Puopolo M, Croes EA, et al. Mortality from Creutzfeldt-Jakob disease and related disorders in Europe, Australia, and Canada. Neurology 2005;64(9):1586–91.
14. Will RG. Epidemiology of Creutzfeldt-Jakob disease. Br Med Bull 1993;49(4):960–70.
15. Will RG, Ironside JW. Sporadic and infectious human prion diseases. Cold Spring Harb Perspect Med 2017;7(1) [pii:a024364].
16. Collins SJ, Sanchez-Juan P, Masters CL, et al. Determinants of diagnostic investigation sensitivities across the clinical spectrum of sporadic Creutzfeldt-Jakob disease. Brain 2006;129(Pt 9):2278–87.
17. Parchi P, Giese A, Capellari S, et al. Classification of sporadic Creutzfeldt-Jakob disease based on molecular and phenotypic analysis of 300 subjects. Ann Neurol 1999;46(2):224–33.
18. Brown P, Brandel JP, Sato T, et al. Iatrogenic Creutzfeldt-Jakob disease, final assessment. Emerg Infect Dis 2012;18(6):901–7.
19. Kim MO, Takada LT, Wong K, et al. Genetic PrP prion diseases. Cold Spring Harb Perspect Biol 2018;10(5) [pii:a033134].
20. Kovacs GG, Puopolo M, Ladogana A, et al. Genetic prion disease: the EUROCJD experience. Hum Genet 2005;118(2):166–74.
21. Luk C, Jones S, Thomas C, et al. Diagnosing sporadic Creutzfeldt-Jakob disease by the detection of abnormal prion protein in patient urine. JAMA Neurol 2016;73(12):1454–60.
22. Brown P, Cathala F, Castaigne P, et al. Creutzfeldt-Jakob disease: clinical analysis of a consecutive series of 230 neuropathologically verified cases. Ann Neurol 1986;20(5):597–602.
23. Brown P, Gibbs CJ Jr, Rodgers-Johnson P, et al. Human spongiform encephalopathy: the National Institutes of Health series of 300 cases of experimentally transmitted disease. Ann Neurol 1994;35(5):513–29.
24. Geschwind MD. Rapidly progressive dementia: prion diseases and other rapid dementias. Continuum (Minneap Minn) 2010;16(2 Dementia):31–56.
25. Will RG, Matthews WB. A retrospective study of Creutzfeldt-Jakob disease in England and Wales 1970-79. I: clinical features. J Neurol Neurosurg Psychiatry 1984;47(2):134–40.

26. Rabinovici GD, Wang PN, Levin J, et al. First symptom in sporadic Creutzfeldt-Jakob disease. Neurology 2006;66(2):286–7.

27. Geschwind MD, Haman A, Miller BL. Rapidly progressive dementia. Neurol Clin 2007;25(3):783–807.

28. Johnson DY, Dunkelberger DL, Henry M, et al. Sporadic Jakob-Creutzfeldt disease presenting as primary progressive aphasia. JAMA Neurol 2013;70(2):254–7.

29. Parchi P, Castellani R, Capellari S, et al. Molecular basis of phenotypic variability in sporadic Creutzfeldt-Jakob disease. Ann Neurol 1996;39(6):767–78.

30. Foutz A, Appleby BS, Hamlin C, et al. Diagnostic and prognostic value of human prion detection in cerebrospinal fluid. Ann Neurol 2017;81(1):79–92.

31. Steinhoff BJ, Zerr I, Glatting M, et al. Diagnostic value of periodic complexes in Creutzfeldt-Jakob disease. Ann Neurol 2004;56(5):702–8.

32. Hsich G, Kenney K, Gibbs CJ, et al. The 14-3-3 brain protein in cerebrospinal fluid as a marker for transmissible spongiform encephalopathies. N Engl J Med 1996;335(13):924–30.

33. Zerr I, Bodemer M, Gefeller O, et al. Detection of 14-3-3 protein in the cerebrospinal fluid supports the diagnosis of Creutzfeldt-Jakob disease. Ann Neurol 1998;43(1):32–40.

34. Geschwind MD, Martindale J, Miller D, et al. Challenging the clinical utility of the 14-3-3 protein for the diagnosis of sporadic Creutzfeldt-Jakob disease. Arch Neurol 2003;60(6):813–6.

35. Chohan G, Pennington C, Mackenzie JM, et al. The role of cerebrospinal fluid 14-3-3 and other proteins in the diagnosis of sporadic Creutzfeldt-Jakob disease in the UK: a 10-year review. J Neurol Neurosurg Psychiatry 2010;81(11):1243–8.

36. Muayqil T, Gronseth G, Camicioli R. Evidence-based guideline: diagnostic accuracy of CSF 14-3-3 protein in sporadic Creutzfeldt-Jakob disease: report of the guideline development subcommittee of the American Academy of Neurology. Neurology 2012;79(14):1499–506.

37. Stoeck K, Sanchez-Juan P, Gawlnecka J, et al. Cerebrospinal fluid biomarker supported diagnosis of Creutzfeldt-Jakob disease and rapid dementias: a longitudinal multicentre study over 10 years. Brain 2012;135(Pt 10):3051–61.

38. Coulthart MB, Jansen GH, Olsen E, et al. Diagnostic accuracy of cerebrospinal fluid protein markers for sporadic Creutzfeldt-Jakob disease in Canada: a 6-year prospective study. BMC Neurol 2011;11:133.

39. Pennington C, Chohan G, Mackenzie J, et al. The role of cerebrospinal fluid proteins as early diagnostic markers for sporadic Creutzfeldt-Jakob disease. Neurosci Lett 2009;455(1):56–9.

40. Lattanzio F, Abu-Rumeileh S, Franceschini A, et al. Prion-specific and surrogate CSF biomarkers in Creutzfeldt-Jakob disease: diagnostic accuracy in relation to molecular subtypes and analysis of neuropathological correlates of p-tau and Abeta42 levels. Acta Neuropathol 2017;133(4):559–78.

41. Huang N, Marie SK, Livramento JA, et al. 14-3-3 protein in the CSF of patients with rapidly progressive dementia. Neurology 2003;61(3):354–7.

42. Chapman T, McKeel DW Jr, Morris JC. Misleading results with the 14-3-3 assay for the diagnosis of Creutzfeldt-Jakob disease. Neurology 2000;55(9):1396–7.

43. Martinez-Yelamos A, Rovira A, Sanchez-Valle R, et al. CSF 14-3-3 protein assay and MRI as prognostic markers in patients with a clinically isolated syndrome suggestive of MS. J Neurol 2004;251(10):1278–9.

44. Martinez-Yelamos A, Saiz A, Sanchez-Valle R, et al. 14-3-3 protein in the CSF as prognostic marker in early multiple sclerosis. Neurology 2001;57:722–4.
45. Rivas E, Sanchez-Herrero J, Alonso M, et al. Miliary brain metastases presenting as rapidly progressive dementia. Neuropathology 2005;25(2):153–8.
46. Satoh J, Yukitake M, Kurohara K, et al. Detection of the 14-3-3 protein in the cerebrospinal fluid of Japanese multiple sclerosis patients presenting with severe myelitis. J Neurol Sci 2003;212(1–2):11–20.
47. Schmidt C, Haik S, Satoh K, et al. Rapidly progressive Alzheimer's disease: a multicenter update. J Alzheimers Dis 2012;30(4):751–6.
48. Jayaratnam S, Khoo AK. Basic D. Rapidly progressive Alzheimer's disease and elevated 14-3-3 proteins in cerebrospinal fluid. Age Ageing 2008;37(4):467–9.
49. van Harten AC, Kester MI, Visser PJ, et al. Tau and p-tau as CSF biomarkers in dementia: a meta-analysis. Clin Chem Lab Med 2011;49(3):353–66.
50. Satoh J, Kurohara K, Yukitake M, et al. The 14-3-3 protein detectable in the cerebrospinal fluid of patients with prion-unrelated neurological diseases is expressed constitutively in neurons and glial cells in culture. Eur Neurol 1999; 41(4):216–25.
51. Forner SA, Takada LT, Bettcher BM, et al. Comparing CSF biomarkers and brain MRI in the diagnosis of sporadic Creutzfeldt-Jakob disease. Neurol Clin Pract 2015;5(2):116–25.
52. Kim MO, Geschwind MD. Clinical update of Jakob-Creutzfeldt disease. Curr Opin Neurol 2015;28(3):302–10.
53. Hamlin C, Puoti G, Berri S, et al. A comparison of tau and 14-3-3 protein in the diagnosis of Creutzfeldt-Jakob disease. Neurology 2012;79(6):547–52.
54. Beaudry P, Cohen P, Brandel JP, et al. 14-3-3 protein, neuron-specific enolase, and S-100 protein in cerebrospinal fluid of patients with Creutzfeldt-Jakob disease. Dement Geriatr Cogn Disord 1999;10(1):40–6.
55. Otto M, Beekes M, Wiltfang J, et al. Elevated levels of serum S100 beta protein in scrapie hamsters. J Neurovirol 1998;4(5):572–3.
56. Rudge P, Hyare H, Green A, et al. Imaging and CSF analyses effectively distinguish CJD from its mimics. J Neurol Neurosurg Psychiatry 2018;89(5):461–6.
57. Skillback T, Rosen C, Asztely F, et al. Diagnostic performance of cerebrospinal fluid total tau and phosphorylated tau in Creutzfeldt-Jakob disease: results from the Swedish Mortality Registry. JAMA Neurol 2014;71(4):476–83.
58. Blennow K, Johansson A, Zetterberg H. Diagnostic value of 14-3-3beta immunoblot and T-tau/P-tau ratio in clinically suspected Creutzfeldt-Jakob disease. Int J Mol Med 2005;16(6):1147–9.
59. Riemenschneider M, Wagenpfeil S, Vanderstichele H, et al. Phospho-tau/total tau ratio in cerebrospinal fluid discriminates Creutzfeldt-Jakob disease from other dementias. Mol Psychiatry 2003;8(3):343–7.
60. Geschwind MD. Rapidly progressive dementia. Continuum (Minneap Minn) 2016;22(2 Dementia):510–37.
61. Atarashi R, Satoh K, Sano K, et al. Ultrasensitive human prion detection in cerebrospinal fluid by real-time quaking-induced conversion. Nat Med 2011;17(2): 175–8.
62. McGuire LI, Peden AH, Orru CD, et al. Real time quaking-induced conversion analysis of cerebrospinal fluid in sporadic Creutzfeldt-Jakob disease. Ann Neurol 2012;72(2):278–85.
63. Franceschini A, Baiardi S, Hughson AG, et al. High diagnostic value of second generation CSF RT-QuIC across the wide spectrum of CJD prions. Sci Rep 2017;7(1):10655.

64. McGuire LI, Poleggi A, Poggiolini I, et al. Cerebrospinal fluid real-time quaking-induced conversion is a robust and reliable test for sporadic Creutzfeldt-Jakob disease: an international study. Ann Neurol 2016;80(1):160–5.

65. Bongianni M, Orru C, Groveman BR, et al. Diagnosis of human prion disease using real-time quaking-induced conversion testing of olfactory mucosa and cerebrospinal fluid samples. JAMA Neurol 2017;74(2):155–62.

66. Satoh K, Takatsuki H, Atarashi R, et al. CSF analysis of patients with human prion disease in a prospective study. Presented at Prion 2016. Tokyo, Japan. May 10–13, 2016.

67. Gold M, Rojiani A, Murtaugh R. A 66-year-old woman with a rapidly progressing dementia and basal ganglia involvement. J Neuroimaging 1997;7(3):171–5.

68. Urbach H, Klisch J, Wolf HK, et al. MRI in sporadic Creutzfeldt-Jakob disease: correlation with clinical and neuropathological data. Neuroradiology 1998;40(2):65–70.

69. Bahn MM, Parchi P. Abnormal diffusion-weighted magnetic resonance images in Creutzfeldt-Jakob disease. Arch Neurol 1999;56(5):577–83.

70. Demaerel P, Heiner L, Robberecht W, et al. Diffusion-weighted MRI in sporadic Creutzfeldt-Jakob disease. Neurology 1999;52(1):205–8.

71. Urbach H. Creutzfeldt-Jakob disease: analysis of the MRI signal. Neuroreport 2000;11(17):L5–6.

72. Matoba M, Tonami H, Miyaji H, et al. Creutzfeldt-Jakob disease: serial changes on diffusion-weighted MRI. J Comput Assist Tomogr 2001;25(2):274–7.

73. Shiga Y, Miyazawa K, Sato S, et al. Diffusion-weighted MRI abnormalities as an early diagnostic marker for Creutzfeldt-Jakob disease. Neurology 2004;I63:443–9.

74. Young GS, Geschwind MD, Fischbein NJ, et al. Diffusion-weighted and fluid-attenuated inversion recovery imaging in Creutzfeldt-Jakob disease: high sensitivity and specificity for diagnosis. AJNR Am J Neuroradiol 2005;26(6):1551–62.

75. Vitali P, Maccagnano E, Caverzasi E, et al. Diffusion-weighted MRI hyperintensity patterns differentiate CJD from other rapid dementias. Neurology 2011;76(20):1711–9.

76. Carswell C, Thompson A, Lukic A, et al. MRI findings are often missed in the diagnosis of Creutzfeldt-Jakob disease. BMC Neurol 2012;12(1):153.

77. Geschwind MD, Kuryan C, Cattaruzza T, et al. Brain MRI in sporadic Jakob-Creutzfeldt disease is often misread. Neurology 2010;74(Supplement 2):A213.

78. Meissner B, Kallenberg K, Sanchez-Juan P, et al. MRI lesion profiles in sporadic Creutzfeldt-Jakob disease. Neurology 2009;72(23):1994–2001.

79. Tian HJ, Zhang JT, Lang SY, et al. MRI sequence findings in sporadic Creutzfeldt-Jakob disease. J Clin Neurosci 2010;17(11):1378–80.

80. Staffaroni AM, Elahi FM, McDermott D, et al. Neuroimaging in dementia. Semin Neurol 2017;37(5):510–37.

81. Caverzasi E, Henry RG, Vitali P, et al. Application of quantitative DTI metrics in sporadic CJD. Neuroimage Clin 2014;4:426–35.

82. Kretzschmar HA, Ironside JW, DeArmond SJ, et al. Diagnostic criteria for sporadic Creutzfeldt-Jakob disease. Arch Neurol 1996;53(9):913–20.

83. Geschwind MD, Josephs KA, Parisi JE, et al. A 54-year-old man with slowness of movement and confusion. Neurology 2007;69(19):1881–7.

84. Zerr I, Kallenberg K, Summers DM, et al. Updated clinical diagnostic criteria for sporadic Creutzfeldt-Jakob disease. Brain 2009;132(Pt 10):2659–68.

85. World Health Organization (WHO). Global surveillance, diagnosis and therapy of human transmissible spongiform encephalopathies: report of a WHO

consultation Geneva, Switzerland 9-11 February 1998. Geneva, Switzerland: World Health Organization; 1998.

86. UK National CJD Research & Surveillance Unit (NCJDRSU). Diagnostic criteria. 2017. Available at: https://www.cjd.ed.ac.uk/surveillance. Accessed July 2, 2018.

87. Takada LT, Kim MO, Cleveland RW, et al. Genetic prion disease: experience of a rapidly progressive dementia center in the United States and a review of the literature. Am J Med Genet B Neuropsychiatr Genet 2017;174(1):36–69.

88. Minikel EV, Vallabh SM, Lek M, et al. Quantifying prion disease penetrance using large population control cohorts. Sci Transl Med 2016;8(322):322ra329.

89. Collinge J, Palmer MS, Sidle KC, et al. Transmission of fatal familial insomnia to laboratory animals. Lancet 1995;346(8974):569–70.

90. Tateishi J, Kitamoto T. Inherited prion diseases and transmission to rodents. Brain Pathol 1995;5(1):53–9.

91. American Red Cross. Eligibility reference material. Eligibility requirements for blood donation. Creutzfeldt-Jakob disease. 2018. Available at: https://www.redcrossblood.org/donate-blood/how-to-donate/eligibility-requirements/eligibility-criteria-alphabetical/eligibility-reference-material.html. Accessed May 1, 2018.

92. Collinge J, Whitfield J, McKintosh E, et al. Kuru in the 21st century–an acquired human prion disease with very long incubation periods. Lancet 2006;367(9528): 2068–74.

93. Mead S, Whitfield J, Poulter M, et al. A novel protective prion protein variant that colocalizes with kuru exposure. N Engl J Med 2009;361(21):2056–65.

94. Collinge J. Molecular neurology of prion disease. J Neurol Neurosurg Psychiatry 2005;76(7):906–19.

95. Britton TC, al-Sarraj S, Shaw C, et al. Sporadic Creutzfeldt-Jakob disease in a 16-year-old in the UK. Lancet 1995;346(8983):1155.

96. Bateman D, Hilton D, Love S, et al. Sporadic Creutzfeldt-Jakob disease in a 18-year-old in the UK. Lancet 1995;346(8983):1155–6.

97. Will RG, Ironside JW, Zeidler M, et al. A new variant of Creutzfeldt-Jakob disease in the UK. Lancet 1996;347(9006):921–5.

98. Spencer MD, Knight RS, Will RG. First hundred cases of variant Creutzfeldt-Jakob disease: retrospective case note review of early psychiatric and neurological features. BMJ 2002;324(7352):1479–82.

99. UK National CJD Research & Surveillance Unit. Creutzfeldt-Jakob disease surveillance in the UK. 25th Annual Report 2016. Available at: https://www.cjd.ed.ac.uk/sites/default/files/report25.pdf. Accessed June 27, 2018.

100. UK National CJD Research & Surveillance Unit. Variant Creutzfeldt-Jakob disease worldwide current data (February 2018). 2018. Available at: https://www.cjd.ed.ac.uk/sites/default/files/worldfigs.pdf. Accessed June 1, 2018.

101. Maheshwari A, Fischer M, Gambetti P, et al. Recent US case of variant Creutzfeldt-Jakob disease-global implications. Emerg Infect Dis 2015;21(5): 750–9.

102. Coulthart MB, Geschwind MD, Qureshi S, et al. A case cluster of variant Creutzfeldt-Jakob disease linked to the Kingdom of Saudi Arabia. Brain 2016; 139(Pt 10):2609–16.

103. Collinge J. Prion diseases of humans and animals: their causes and molecular basis. Annu Rev Neurosci 2001;24:519–50.

104. Scott MR, Will R, Ironside J, et al. Compelling transgenetic evidence for transmission of bovine spongiform encephalopathy prions to humans. Proc Natl Acad Sci U S A 1999;96(26):15137–42.

105. Pattison J. The emergence of bovine spongiform encephalopathy and related diseases. Emerg Infect Dis 1998;4(3):390–4.
106. Bruce ME, Will RG, Ironside JW, et al. Transmissions to mice indicate that 'new variant' CJD is caused by the BSE agent. Nature 1997;389(6650):498–501.
107. Hill AF, Desbruslais M, Joiner S, et al. The same prion strain causes vCJD and BSE. Nature 1997;389(6650):448–50, 526.
108. Will RG, Matthews WB. Evidence for case-to-case transmission of Creutzfeldt-Jakob disease. J Neurol Neurosurg Psychiatry 1982;45(3):235–8.
109. Zeidler M, Sellar RJ, Collie DA, et al. The pulvinar sign on magnetic resonance imaging in variant Creutzfeldt-Jakob disease. Lancet 2000;355(9213):1412–8.
110. Petzold GC, Westner I, Bohner G, et al. False-positive pulvinar sign on MRI in sporadic Creutzfeldt-Jakob disease. Neurology 2004;62(7):1235–6.
111. Schmidt C, Plickert S, Summers D, et al. Pulvinar sign in Wernicke's encephalopathy. CNS Spectr 2010;15(4):215–8.
112. Stone R, Archer JS, Kiernan M. Wernicke's encephalopathy mimicking variant Creutzfeldt-Jakob disease. J Clin Neurosci 2008;15(11):1308–10.
113. Renard D, Castelnovo G, Campello C, et al. Thalamic lesions: a radiological review. Behav Neurol 2014;2014:154631.
114. Mead S, Rudge P. CJD mimics and chameleons. Pract Neurol 2017;17(2):113–21.
115. Mihara M, Sugase S, Konaka K, et al. The "pulvinar sign" in a case of paraneoplastic limbic encephalitis associated with non-Hodgkin's lymphoma. J Neurol Neurosurg Psychiatry 2005;76(6):882–4.
116. Gamache PL, Gagnon MM, Savard M, et al. Pulvinar sign in a case of anti-HU paraneoplastic encephalitis. Neuroradiol J 2016;29(6):436–9.
117. Dabadghao VS, Ostwal P, Sharma SK, et al. Pulvinar sign in acute disseminated encephalomyelitis. Ann Indian Acad Neurol 2014;17(2):214–6.
118. Collie DA, Summers DM, Sellar RJ, et al. Diagnosing variant Creutzfeldt-Jakob disease with the pulvinar sign: MR imaging findings in 86 neuropathologically confirmed cases. AJNR Am J Neuroradiol 2003;24(8):1560–9.
119. Haik S, Brandel JP, Oppenheim C, et al. Sporadic CJD clinically mimicking variant CJD with bilateral increased signal in the pulvinar. Neurology 2002;58(1):148–9.
120. Martindale J, Geschwind MD, De Armond S, et al. Sporadic Creutzfeldt-Jakob disease mimicking variant Creutzfeldt-Jakob disease. Arch Neurol 2003;60(5):767–70.
121. Yamada M, Variant CJD Working Group, Creutzfeldt-Jakob Disease Surveillance Committee, Japan. The first Japanese case of variant Creutzfeldt-Jakob disease showing periodic electroencephalogram. Lancet 2006;367(9513):874.
122. Zeidler M, Johnstone EC, Bamber RW, et al. New variant Creutzfeldt-Jakob disease: psychiatric features. Lancet 1997;350(9082):908–10.
123. Binelli S, Agazzi P, Giaccone G, et al. Periodic electroencephalogram complexes in a patient with variant Creutzfeldt-Jakob disease. Ann Neurol 2006;59(2):423–7.
124. Green AJ, Thompson EJ, Stewart GE, et al. Use of 14-3-3 and other brain-specific proteins in CSF in the diagnosis of variant Creutzfeldt-Jakob disease. J Neurol Neurosurg Psychiatry 2001;70(6):744–8.
125. Goodall CA, Head MW, Everington D, et al. Raised CSF phospho-tau concentrations in variant Creutzfeldt-Jakob disease: diagnostic and pathological implications. J Neurol Neurosurg Psychiatry 2006;77(1):89–91.

126. Diack AB, Head MW, McCutcheon S, et al. Variant CJD. 18 years of research and surveillance. Prion 2014;8(4):286–95.
127. Parchi P, Saverioni D. Molecular pathology, classification, and diagnosis of sporadic human prion disease variants. Folia Neuropathol 2012;50(1):20–45.
128. Wadsworth JD, Collinge J. Molecular pathology of human prion disease. Acta Neuropathol 2011;121(1):69–77.
129. Wadsworth JD, Joiner S, Hill AF, et al. Tissue distribution of protease resistant prion protein in variant Creutzfeldt-Jakob disease using a highly sensitive immunoblotting assay. Lancet 2001;358(9277):171–80.
130. Hill AF, Zeidler M, Ironside J, et al. Diagnosis of new variant Creutzfeldt-Jakob disease by tonsil biopsy. Lancet 1997;349(9045):99–100.
131. Heath CA, Cooper SA, Murray K, et al. Validation of diagnostic criteria for variant Creutzfeldt-Jakob disease. Ann Neurol 2010;67(6):761–70.
132. Mok T, Jaunmuktane Z, Joiner S, et al. Variant Creutzfeldt-Jakob disease in a patient with heterozygosity at PRNP Codon 129. N Engl J Med 2017;376(3):292–4.
133. Kaski D, Mead S, Hyare H, et al. Variant CJD in an individual heterozygous for PRNP codon 129. Lancet 2009;374(9707):2128.
134. Knight R. The risk of transmitting prion disease by blood or plasma products. Transfus Apher Sci 2010;43(3):387–91.
135. Wroe SJ, Pal S, Siddique D, et al. Clinical presentation and pre-mortem diagnosis of variant Creutzfeldt-Jakob disease associated with blood transfusion: a case report. Lancet 2006;368(9552):2061–7.
136. Llewelyn CA, Hewitt PE, Knight RS, et al. Possible transmission of variant Creutzfeldt-Jakob disease by blood transfusion. Lancet 2004;363(9407): 417–21.
137. Health Protection Agency. Fourth case of transfusion-associated variant-CJD infection. Health Protection Report: weekly report 2007;1(3):2–3.
138. Ironside JW. Variant Creutzfeldt-Jakob disease: an update. Folia Neuropathol 2012;50(1):50–6.
139. Peden AH, Head MW, Ritchie DL, et al. Preclinical vCJD after blood transfusion in a PRNP codon 129 heterozygous patient. Lancet 2004;364(9433):527–9.
140. Peden A, McCardle L, Head MW, et al. Variant CJD infection in the spleen of a neurologically asymptomatic UK adult patient with haemophilia. Haemophilia 2010;16(2):296–304.
141. Crowder LA, Schonberger LB, Dodd RY, et al. Creutzfeldt-Jakob disease lookback study: 21 years of surveillance for transfusion transmission risk. Transfusion 2017;57(8):1875–8.
142. Dorsey K, Zou S, Schonberger LB, et al. Lack of evidence of transfusion transmission of Creutzfeldt-Jakob disease in a US surveillance study. Transfusion 2009;49(5):977–84.
143. Zou S, Fang CT, Schonberger LB. Transfusion transmission of human prion diseases. Transfus Med Rev 2008;22(1):58–69.
144. Hill AF, Butterworth RJ, Joiner S, et al. Investigation of variant Creutzfeldt-Jakob disease and other human prion diseases with tonsil biopsy samples. Lancet 1999;353(9148):183–9.
145. Frosh A, Smith LC, Jackson CJ, et al. Analysis of 2000 consecutive UK tonsillectomy specimens for disease-related prion protein. Lancet 2004;364(9441): 1260–2.
146. Hilton DA, Fathers E, Edwards P, et al. Prion immunoreactivity in appendix before clinical onset of variant Creutzfeldt-Jakob disease. Lancet 1998; 352(9129):703–4.

147. Gill ON, Spencer Y, Richard-Loendt A, et al. Prevalent abnormal prion protein in human appendixes after bovine spongiform encephalopathy epizootic: large scale survey. BMJ 2013;347:f5675.

148. Moda F, Gambetti P, Notari S, et al. Prions in the urine of patients with variant Creutzfeldt-Jakob disease. N Engl J Med 2014;371(6):530–9.

149. Edgeworth JA, Farmer M, Sicilia A, et al. Detection of prion infection in variant Creutzfeldt-Jakob disease: a blood-based assay. Lancet 2011;377(9764): 487–93.

150. Jackson GS, Burk-Rafel J, Edgeworth J, et al. Population screening for variant Creutzfeldt-Jakob disease using a novel blood test: diagnostic accuracy and feasibility study. JAMA Neurol 2014;71(4):421–8.

151. Hilton DA, Ghani AC, Conyers L, et al. Prevalence of lymphoreticular prion protein accumulation in UK tissue samples. J Pathol 2004;203(3):733–9.

152. Salmon R. How widespread is variant Creutzfeldt-Jakob disease? BMJ 2013; 347:f5994.

153. de Marco MF, Linehan J, Gill ON, et al. Large-scale immunohistochemical examination for lymphoreticular prion protein in tonsil specimens collected in Britain. J Pathol 2010;222(4):380–7.

154. Duffy P, Wolf J, Collins G, et al. Letter: possible person-to-person transmission of Creutzfeldt-Jakob disease. N Engl J Med 1974;290(12):692–3.

155. Bonda DJ, Manjila S, Mehndiratta P, et al. Human prion diseases: surgical lessons learned from iatrogenic prion transmission. Neurosurg Focus 2016;41(1): E10.

156. Abrams JY, Schonberger LB, Belay ED, et al. Lower risk of Creutzfeldt-Jakob disease in pituitary growth hormone recipients initiating treatment after 1977. J Clin Endocrinol Metab 2011;96(10):E1666–9.

157. Healy DL, Evans J. Creutzfeldt-Jakob disease after pituitary gonadotrophins. BMJ 1993;307(6903):517–8.

158. Boyd A, Fletcher A, Lee JS, et al. Transmissible spongiform encephalopathies in Australia. Commun Dis Intell Q Rep 2001;25(4):248–52.

159. Centers for Disease Control and Prevention (CDC). Creutzfeldt-Jakob disease associated with cadaveric dura mater grafts – Japan, January 1979-May 1996. MMWR Morb Mortal Wkly Rep 1997;46(45):1066–9.

160. Noguchi-Shinohara M, Hamaguchi T, Kitamoto T, et al. Clinical features and diagnosis of dura mater graft associated Creutzfeldt Jakob disease. Neurology 2007;69(4):360–7.

161. Yamada M, Noguchi-Shinohara M, Hamaguchi T, et al. Dura mater graft-associated Creutzfeldt-Jakob disease in Japan: clinicopathological and molecular characterization of the two distinct subtypes. Neuropathology 2009;29(5): 609–18.

162. Kobayashi A, Matsuura Y, Mohri S, et al. Distinct origins of dura mater graft-associated Creutzfeldt-Jakob disease: past and future problems. Acta Neuropathol Commun 2014;2:32.

163. Heckmann JG, Lang CJ, Petruch F, et al. Transmission of Creutzfeldt-Jakob disease via a corneal transplant. J Neurol Neurosurg Psychiatry 1997;63(3): 388–90.

164. Hammersmith KM, Cohen EJ, Rapuano CJ, et al. Creutzfeldt-Jakob disease following corneal transplantation. Cornea 2004;23(4):406–8.

165. Maddox RA, Belay ED, Curns AT, et al. Creutzfeldt-Jakob disease in recipients of corneal transplants. Cornea 2008;27(7):851–4.

166. Brown P, Preece M, Brandel JP, et al. Iatrogenic Creutzfeldt-Jakob disease at the millennium. Neurology 2000;55(8):1075–81.
167. Creange A, Gray F, Cesaro P, et al. Creutzfeldt-Jakob disease after liver transplantation. Ann Neurol 1995;38(2):269–72.
168. Gilch S, Chitoor N, Taguchi Y, et al. Chronic wasting disease. Top Curr Chem 2011;305:51–77.
169. Haley NJ, Hoover EA. Chronic wasting disease of cervids: current knowledge and future perspectives. Annu Rev Anim Biosci 2015;3:305–25.
170. Saunders SE, Bartelt-Hunt SL, Bartz JC. Occurrence, transmission, and zoonotic potential of chronic wasting disease. Emerg Infect Dis 2012;18(3):369–76.
171. Kim TY, Shon HJ, Joo YS, et al. Additional cases of chronic wasting disease in imported deer in Korea. J Vet Med Sci 2005;67(8):753–9.
172. Mathiason CK. Chapter twelve - scrapie, CWD, and transmissible mink encephalopathy. In: Legname G, Vanni S, editors. Progress in molecular biology and translational science, vol. 150. Cambridge (MA): Academic Press; 2017. p. 267–92.
173. Tamguney G, Miller MW, Wolfe LL, et al. Asymptomatic deer excrete infectious prions in faeces. Nature 2009;461(7263):529–32.
174. Haley NJ, Seelig DM, Zabel MD, et al. Detection of CWD prions in urine and saliva of deer by transgenic mouse bioassay. PLoS One 2009;4(3):e4848.
175. Race B, Williams K, Orru CD, et al. Lack of transmission of chronic wasting disease to cynomolgus macaques. J Virol 2018. [Epub ahead of print].
176. Zanusso G, Ferrari S, Cardone F, et al. Detection of pathologic prion protein in the olfactory epithelium in sporadic Creutzfeldt-Jakob disease. N Engl J Med 2003;348(8):711–9.
177. Tabaton M, Monaco S, Cordone MP, et al. Prion deposition in olfactory biopsy of sporadic Creutzfeldt-Jakob disease. Ann Neurol 2004;55(2):294–6.
178. Collins S, Law MG, Fletcher A, et al. Surgical treatment and risk of sporadic Creutzfeldt-Jakob disease: a case-control study. Lancet 1999;353(9154):693–7.
179. de Pedro-Cuesta J, Bleda MJ, Rabano A, et al. Classification of surgical procedures for epidemiologic assessment of sporadic Creutzfeldt-Jakob disease transmission by surgery. Eur J Epidemiol 2006;21(8):595–604.
180. Ward HJ, Everington D, Cousens SN, et al. Risk factors for sporadic Creutzfeldt-Jakob disease. Ann Neurol 2008;63(3):347–54.
181. Ward HJ, Knight RS. Surgery and risk of sporadic Creutzfeldt-Jakob disease. Neuroepidemiology 2008;31(4):241–2.
182. Zou WQ, Puoti G, Xiao X, et al. Variably protease-sensitive prionopathy: a new sporadic disease of the prion protein. Ann Neurol 2010;68(2):162–72.
183. Orru CD, Yuan J, Appleby BS, et al. Prion seeding activity and infectivity in skin samples from patients with sporadic Creutzfeldt-Jakob disease. Sci Transl Med 2017;9(417).
184. Beekes M, Baldauf E, Diringer H. Sequential appearance and accumulation of pathognomonic markers in the central nervous system of hamsters orally infected with scrapie. J Gen Virol 1996;77(Pt 8):1925–34.
185. Andreoletti O, Simon S, Lacroux C, et al. PrPSc accumulation in myocytes from sheep incubating natural scrapie. Nat Med 2004;10(6):591–3.
186. World Health Organization (WHO). WHO guidelines on tissue infectivity distribution in transmissible spongiform encephalopathies; report of the WHO consultation in Geneva 14-16 September 2005. Geneva, Switzerland: Quality and Safety of Plasma Derivatives and Related Substances Department of Medicines Policy and Standards Health Technology and Pharmaceuticals Cluster, World Health Organization; 2006. 92-4-154701-4.

187. UCSF Medical Center. Policies and procedures for patients with suspected or confirmed human prion disease (E.G., Creutzfeldt-Jakob Disease [CJD]). Hospital epidemiology and infection control 2012. Available at: http://infectioncontrol. ucsfmedicalcenter.org/sites/infectioncontrol.ucsfmedicalcenter.org/files/Sec%204. 2%20Human%20Prion%20Policy.pdf. Accessed June 3, 2016.

188. World Health Organization (WHO). WHO infection control guidelines for transmissible spongiform encephalopathies: report of a WHO consultation Geneva, Switzerland, 23-26 March 1999. Presented at World Health Organization: Communicable Disease Surveillance and Control. Geneva, Switzerland, February 9-11, 1999.

189. UK National Health Service Advisory Committee on Dangerous Pathogens; Spongiform Encephalopathy Advisory Committee. Transmissible spongiform encephalopathy agents: safe working and the prevention of infection. Part 4 infection prevention and control of CJD and variant CJD in healthcare and community settings. 2015. London, UK. Available at: https://assets.publishing. service.gov.uk/government/uploads/system/uploads/attachment_data/file/427854/ Infection_controlv3.0.pdf. Accessed June 21, 2018.

190. Australian Government Department of Public Health. Infection control guidelines: Creutzfeldt-Jakob disease. 2013; CJD and prion infection control guidelines. Available at: http://www.health.gov.au/internet/main/publishing.nsf/ content/icg-guidelines-index.htm. Accessed July 18, 2018.

191. Cervenakova L. Creutzfeldt-Jakob disease and blood transfusion: safe or not safe? Transfusion 2017;57(8):1851-3.

192. Urwin PJ, Mackenzie JM, Llewelyn CA, et al. Creutzfeldt-Jakob disease and blood transfusion: updated results of the UK transfusion medicine epidemiology review study. Vox Sang 2016;110(4):310-6.

193. Heinemann U, Krasnianski A, Meissner B, et al. Creutzfeldt-Jakob disease in Germany: a prospective 12-year surveillance. Brain 2007;130(Pt 5):1350-9.

194. Heinemann U, Krasnianski A, Meissner B, et al. Brain biopsy in patients with suspected Creutzfeldt-Jakob disease. J Neurosurg 2008;109(4):735-41.

195. Chitravas N, Jung RS, Kofskey DM, et al. Treatable neurological disorders misdiagnosed as Creutzfeldt-Jakob disease. Ann Neurol 2011;70(3):437-44.

196. Prusiner SB. Cell biology. A unifying role for prions in neurodegenerative diseases. Science 2012;336(6088):1511-3.

197. Jucker M, Walker LC. Self-propagation of pathogenic protein aggregates in neurodegenerative diseases. Nature 2013;501(7465):45-51.

198. Prusiner SB. Prions. Proc Natl Acad Sci U S A 1998;95(23):13363-83.

199. Ren PH, Lauckner JE, Kachirskaia I, et al. Cytoplasmic penetration and persistent infection of mammalian cells by polyglutamine aggregates. Nat Cell Biol 2009;11(2):219-25.

200. Cucchiaroni ML, Viscomi MT, Bernardi G, et al. Metabotropic glutamate receptor 1 mediates the electrophysiological and toxic actions of the cycad derivative beta-N-Methylamino-L-alanine on substantia nigra pars compacta DAergic neurons. J Neurosci 2010;30(15):5176-88.

201. Munch C, O'Brien J, Bertolotti A. Prion-like propagation of mutant superoxide dismutase-1 misfolding in neuronal cells. Proc Natl Acad Sci U S A 2011; 108(9):3548-53.

202. Furukawa Y, Kaneko K, Nukina N. Molecular properties of TAR DNA binding protein-43 fragments are dependent upon its cleavage site. Biochim Biophys Acta 2011;1812(12):1577-83.

203. Prusiner SB. Biology and genetics of prions causing neurodegeneration. Annu Rev Genet 2013;47:601–23.

204. Kane MD, Lipinski WJ, Callahan MJ, et al. Evidence for seeding of beta -amyloid by intracerebral infusion of Alzheimer brain extracts in beta -amyloid precursor protein-transgenic mice. J Neurosci 2000;20(10):3606–11.

205. Eisele YS, Obermuller U, Heilbronner G, et al. Peripherally applied Abeta-containing inoculates induce cerebral beta-amyloidosis. Science 2010; 330(6006):980–2.

206. Eisele YS, Bolmont T, Heikenwalder M, et al. Induction of cerebral beta-amyloidosis: intracerebral versus systemic Abeta inoculation. Proc Natl Acad Sci U S A 2009;106(31):12926–31.

207. Meyer-Luehmann M, Coomaraswamy J, Bolmont T, et al. Exogenous induction of cerebral beta-amyloidogenesis is governed by agent and host. Science 2006;313:1781–4.

208. Jucker M, Walker LC. Pathogenic protein seeding in Alzheimer disease and other neurodegenerative disorders. Ann Neurol 2011;70(4):532–40.

209. Hamaguchi T, Eisele YS, Varvel NH, et al. The presence of Abeta seeds, and not age per se, is critical to the initiation of Abeta deposition in the brain. Acta Neuropathol 2012;123(1):31–7.

210. Cali I, Cohen ML, Hasmall yi US, et al. Iatrogenic Creutzfeldt-Jakob disease with Amyloid-beta pathology: an international study. Acta Neuropathol Commun 2018;6(1):5.

211. Tousseyn T, Bajsarowicz K, Sanchez H, et al. Prion disease induces Alzheimer disease-like neuropathologic changes. J Neuropathol Exp Neurol 2015;74(9): 873–88.

212. Jaunmuktane Z, Mead S, Ellis M, et al. Evidence for human transmission of amyloid-beta pathology and cerebral amyloid angiopathy. Nature 2015; 525(7568):247–50.

213. Jucker M, Walker LC. Neurodegeneration: amyloid-beta pathology induced in humans. Nature 2015;525(7568):193–4.

214. Frost B, Diamond MI. The expanding realm of prion phenomena in neurodegenerative disease. Prion 2009;3(2):74–7.

215. Lasagna-Reeves CA, Castillo-Carranza DL, Sengupta U, et al. Alzheimer brain-derived tau oligomers propagate pathology from endogenous tau. Sci Rep 2012;2:700.

216. Clavaguera F, Akatsu H, Fraser G, et al. Brain homogenates from human tauopathies induce tau inclusions in mouse brain. Proc Natl Acad Sci U S A 2013; 110(23):9535–40.

217. Annus A, Csati A, Vecsei L. Prion diseases: new considerations. Clin Neurol Neurosurg 2016;150:125–32.

218. Sandberg MK, Al-Doujaily H, Sharps B, et al. Prion propagation and toxicity in vivo occur in two distinct mechanistic phases. Nature 2011;470(7335):540–2.

219. Jarrett JT, Berger EP, Lansbury PT. The C-terminus of the beta-protein is critical in amyloidogenesis. Ann N Y Acad Sci 1993;695(695):144–8.

220. Kordower JH, Chu Y, Hauser RA, et al. Lewy body-like pathology in long-term embryonic nigral transplants in Parkinson's disease. Nat Med 2008;14(5):504–6.

221. Kordower JH, Chu Y, Hauser RA, et al. Transplanted dopaminergic neurons develop PD pathologic changes: a second case report. Mov Disord 2008; 23(16):2303–6.

222. Li JY, Englund E, Holton JL, et al. Lewy bodies in grafted neurons in subjects with Parkinson's disease suggest host-to-graft disease propagation. Nat Med 2008;14(5):501–3.
223. Watts JC, Giles K, Oehler A, et al. Transmission of multiple system atrophy prions to transgenic mice. Proc Natl Acad Sci U S A 2013;110(48):19555–60.
224. Prusiner SB, Woerman AL, Mordes DA, et al. Evidence for alpha-synuclein prions causing multiple system atrophy in humans with parkinsonism. Proc Natl Acad Sci U S A 2015;112(38):E5308–17.
225. Stopschinski BE, Diamond MI. The prion model for progression and diversity of neurodegenerative diseases. Lancet Neurol 2017;16(4):323–32.
226. Hufnagel A, Weber J, Marks S, et al. Brain diffusion after single seizures. Epilepsia 2003;44(1):54–63.
227. Milligan TA, Zamani A, Bromfield E. Frequency and patterns of MRI abnormalities due to status epilepticus. Seizure 2009;18(2):104–8.
228. Burdette JH, Elster AD, Ricci PE. Acute cerebral infarction: quantification of spin-density and T2 shine-through phenomena on diffusion-weighted MR images. Radiology 1999;212(2):333–9.
229. Cochius JI, Burns RJ, Blumbergs PC, et al. Creutzfeldt-Jakob disease in a recipient of human pituitary-derived gonadotrophin. Aust N Z J Med 1990;20(4):592–3.
230. Cochius JI, Hyman N, Esiri MM. Creutzfeldt-Jakob disease in a recipient of human pituitary-derived gonadotrophin: a second case. J Neurol Neurosurg Psychiatry 1992;55(11):1094–5.
231. el Hachimi KH, Chaunu MP, Cervenakova L, et al. Putative neurosurgical transmission of Creutzfeldt-Jakob disease with analysis of donor and recipient: agent strains. C R Acad Sci III 1997;320(4):319–28.

UNITED STATES POSTAL SERVICE® — Statement of Ownership, Management, and Circulation
(All Periodicals Publications Except Requester Publications)

1. Publication Title	2. Publication Number		3. Filing Date
NEUROLOGIC CLINICS	000 – 712		9/18/2018

4. Issue Frequency	5. Number of Issues Published Annually	6. Annual Subscription Price
FEB, MAY, AUG, NOV	4	$312.00

7. Complete Mailing Address of Known Office of Publication (Not printer) (Street, city, county, state, and ZIP+4®)

ELSEVIER INC.
230 Park Avenue, Suite 800
New York, NY 10169

Contact Person: STEPHEN R. BUSHING
Telephone (Include area code): 215-235-3688

8. Complete Mailing Address of Headquarters or General Business Office of Publisher (Not printer)

ELSEVIER INC.
230 Park Avenue, Suite 800
New York, NY 10169

9. Full Names and Complete Mailing Addresses of Publisher, Editor, and Managing Editor (Do not leave blank)

Publisher (Name and complete mailing address)

TAYLOR E. BALL, ELSEVIER INC.
1600 JOHN F KENNEDY BLVD. SUITE 1800
PHILADELPHIA, PA 19103-2899

Editor (Name and complete mailing address)

STACY EASTMAN, ELSEVIER INC.
1600 JOHN F KENNEDY BLVD. SUITE 1800
PHILADELPHIA, PA 19103-2899

Managing Editor (Name and complete mailing address)

PATRICK MANLEY, ELSEVIER INC.
1600 JOHN F KENNEDY BLVD. SUITE 1800
PHILADELPHIA, PA 19103-2899

10. Owner (Do not leave blank. If the publication is owned by a corporation, give the name and address of the corporation immediately followed by the names and addresses of all stockholders owning or holding 1 percent or more of the total amount of stock. If not owned by a corporation, give the names and addresses of the individual owners. If owned by a partnership or other unincorporated firm, give its name and address as well as those of each individual owner. If the publication is published by a nonprofit organization, give its name and address.)

Full Name	Complete Mailing Address
WHOLLY OWNED SUBSIDIARY OF REED/ELSEVIER, US HOLDINGS	1600 JOHN F KENNEDY BLVD. SUITE 1800 PHILADELPHIA, PA 19103-2899

11. Known Bondholders, Mortgagees, and Other Security Holders Owning or Holding 1 Percent or More of Total Amount of Bonds, Mortgages, or Other Securities. If none, check box ▶ ☑ None

Full Name	Complete Mailing Address
N/A	

12. Tax Status (For completion by nonprofit organizations authorized to mail at nonprofit rates) (Check one)
The purpose, function, and nonprofit status of this organization and the exempt status for federal income tax purposes:
☑ Has Not Changed During Preceding 12 Months
☐ Has Changed During Preceding 12 Months (Publisher must submit explanation of change with this statement)

PS Form 3526, July 2014 [Page 1 of 4 (see instructions page 4)] PSN: 7530-01-000-9931   PRIVACY NOTICE: See our privacy policy on www.usps.com.

---

13. Publication Title	14. Issue Date for Circulation Data Below
NEUROLOGIC CLINICS	MAY 2018

15. Extent and Nature of Circulation			Average No. Copies Each Issue During Preceding 12 Months	No. Copies of Single Issue Published Nearest to Filing Date
a. Total Number of Copies (Net press run)			207	309
b. Paid Circulation (By Mail and Outside the Mail)	(1)	Mailed Outside-County Paid Subscriptions Stated on PS Form 3541 (Include paid distribution above nominal rate, advertiser's proof copies, and exchange copies)	100	154
	(2)	Mailed In-County Paid Subscriptions Stated on PS Form 3541 (Include paid distribution above nominal rate, advertiser's proof copies, and exchange copies)	0	0
	(3)	Paid Distribution Outside the Mails Including Sales Through Dealers and Carriers, Street Vendors, Counter Sales, and Other Paid Distribution Outside USPS®	55	76
	(4)	Paid Distribution by Other Classes of Mail Through the USPS (e.g., First-Class Mail®)	0	0
c. Total Paid Distribution (Sum of 15b (1), (2), (3), and (4))		▶	155	230
d. Free or Nominal Rate Distribution (By Mail and Outside the Mail)	(1)	Free or Nominal Rate Outside-County Copies included on PS Form 3541	41	64
	(2)	Free or Nominal Rate In-County Copies Included on PS Form 3541	0	0
	(3)	Free or Nominal Rate Copies Mailed at Other Classes Through the USPS (e.g., First-Class Mail)	0	0
	(4)	Free or Nominal Rate Distribution Outside the Mail (Carriers or other means)	0	0
e. Total Free or Nominal Rate Distribution (Sum of 15d (1), (2), (3) and (4))		▶	41	64
f. Total Distribution (Sum of 15c and 15e)		▶	196	294
g. Copies not Distributed (See Instructions to Publishers #4 (page #3))		▶	11	15
h. Total (Sum of 15f and g)		▶	207	309
i. Percent Paid (15c divided by 15f times 100)		▶	79.08%	78.23%

* If you are claiming electronic copies, go to line 16 on page 3. If you are not claiming electronic copies, skip to line 17 on page 3.

16. Electronic Copy Circulation		Average No. Copies Each Issue During Preceding 12 Months	No. Copies of Single Issue Published Nearest to Filing Date
a. Paid Electronic Copies	▶	0	0
b. Total Paid Print Copies (Line 15c) + Paid Electronic Copies (Line 16a)	▶	155	230
c. Total Print Distribution (Line 15f) + Paid Electronic Copies (Line 16a)	▶	196	294
d. Percent Paid (Both Print & Electronic Copies) (16b divided by 16c × 100)	▶	79.08%	78.23%

☑ I certify that 50% of all my distributed copies (electronic and print) are paid above a nominal price.

17. Publication of Statement of Ownership
☑ If the publication is a general publication, publication of this statement is required. Will be printed in the NOVEMBER 2018 issue of this publication.   ☐ Publication not required.

18. Signature and Title of Editor, Publisher, Business Manager, or Owner

STEPHEN R. BUSHING - INVENTORY DISTRIBUTION CONTROL MANAGER

Date: 9/18/2018

I certify that all information furnished on this form is true and complete. I understand that anyone who furnishes false or misleading information on this form or who omits material or information requested on the form may be subject to criminal sanctions (including fines and imprisonment) and/or civil sanctions (including civil penalties).

PS Form 3526, July 2014 (Page 3 of 4)   PRIVACY NOTICE: See our privacy policy on www.usps.com

Moving?

Make sure your subscription moves with you!

To notify us of your new address, find your **Clinics Account Number** (located on your mailing label above your name), and contact customer service at:

Email: journalscustomerservice-usa@elsevier.com

800-654-2452 (subscribers in the U.S. & Canada)
314-447-8871 (subscribers outside of the U.S. & Canada)

Fax number: 314-447-8029

Elsevier Health Sciences Division
Subscription Customer Service
3251 Riverport Lane
Maryland Heights, MO 63043

*To ensure uninterrupted delivery of your subscription, please notify us at least 4 weeks in advance of move.

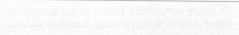

Printed and bound by CPI Group (UK) Ltd, Croydon, CR0 4YY

07/10/2024

01040501-0004